Fear and Anxiety

The Benefits of Translational Research

Fear and Anxiety

The Benefits of Translational Research

Edited by

Jack M. Gorman, M.D.

American Psychopathological Association

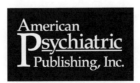

Washington, DC
London, England

Copyright © 2004 American Psychiatric Publishing, Inc.
ALL RIGHTS RESERVED

Manufactured in the United States of America on acid-free paper
08 07 06 05 04   5 4 3 2 1
First Edition

Typeset in Baskerville, Adobe Systems, Inc., and HelveticaNeueCondensed, Adobe Systems, Inc.

American Psychiatric Publishing, Inc.
1000 Wilson Boulevard
Arlington, VA 22209-3901
www.appi.org

Library of Congress Cataloging-in-Publication Data
Fear and anxiety : the benefits of translational research / edited by Jack M.
   Gorman.
     p. ; cm.
   Includes bibliographical references and index.
   ISBN 1-58562-149-8 (alk. paper)
    1. Anxiety. 2. Fear. I. Gorman, Jack M.
   RC531.F43 2003
   616.85′22—dc22   2003057890

British Library Cataloguing in Publication Data
A CIP record is available from the British Library.

Contents

Contributors

Laura B. Allen, M.A.
Doctoral student in clinical psychology, Center for Anxiety and Related Disorders, Boston, Massachusetts

David G. Amaral, Ph.D.
Professor, Department of Psychiatry and Behavioral Science, Center for Neuroscience, California National Primate Research Center and the M.I.N.D. Institute, University of California, Davis, California

Silviu A. Bacanu, Ph.D.
Research Assistant Professor, Department of Psychiatry, University of Pittsburgh, Pittsburgh, Pennsylvania

David H. Barlow, Ph.D.
Director, Center for Anxiety and Related Disorders, Boston, Massachusetts

Gerard E. Bruder, Ph.D.
Professor of Clinical Psychology, Department of Psychiatry, College of Physicians and Surgeons, Columbia University; Acting Chief, Department of Biopsychology, New York State Psychiatric Institute, New York, New York

Judy L. Cameron, Ph.D.
Professor, Department of Psychiatry, University of Pittsburgh, Pittsburgh, Pennsylvania; and Senior Scientist, Divisions of Neuroscience and Reproductive Science, Oregon National Primate Research Center, Oregon Health and Science University, Beaverton, Oregon

Kristine D. Coleman, Ph.D.
Assistant Scientist, Divisions of Animal Resources and Reproductive Science, Oregon National Primate Research Center, Oregon Health and Science University, Beaverton, Oregon

Jeremy D. Coplan, M.D.

Professor of Psychiatry; Chief, Division of Neuropsychopharmacology; and Co-Director, Primate Behavioral Laboratory, State University of New York, Downstate Medical Center, Brooklyn, New York

Ronald E. Dahl, M.D.

Professor, Department of Psychiatry, University of Pittsburgh, Pittsburgh, Pennsylvania

Michael D. De Bellis, M.D., M.P.H.

Professor of Psychiatry and Behavioral Sciences and Director, Healthy Childhood Brain Development and Developmental Traumatology Research Program, Department of Psychiatry and Behavioral Sciences, Duke University Medical Center, Durham, North Carolina

Bernard J. Devlin, Ph.D.

Assistant Professor, Department of Psychiatry, University of Pittsburgh, Pittsburgh, Pennsylvania

Jack M. Gorman, M.D.

Chair, Department of Psychiatry, Mt. Sinai School of Medicine, New York, New York

Christian Grillon, Ph.D.

Chief, Unit of Affective Psychophysiology, National Institute of Mental Health/Mood and Anxiety Disorders Program, Bethesda, Maryland

David Gutman, M.D.

Assistant Clinical Professor of Psychiatry, Columbia University College of Physicians and Surgeons, New York, New York

Joy Hirsch, Ph.D.

Professor, Department of Radiology, and Director, fMRI Research Center, Center for Neurobiology and Behavior, Columbia University, New York, New York

Luke R. Johnson, Ph.D.

Research Scientist, Center for Neural Science, New York University, New York, New York

Justine M. Kent, M.D.

Assistant Professor of Clinical Psychiatry, Columbia University College of Physicians and Surgeons, New York, New York

Joseph E. LeDoux, Ph.D.
Henry and Lucy Moses Professor of Science, Center for Neural Science, New York University, New York, New York

Ana Maria Magarinos, Ph.D.
Research Associate, Harold and Margaret Milliken Hatch Laboratory of Neuro-endocrinology, The Rockefeller University, New York, New York

Xiangling Mao, M.S.
Staff Associate, Department of Radiology, Columbia University College of Physicians and Surgeons, Neurological Institute of New York, New York, New York

Sanjay J. Mathew, M.D.
Fellow, Department of Psychiatry, Columbia University College of Physicians and Surgeons, New York State Psychiatric Institute, New York, New York

Bruce S. McEwen, Ph.D.
Alfred E. Mirsky Professor and Head, Harold and Margaret Milliken Hatch Laboratory of Neuroendocrinology, The Rockefeller University, New York, New York

Kathleen R. Merikangas, Ph.D.
Senior Investigator and Chief, Section on Developmental Genetic Epidemiology, National Institute of Mental Health/Mood and Anxiety Disorders Program, Bethesda, Maryland

Yoko Nomura, Ph.D.
Research Scientist, Division of Clinical and Genetic Epidemiology, New York State Psychiatric Institute, New York, New York

Carol S. North, M.D., M.P.E.
Professor, Department of Psychiatry, Washington University School of Medicine, St. Louis, Missouri

Anca D. Paunica, M.D.
PGY4 Psychiatry Resident, Department of Psychiatry, State University of New York, Downstate Medical Center, Brooklyn, New York

Daniel S. Pine, M.D.
Chief, Section on Development and Affective Neuroscience, National Institute of Mental Health/Mood and Anxiety Disorders Program, Bethesda, Maryland

Jeffrey A. Rogers, Ph.D.
Scientist, Southwest National Primate Research Center, San Antonio, Texas

Leonard A. Rosenblum, Ph.D.
Professor of Psychiatry and Co-Director, Primate Behavioral Laboratory, Department of Psychiatry, State University of New York, Downstate Medical Center, Brooklyn, New York

Neal D. Ryan, M.D.
Professor, Department of Psychiatry, University of Pittsburgh, Pittsburgh, Pennsylvania

Dikoma C. Shungu, Ph.D.
Associate Professor of Radiology, Columbia University College of Physicians and Surgeons, Neurological Institute of New York, New York, New York

Gregory M. Sullivan, M.D.
Assistant Professor of Clinical Psychiatry, Department of Psychiatry, Columbia University, New York, New York

Craig E. Tenke, Ph.D.
Research Scientist, Department of Biopsychology, New York State Psychiatric Institute, New York, New York

Virginia Warner, M.P.H.
Research Scientist, Division of Clinical and Genetic Epidemiology, New York State Psychiatric Institute, New York, New York

Myrna M. Weissman, Ph.D.
Professor of Epidemiology in Psychiatry, College of Physicians and Surgeons and Mailman School of Public Health, Columbia University; Chief, Division of Clinical and Genetic Epidemiology, New York State Psychiatric Institute, New York, New York

Priya Wickramaratne, Ph.D.
Associate Professor of Psychiatry (in Biostatistics), Department of Psychiatry, College of Physicians and Surgeons, Division of Biostatistics, Mailman School of Public Health, Columbia University; Division of Clinical and Genetic Epidemiology, New York State Psychiatric Institute, New York, New York

Douglas E. Williamson, Ph.D.
Assistant Professor, Department of Psychiatry, University of Pittsburgh, Pittsburgh, Pennsylvania

Preface

Jack M. Gorman, M.D.

Perhaps scientists always believe that theirs is an age of never-before-realized promise and progress, and the unbridled enthusiasm of those of us who work in the area of mental health and illness research may one day seem like another of history's examples of wishful thinking. Nonetheless, there are many reasons to assert that the large field encompassed by brain science is indeed undergoing an era of unprecedented developments. That sense was wonderfully reinforced at the 92nd annual meeting of the American Psychopathological Association in March 2002. The topic was fear and anxiety, emotions and behaviors ubiquitous to human and nonhuman life. Three types of evidence were presented: basic neuroscience, neuroimaging of both animals and humans, and careful clinical observation. The result was a true ability to "translate" the work of basic, preclinical, and clinical investigators into common themes, hypotheses, and even concrete conclusions. From this derives our current state of optimism: Never before in the history of psychiatry and psychology have we been able to call on a basic science relevant to the clinical illnesses we are charged with treating. Finally, as occurs in all other specialties of medicine, laboratory and clinical scientists can work together to solve an overriding problem and make headway toward understanding disorders of emotion, behavior, and cognition.

To be sure, the study of fear and anxiety lends itself to this kind of translational approach. It is difficult (although by no means impossible) to conceive of convincing animal models for depression or psychosis. Animals by and large do not commit suicide, starve themselves, or attend to imaginary voices. Fear and avoidance, on the other hand, can reliably be observed, quantified, and manipulated in almost all species. What is remarkable, as the chapters in this volume reveal, is that the neural circuits responsible for the acquisition and expression of fear appear to be conserved throughout phylogeny, at least from rodents through nonhuman primates to humans. Hence, what is discovered about the neuroanatomy and physiology of fear in a mouse can be usefully translated to a human with an anxiety disorder. Such knowledge surely represents a breakthrough in both neuroscience and mental health research.

At the basic level, we have several papers that focus on a particular type of fear: conditioned fear. This example of classical or Pavlovian conditioning has been elegantly studied in laboratories such as those of Joseph LeDoux of New York University. He and others have convincingly documented that the amygdala is the essential brain structure necessary for an animal to exhibit conditioned fear, and the hippocampus is required for contextual memory of conditioned fear. Two objections have been raised with respect to the relevance of this research to human fear. First, it focuses on only one particular type of fear, the conditioned type. As LeDoux has often made clear, this type of fear was chosen because it is tractable to laboratory study. There is much debate about the extent to which fears in humans are learned and whether pathological fear states, such as panic attacks and phobias, represent conditioned phenomena. Nevertheless, as other studies show, the applicability of anatomical and physiological findings from studies of conditioned fear to other forms of fear is actually quite robust. Second, the present model of "fear circuitry" has been called unduly "amygdalocentric." I find this criticism unfair. The data clearly show that the amygdala is essential for the acquisition and expression of conditioned fear, but most investigators in the field have pointed to multiple other brain structures involved, including (but not limited to) the hippocampus, brainstem, prefrontal cortex, and ventral striatum. Once again, the validity lies to some degree in the applicability. Human neuroimaging studies persistently show that although many areas of the brain are activated when an individual experiences fear, the amygdala is the area most consistently energized.

Several of the papers in this volume do indeed add to the mounting literature that the amygdala is an area of the brain that is important in fear responses of nonhuman and human primates. When nonanxious volunteers are shown masked fearful faces, for example, most studies show amygdala activation. It appears that patients with anxiety disorders such as posttraumatic stress disorder (PTSD), social anxiety disorder, and panic disorder have a lower threshold for amygdala activation than control subjects, so that fear cues apparently not capable of registering an amygdala response in most individuals do so in anxious patients.

As if anxiety and fear were not sufficient cause for concern among patients with anxiety disorders, several papers in this volume present the possibility, based on both animal studies and clinical studies in children and adults, that chronic exposure to fear may have deleterious effects on the structural integrity of the brain. The hippocampus appears to be particularly vulnerable to this stress effect, and reports of smaller hippocampal volume in patients with depression and PTSD, although controversial, suggest that this is a matter of concern. Furthermore, animal and clinical studies suggest that damage from stress may not be limited to the hippocampus but may also occur in regions of the prefrontal cortex, such as the anterior cingulate.

Just as translational research can give rise to concerns that observed negative changes in animal brains might apply to humans, the same strategy can suggest advantageous interventions. Thus, both psychosocial and psychopharmacological approaches are effective in reversing anxiety disorders and may even reverse some of the brain changes. What is perhaps of greatest interest is the way in which the mutually beneficial approaches to treatment—psychotherapy and medication—can be understood as complementary when one refers to the basic scientists' models of brain function underlying fear and anxiety. Rather than being antagonistic, as they once appeared to be, the cognitive-behavioral and pharmacological approaches to treating anxiety are now understood as addressing different parts of the same fear circuitry. For psychopharmacologists like me, this means that cognitive-behavioral psychotherapy can be viewed as a very effective drug.

I would like to thank all of the people who helped make the APPA meeting so successful, including Charles Zorumski, William Eaton, Ezra Susser, Linda Cottler, John Helzer, Nina Schooler, Eliot Gershon, Kathleen Merikangas, Andrew Skodol, and Gary Heiman. Also, Christopher Tulysewski was immensely helpful in both planning the meeting and organizing this book. Most of all, I want to thank the great group of scientists who gave their time to present lectures and write chapters. I firmly believe that the synthesis of knowledge represented in this book does indeed justify our belief that psychiatric research is at last in a period in which unprecedented insight will be gained and progress toward better treatments made.

Synaptic Self

Conditioned Fear, Developmental Adversity, and the Anxious Individual

Gregory M. Sullivan, M.D.
Joseph E. LeDoux, Ph.D.

Neuroscience research has revealed a great deal about the brain mechanisms underlying perception, cognition, emotion, memory, and behavior. Yet for neuroscience to offer an understanding of self, we need to know how these brain processes work interactively to make us who we are. It is therefore important to have a firm foundation in each of these more basic processes and to establish the features they share. The brain carries out its business by transferring information across the synapses that lie between neurons. Therefore, synapses can be considered the most basic units of the brain's wiring. Both our genetic code and our experiences determine the microanatomy and activity of individual synapses. Understanding exactly how nature and nurture determine synaptic structure and activity is therefore critical to understanding our minds, our personalities, and our behaviors. Synapses are the basic units of the self.

A recent trend in psychiatry has been to integrate neuroscience research in the efforts to delineate brain circuits that mediate particular pathological behavioral patterns. Research in anxiety disorders is no exception to this trend, and focus has been placed on the role of the fear system. Fear is a central constituent of the anxiety disorders. For example, intense, overwhelming fear characterizes most panic attacks; agoraphobics fear and avoid particular places or situations; social anxiety disorder involves excessive fear of being observed by others; and generalized anxiety is characterized by fear of future events and the negative consequences of actions. Fear is adaptive to the extent that it determines the most appropriate behavioral response to a threat. Yet in anxiety disorders, the level of fear appears to be pathological. The occurrence of fear is not in synchrony with true threat, and the activation of fear interferes with other brain processes essential for psychological homeostasis. Therefore, there is reason to suspect that information processing through, or dependent on, the brain's fear system may be different in individuals suffering from pathological anxiety. Understanding what is happening at the synaptic level in the fear system may ultimately assist us in understanding the neuropathologies of the anxiety disorders.

Approaching anxiety from a neurobiological perspective also offers an opportunity to illustrate three shifts in emphasis that should facilitate the development of a neuroscience of self. First, we need to know how systems that mediate perceptions, memories, and emotions work interactively. Symptoms of anxiety disorders clearly suggest involvement of all of these systems. Second, we must understand the roles of both conscious and nonconscious processes. Neuroscience and psychiatry were both formerly plagued by the conception that to understand emotions you must understand how consciousness is generated. More recently, this conception has been dispensed with, replaced by the more parsimonious view that conscious cognition is simply one component of a vast network of processes that occur between stimulus perception and behavioral response. Understanding these nonconscious processes will also lay the foundation for understanding how consciousness is generated. From this perspective, empirical investigation of emotions and emotional disorders is not so daunting as to discourage neurobiological investigation. Third, learning and memory must be considered alongside genetic makeup, and evidence suggests that nurture has substantial effects on the phenotypic expression of anxiety. These shifts in emphasis should bring us to an exciting stage in neuroscience in which we can begin to approach what generates our minds, what shapes our personalities, and, essentially, what makes up our selves.

THE FEAR SYSTEM: FROM CIRCUITS TO SYNAPSES

Fear is perhaps the most basic emotion. It occurs when we encounter stimuli that predict danger. Regardless of whether the danger is real or imagined, the consequences are the same: The system designed through evolution to cope with danger becomes activated. Much has been learned about the anatomical and functional organization of this system through work in animal models, and recently the findings have been shown to be applicable to the human brain.

Activation of the fear system leads to what Walter Cannon described as the "fight or flight" response (Cannon 1914). This response may be more appropriately termed the *freeze-fight-flight response,* because freezing often occurs, if only briefly, in the presence of stimuli interpreted as harmful. Some stimuli, termed *prepared* stimuli, are capable of activating this system naturally, through the brain's hardwiring. For example, our primate ancestors were preyed on by snakes, and the human fear system is biologically prepared to respond to snakes. It is not that all humans have snake phobias, but rather that snakes represent very potent stimuli that can easily activate the fear system in humans. It appears that an individual's degree of fear response to snakes depends on both genetic variation and prior experience. Yet most stimuli arousing fear and other emotions in humans are not hardwired. Instead, they come to arouse fear solely through learning, and they persist through encoding into memory.

Ivan Pavlov first described how an initially neutral, innocuous stimulus, termed the *conditioned stimulus* (CS), could acquire emotional properties if it occurs simultaneously with a biologically significant event, termed the *unconditioned stimulus* (US; Pavlov 1927). For example, a rat can be exposed to a sound, and before the sound finishes, it can be given a mild electrical shock. This is known as Pavlovian or classical conditioning. Once a relationship between the CS and the US is learned, the physiological and behavioral responses that are hardwired for response to the US come under control of the CS. In fact, after only one CS-US pairing, it can be demonstrated that the animal has learned to respond to the sound alone with an array of stereotyped, species-specific defensive responses. These measurable responses include defensive postures (freezing), autonomic arousal (heart rate and blood pressure changes), decreased pain sensitivity (i.e., hypoalgesia), potentiation of reflexes (e.g., fear-potentiated startle and eyeblink response), and endocrine activation (corticosteroid and epinephrine release).

Research efforts subsequent to Pavlov consistently pointed to a structure known as the *amygdala* as a neuroanatomical locus essential for the acquisition and expression of conditioned fear responses. The amygdala is a region in the medial temporal lobe that is made up of structurally and functionally heterogeneous nuclei (Pitkänen et al. 1997; Swanson and Petrovich 1998). By the early 1990s a relatively clear picture of the neurocircuitry of conditioned fear had been established (Davis 1992; Fanselow 1994; Kapp et al. 1992; LeDoux 1992). It is generally agreed that conditioned fear is dependent on the transmission of information about the CS and the

US to the amygdala, and that the output pathways from the amygdala control the autonomic, endocrine, and behavioral responses. Other brain regions to which the amygdala connects mediate the individual components of the fear response. The areas of the amygdala identified as relevant to fear conditioning are the lateral, basal, accessory basal, and central nuclei. Studies in several species, including rats, cats, and nonhuman primates, are in general agreement about the essential connections between these nuclei necessary for fear conditioning (Amaral et al. 1992; Cassell et al. 1999; Pare et al. 1995; Pitkänen et al. 1997).

In the case of auditory conditioning, where a tone and a mild shock overlap in time, the tone CS information proceeds from the ear through the brainstem to the auditory relay in the thalamus (LeDoux 1996). From there the information is relayed through two different pathways, one directly to the amygdala and another to auditory cortex. The auditory cortical region also has projections to the amygdala. A fast, monosynaptic thalamus-amygdala pathway (12 ms) and a slower, polysynaptic thalamus-cortex-amygdala pathway (30–40 ms) thus converge on the lateral nucleus (see Figure 1–1). The direct thalamus-amygdala pathway, termed the "low road," is believed to provide a rapid yet crude representation of environmental stimuli, allowing fast response to potential danger. The slower pathway through the auditory cortex, termed the "high road," provides a delayed but more complex representation processed through cortex that may provide for a more appropriate response (Mascagni et al. 1993; Romanski and LeDoux 1993). As a result of this arrangement, the amygdala can be activated in parallel with the cortex, allowing a response to danger at the same time or even before we know, through cortical processing, to what we are responding.

Sensory modalities in addition to hearing also have nerve pathways terminating mainly in the lateral nucleus (Amaral et al. 1992; LeDoux et al. 1990b; Mascagni et al. 1993; McDonald 1998). US information must also reach the amygdala. Such information is relayed through spinothalamic tract afferents to thalamic areas (LeDoux 1987) that then project to the lateral nucleus (LeDoux et al. 1990a). Cells in the lateral nucleus respond to activity in pain receptors, with some of these cells shown also to respond to auditory input (Romanski and LeDoux 1993). Afferent neurons that form the synapses to neurons in the lateral nucleus use the neurotransmitter glutamate to activate postsynaptic receptors of the lateral nucleus neurons.

The central nucleus is considered the main output station of the amygdala, because it is critical to the *expression* of the conditioned fear response (Davis 1992; Kapp et al. 1992; LeDoux et al. 1988; Maren and Fanselow 1996). The central nucleus sends projections to regions that

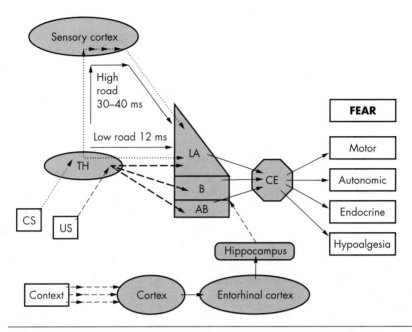

FIGURE 1–1   Pathways to the amygdala for cue-conditioned stimulus (CS, *dotted lines*) information, unconditioned stimulus (US, *large dashed lines*) information, and contextual (*small dashed lines*) information.

TH = thalamus, LA = lateral nucleus of amygdala, B = basal nucleus of amygdala, AB = accessory basal nucleus of amygdala, CE = central nucleus of amygdala. CE receives projections from LA, B, and AB and projects to areas mediating specific components of the fear response (*solid lines*).

mediate the specific components of a fear response. The central nucleus projections to the periaqueductal gray (PAG) are involved in freezing behavior and pain modulation; those through the stria terminalis and directly from the central nucleus to the paraventricular nucleus of the hypothalamus appear to mediate hypothalamic-pituitary-adrenal (HPA) axis activation; and those to the parabrachial nucleus, lateral hypothalamus, and dorsal motor nucleus of the vagus are involved in autonomic responses such as cardiovascular and respiratory alterations (see Figure 1–1; Davis 1992; LeDoux et al. 1988; Manning 1998; van de Kar et al. 1991).

Long-term potentiation (LTP) is a widely studied model for the cellular mechanisms underlying the establishment of stable memories. LTP is defined as a long-lasting increase in the efficiency of transmission though a synapse that results from high-frequency stimulation of the afferent fibers to the synapse. Electrical stimulation of the glutamatergic pathway from the thalamus to the lateral nucleus results in LTP of synapses in the lateral nucleus, and establishment of LTP in this pathway involves activation of voltage-gated calcium ion channels on the postsynaptic neuron (Weiss-kopf et al. 1999). If an LTP-like process is indeed central to the establishment of long-term fear memories, it would be predicted that intracellular inhibitors of LTP would also inhibit long-term fear memories. This has been shown to be true by both systemic injection and local amygdala infusion of inhibitors of protein kinase second-messenger pathways or protein synthesis. In fact, inhibition of protein synthesis, protein kinase A (PKA), and extracellular signal-regulated kinase/mitogen-activated protein (ERK/MAP) kinase activity, treatments known to block LTP (Huang and Kandel 1998; Huang et al. 1996, 2000), all interfere with consolidation of long-term fear memory while leaving short-term memory intact (Schafe and LeDoux 2000; Schafe et al. 1999, 2000).

There is a growing body of evidence suggesting that fear memory is encoded by changes in the microanatomy of synapses in the amygdala. Such encoding appears to require a cascade of cellular events initially set off by the coincident activation of postsynaptic cells by presynaptic afferents carrying CS *and* US sensory information. More specifically, this cascade involves activation of postsynaptic receptors, ion flow through membrane channels, action potentials, activation of second-messenger systems, new protein synthesis (possibly including neurotrophic proteins such as brain-derived neurotrophic factor [BDNF]), and, ultimately, microstructural changes in the synapse. Figure 1–2 shows a representative synapse between a presynaptic neuron carrying CS information and a postsynaptic neuron of the amygdala. One of the postsynaptic receptors for glutamate is termed the *N*-methyl-D-aspartate (NMDA) receptor. Recently, utilizing an inhibitor of the NR2B subunit of the NMDA receptor known as ifen-prodil, it has been shown that the NR2B subunit is involved in acquisition of fear memory but not consolidation into long-term memory (Rodrigues et al. 2001). In other words, the NR2B subunit appears to be involved in the synaptic plasticity required for transient changes in transmission that occur during learning, but not in the protein synthesis–dependent changes that occur in the hours after learning and that lead to microstructural changes in the synaptic architecture that sustain long-term plasticity.

The lateral nucleus certainly meets the minimal criteria for a cell group to be a site of essential plasticity. That is, damage to the lateral nucleus prevents conditioning to a cue, afferents carrying CS and US information converge on the same cells in the lateral nucleus, neural activity in the lateral nucleus changes during conditioning, and neural activity in the lateral nucleus is necessary for conditioning to take place. The more dorsal region of the dorsal portion of the lateral nucleus contains cells with converging

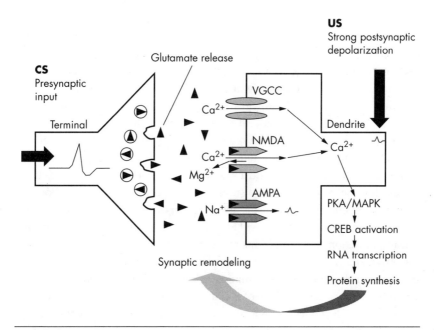

FIGURE 1–2   Model of synaptic plasticity.

Concurrent action potentials are generated in the presynaptic neuron, relaying conditioned stimulus (CS) information, and the postsynaptic neuron, generated by a neuron relaying unconditioned stimulus (US) information synapsing elsewhere (not shown) on the postsynaptic neuron. Although the presynaptic neuron can activate the α-amino-3-hydroxy-5-methyl-4-isoxazole propionic acid (AMPA) receptor without a postsynaptic depolarization, the N-methyl-D-aspartate (NMDA) receptor can be opened only by a postsynaptic depolarization, unblocking its pore of magnesium ion (Mg^{2+}), allowing a large calcium (Ca^{2+}) influx through both the NMDA receptors and the L-type voltage-gated calcium channels (VGCC). Only through this mechanism can activation of the second-messenger cascade occur, resulting in new protein synthesis and synaptic remodeling. Na^+ = sodium ion, PKA = cyclic AMP–dependent protein kinase, MAPK = mitogen-activated protein kinase, CREB = cyclic AMP response element binding protein.

sensory inputs that demonstrate transient plastic changes, termed *trigger cells* (Repa et al. 2001). Cells in the more ventral region of the dorsal portion of the lateral nucleus demonstrate long-lasting plastic changes; these are termed *storage cells*. It appears that these storage cells relay information to the medial portion of the lateral nucleus, and from there information is relayed to the central nucleus.

In addition to auditory fear conditioning, it has been well demonstrated that an association can be learned between a foot shock and a representation of the environment (the context) in which the foot shock was received. A rat that is placed back in the environment in which it had previously been conditioned will respond with the same stereotyped fear responses described for auditory conditioning. This is known as contextual fear conditioning. Recent evidence indicates that auditory and contextual fear conditioning occur by different intra-amygdala pathways. Whereas an auditory CS depends on a pathway that includes the lateral nucleus, conditioning to the context depends not only on different amygdala nuclei but also on the hippocampus (Blanchard et al. 1970; Frankland et al. 1998; Kim and Fanselow 1992; Maren et al. 1997; Phillips and LeDoux 1992). There is evidence that the ventral hippocampus (CA1 and subiculum), utilizing information about the context from entorhinal cortex, is necessary for providing a representation of the context to the amygdala (see Figure 1–1; LeDoux et al. 1990a). This hippocampal region has projections to the basal and accessory basal nuclei of the amygdala (Canteras and Swanson 1992), and contextual conditioning is disrupted if these areas are damaged (Majidishad et al. 1996; Maren and Fanselow 1995). As in the case of auditory fear conditioning, the information is ultimately relayed to the central nucleus for output of the fear response. It is also important to note that thalamic stimulation induces LTP in the lateral nucleus, whereas stimulation of cortical areas that receive inputs from auditory cortex and that project to the amygdala induces LTP in the basal nucleus; this suggests that the lateral nucleus mediates simple representations of the environment whereas the basal nucleus may serve as an amygdaloid sensory interface for complex stimulus information (Yaniv et al. 2001).

There is evidence that the prefrontal cortex (PFC) also plays a critical role in the normal acquisition, expression, and extinction of fear responses. Lesions of the dorsal portion of the medial PFC enhance fear reactivity to CS and context during both acquisition and extinction (Morgan and LeDoux 1995), whereas lesions to the ventral portion of the medial PFC prolong fear responses to the CS during extinction involving multiple presentations of the CS (Morgan et al. 1993). On the other hand, lesions to the ventrolateral PFC reduce fear responses to contextual stimuli without affecting CS acquisition and without an effect on response extinction (Morgan and LeDoux 1999). It has been demonstrated that PFC neurons reduce their spontaneous activity in the presence of a tone CS as a function of the degree of fear, and this depression in activity is related to amygdala activity but not to the freezing response itself (Garcia et al. 1999). This suggests that in the presence of threatening stimuli, the amygdala controls not only fear expression but also PFC activity.

Given the amygdala's role in fear responses, it is reasonable to speculate that this structure may be involved in the pathological fear that occurs in humans with anxiety disorders such as panic disorder, generalized anxiety disorder, social anxiety disorder, and posttraumatic stress disorder (PTSD). For example, pathological fear could result if the amygdala were overly sensitive. That is, a stimulus that is only mildly, or not at all, threatening to most people might be perceived as threatening if amygdala neurons were excessively sensitive. Alternatively, pathological fear might also come about if the amygdala were overreactive, such that it detects the same degree of threat as in other people but, upon detection of threat, responds excessively, producing an exaggerated fear response. To illustrate how the amygdala might become pathologically sensitive or overly reactive, we need to consider the interactions between the hippocampus, amygdala, and prefrontal cortex. As described earlier, hippocampal damage disrupts conditioning to context, and damage to the medial PFC, which includes the infra- and prelimbic regions and portions of the anterior cingulate cortex, leads to problems with fear regulation. That is, fear responses are either exaggerated (in the case of anterior cingulate damage) or difficult to extinguish (in the case of infra- and prelimbic damage). Extinction is of particular interest in connection with psychotherapies for fear and avoidance, because it is the process by which the brain learns that a stimulus or context no longer predicts harm.

The stress hormone cortisol (corticosterone in the rodent) has differential effects on the amygdala, hippocampus, and PFC, and these effects are relevant to the origin and maintenance of pathological fear. Cortisol released by the adrenal glands into the bloodstream binds to receptors on neurons in each of these three brain regions. Cortisol is known to impair hippocampal and medial prefrontal cortex function, but to enhance amygdala function. Given such effects, it is possible to speculate how pathological fear could arise. By impairing the hippocampus, cortisol could promote a loss of contextual restraint on fear. By impairing the medial PFC, cortisol could lead to poor ability to modulate the degree of fear reactivity, or the appropriateness of expressing fear in the face of changes in the meaning of a stimulus. Therefore, through enhanced amygdala function, one could become overly sensitive or overly reactive to threats.

THE HUMAN AMYGDALA

Much evidence has accumulated suggesting similar function of the amygdala in man as in animal in establishing emotional valence to stimuli, predicting adversity, and coordinating the fear response. Direct electrical stimulation of the amygdala in conscious humans has been reported to elicit fear and changes in autonomic measures as well as symptoms common to anxiety disorders, including subjective anxiety and depersonalization (Halgren 1981). Neuroimaging studies indicate amygdala involvement in human conditioned fear as well as in conscious and unconscious responses to fearful facial expressions (Buchel et al. 1998; LaBar et al. 1998; Morris et al. 1999; Whalen et al. 1998). Patients with amygdala damage have deficits in the perception of the emotional meaning of faces, particularly fearful faces (Adolphs et al. 1995; Calder et al. 1996). For example, compared with judgments of trustworthiness and approachability by healthy control subjects, individuals with bilateral amygdala damage have a poor ability to judge unfamiliar faces as not trustworthy or not approachable (Adolphs et al. 1998). Similar results have been reported for the perception of emotions in voices (Scott et al. 1997). In addition, patients with bilateral amygdala lesions (Bechara et al. 1995) or damage to the greater temporal lobe areas including amygdala (LaBar et al. 1995) have deficits in their fear conditioning ability. There is evidence in the human of the importance of the direct thalamo-amygdala pathway: Activity of the amygdala during fear conditioning has the strongest cross-correlation with activity of subcortical areas (thalamic and collicular) rather than cortical areas (Morris et al. 1999). Thus, current evidence points to a phylogenetic conservation of function of the amygdala in the human when considered in conjunction with what has been learned from animal work.

CONSCIOUS AND NONCONSCIOUS MEMORIES

Conscious recollection of an event requires an intact temporal lobe memory system, including the hippocampus and related cortical areas (Squire et al. 1993). Such consciously recalled memories are termed *explicit* or declarative memories. Fear conditioning, on the other hand, involves one of several *implicit* memory systems in that it does not depend on the hippocampal memory system or on conscious recall of the event. For example, the details a person can recall of a traumatic car accident require the hippocampal-dependent explicit memory system. On the other hand, a reminder of the event, such as a similar crashing noise, can elicit a strong emotional response with associated physical sensations. This type of implicit memory response is amygdala mediated. At the time of an adverse event, implicitly and explicitly processed information both presumably reach working memory and are part of the immediate conscious experience. Reactivation of such memory systems can again result in a unified conscious experience, but animal studies and studies of humans with rare hippocampal and amygdala lesions indicate that these are two distinct memory systems operating in parallel. For example, a study of human subjects with damage in these regions showed that a subject with selective bilateral amygdala damage could not condition to fear but could express declarative facts about the conditioning procedure (Bechara et al. 1995). In contrast, a subject with selective bilateral hippocampal damage could condition to fear but was unable to express declarative facts, and a patient with bilateral damage in both areas could neither condition nor express facts about the procedure.

As noted previously, functional imaging studies have shown that the amygdala is activated during fear conditioning (Labar et al. 1998; Morris et al. 1998). Some studies have used an experimental technique known as masking that allows isolation of the implicit fear memory systems from explicit memory in the human. In this procedure, subjects are exposed to a picture that has previously been paired with an aversive stimulus such as an electric shock. If this exposure is extremely brief, on the order of tens of milliseconds, and is followed by a neutral picture to which conditioning was not carried out, the subject develops conscious awareness only of the second picture. It has been shown that subjects who have been conditioned to pictures of fear-relevant stimuli, such as snakes, spiders, and angry faces, have an electrodermal response and enhanced neural activity in the amygdala to the masked picture despite no conscious awareness of the presentation of the conditioned picture (Morris et al. 1998, 1999; Whalen et al. 1998). Such nonconscious processing and autonomic fear response to the masked picture may be a result of the subcortical, direct thalamo-amygdala pathway, whereas explicit information processed by cortex is temporally inadequate to produce an explicit memory response or is superseded by cortical processing of the second, neutral picture.

DEVELOPMENTAL SCULPTING OF THE FEAR SYSTEM AND THE STRESS RESPONSE THRESHOLD

In attempts to understand human personality and behavior, the nature versus nurture argument has largely been replaced by the assumption that both the genetic code and the developmental environment contribute to emotional processing. For the purpose of this review, we will describe only the impact of the developmental component on fear, the stress response, and anxiety-related behaviors.

Handling is a laboratory procedure in which rat pups are taken from their dams by their human caregivers for short periods of time (about 15 minutes) and then returned. Handled pups have long been noted to appear more resilient in the face of stress and exhibit fewer anxiety-related behaviors. Rigorous investigation of this phenomenon has confirmed that the environmental manipulation reduces the level of stress response throughout the life of the animals. The manipulation leads to receptor changes resulting in increased sensitivity to glucocorticoid feedback at the level of the hippocampus, which essentially sets a higher threshold for HPA axis activation (Liu et al. 1997). It also results in reduced benzodiazepine receptor density at the level of the amygdala and locus ceruleus (Caldji et al. 1998). In contrast to the handling effect, maternal deprivation (achieved by extending the 15 minutes to 180 minutes) results in heightened response to stress (Caldji et al. 2000; Liu et al. 2000). Messenger RNA for the corticotropin-releasing factor (CRF) is increased in the central nucleus, whereas the glucocorticoid receptor to mineralocorticoid ratio in the hippocampus favors decreased feedback inhibition of the HPA axis. Remarkably, paroxetine, a selective serotonin reuptake inhibitor (SSRI), given for 21 days appears to normalize the observed changes (Huot et al. 2001). In related studies in the precocial rodent, maternal separation and early social deprivation results in altered monoaminergic innervation in areas of PFC, including medial PFC and another region of the PFC, the anterior cingulate cortex (ACC) (Braun et al. 2000). Apparently, the thresholds for activation of these regions are shaped by the developmental environment.

A lowered threshold for stress response, due to an interaction of genetics and developmental environment, may result in a potentiated fear system. For example, corticosteroids administered to rats in doses mimicking those seen under stress results in potentiation of freezing behavior to a tone CS (Corodimas et al. 1994). Direct corticosterone administration to the rat amygdala increases CRF mRNA in the central nucleus and anxiety-like behavior on the elevated plus maze (Shepard et al. 2000). And when the placental "barrier" to maternal steroids is inhibited (by inactivation of placental 11beta-hydroxysteroid dehydrogenase), the offspring of the experimental group have increased CRF and glucocorticoid mRNA in the paraventricular nucleus and increased glucocorticoid receptor mRNA in the lateral, basal, and central nuclei of the amygdala (Welberg et al. 2000). Conversely, removal of the adrenal glands during the nursing period of rat pups impairs the development of normal behavioral inhibition (Takahashi and Rubin 1993). Also, social isolation, a stressful event for adult rats, increases the generalization of fear response such that tones that normally would not cause significant freezing due to difference in frequency from the CS instead elicit a similar degree of freezing as the CS (Rudy and Pugh

1996). The hippocampus, on the other hand, appears to be differentially affected by stress. Stress has been shown to impair the anatomy, physiology, and behavioral functions of the hippocampus (McEwen and Sapolsky 1995; Sapolsky 1996). Social isolation, which has no effect on the magnitude of auditory conditioning, has been shown to decrease the level of contextually elicited fear conditioning (Rudy 1996; Rudy and Pugh 1996). This is conceivably due to an impaired ability of the hippocampus to create a representation of the context. Yet caution must be exercised in interpreting these data because an alternative stress, restraint stress, has been shown to enhance freezing to context despite dendritic atrophy in the CA3 region of the hippocampus (Conrad et al. 1999).

It should be kept in mind that every simple association between a cue and adversity is acquired in a context. In a situation in which there are multiple CSs, behavioral research indicates conditioning occurs to the CSs that provide the most reliable and nonredundant information about the occurrence of the US (Rescorla 1988). *Occasion setters* are stimuli that in and of themselves do not evoke a conditioned response but may influence behavior in the presence of a CS (Holland 1983). To the degree that a context associated with nonadversity can act as an occasion setter that decreases the fear response to a CS, hippocampal dysfunction due to stress could theoretically result in loss of differential contextual control over discrete fear conditioning. Therefore, a lower threshold for a stress response may result in heightened fear responding by increasing the level of fear response, increasing the generalization to other cues, and interfering with the contextual specificity of a response.

The nonhuman primate has been studied for potential connections between the early environment during rearing and the development of anxiety-like behaviors. Rosenblum and co-workers have shown that subtle manipulations of the early psychosocial environment of infant bonnet macaques result in anxiety-related behavioral profiles in youth and adult life (Rosenblum and Paully 1984). In a paradigm utilizing nursing mothers and their infants, the mothers are subjected to unpredictable demands when foraging for food, as opposed to predictable low-demand and predictable high-demand control environments. The unpredictable foraging requirements result in adversely altered behavior toward the infant (Rosenblum et al. 1994). By following these infants longitudinally, it has been found that they have heightened anxiety-related behaviors throughout development. This includes increased behavioral inhibition in response to separation, to fear stimuli, and to new social groups and environments. Such behavior is analogous to children described by Jerome Kagan as behaviorally inhibited to the unfamiliar (Kagan et al. 1987). Pharmacological challenge studies of these monkeys using yohimbine, an α_2-adrenergic antagonist, and mCPP, which has mixed agonist and antagonist activity on serotonergic receptors, were carried out when the offspring were 4.5–5.5 years old. They were found to be behaviorally hyperresponsive to the noradrenergic challenge and hyporesponsive to the serotonergic challenge compared with control subjects (Rosenblum et al. 1994). Remarkably, the cerebrospinal fluid (CSF) of these monkeys had CRF levels that were persistently elevated whereas CSF cortisol levels were depressed (Coplan et al. 1996, 1998). There were also significant correlations between CSF CRF and heightened CSF levels of serotonin and dopamine metabolites and the growth hormone axis peptide somatostatin. One theory explaining such lasting biochemical abnormalities is that increased adversity in the mother-infant interaction results in CRF overexpression, which secondarily results in alteration in other systems relevant to stress and anxiety, such as the amygdala, hippocampus, and locus ceruleus.

Kagan and co-workers have carried out prospective studies in humans that, taken with the aforementioned developmental data, suggest even stronger links between the fear system and anxiety. The level of response manifested in 4-month-old infants to unfamiliar stimuli has been correlated with subdued and fearful behavior in early childhood (Kagan et al. 1998). Further, those children identified as behaviorally inhibited at 21 months who remain inhibited at three follow-ups in their first decade of life have higher rates of anxiety disorders than children who were not consistently inhibited (Hirshfeld et al. 1992). Kagan and co-workers have utilized physiological measures that would be expected to come under control of the amygdala. For example, lower heart rate variability, greater muscle tension, higher urinary norepinephrine (and its metabolites), and higher salivary cortisol level all correlated with behavioral inhibition (Kagan et al. 1987). Inhibition of normal activity, such as exploration of a new environment, could also conceivably come under the control of an activated amygdala. For example, once a rat has been fear-conditioned to a context, the normal exploratory behavior that the animal would express if placed for the first time in the conditioning box is instead inhibited due to competition with the contextual freezing response. Such inhibition was investigated in an experiment that sought to identify whether conditioned freezing and suppression of ongoing activity constituted a single process or more than one process. Rats can be trained to bar-press for food, so the competition between context-induced freezing and bar pressing can be measured. Lesions of the PAG that block freezing behavior were found to have no effect on suppression of bar pressing (Amorapanth et al. 1999). Therefore, suppression is mediated not by the PAG but rather by some other process that is mediated by the fear system. Thus, just as the fear system may mediate the level of a child's physiological reactivity to novelty, it may also mediate the cessation of normal exploratory activity expected in such situations.

It is important to point out that the pathway from the lateral nucleus to the central nucleus that initiates defensive freezing and associated autonomic and endocrine reactions can be redirected (Amorapanth et al. 2000). Rats trained in a classical conditioning paradigm can be subsequently trained in an "escape from fear" (EFF) paradigm. In the EFF task, the same tone CS reinforces a locomotor response that results in termination of the CS. Lesions of the lateral nucleus block both acquisition of the conditioned fear response and the CS reinforcement of a motor response in the EFF task. Central nucleus lesions block conditioned fear but not the motor response, and basal nucleus lesions block the motor response but not conditioned fear. This new learning does not occur if the rat remains passive; it is the success in terminating the CS that reinforces the motor response. The shift from passive to active coping may be the neurological correlate of "getting on with life," a behavioral shift that appears compromised in people suffering from anxiety disorders.

MOLECULAR TARGETS IN THE FEAR SYSTEM

If the links between the fear system and pathological anxiety states are indeed real, the mechanisms of current and future treatments for anxiety disorders may be explained by activity at the level of the synapse (see Figure 1–3). For example, the SSRIs are efficacious in panic disorder, social anxiety disorder, generalized anxiety disorder, and, to a certain degree, PTSD. These agents may be acting by alteration of activity of brainstem (raphe) serotonergic neurons that synapse on gamma-aminobutyric acid (GABA)-ergic interneurons in the amygdala. Similarly, benzodiazepines may be efficacious in particular anxiety disorders by directly stimulating these GABAergic interneurons in the amygdala, dampening glutamatergic transmission through amygdala nuclei. Agents with activity at metabotropic glutamate receptors may dampen glutamatergic transmission of neurons synapsing in the amygdala by altering activity at the synaptic ionotropic glutamatergic receptors. And particular amygdalofugal pathways, such as those to the locus ceruleus, are known to involve neurons that co-express CRF. Therefore, inhibitors of CRF receptors, which are currently in the drug development pipeline, may be an alternative, and possibly more specific, approach to dampening fear and anxiety responses. These four types of agents all influence change at the receptor level. As knowledge increases about the intracellular processes, gene activation, and neurotrophic factors, novel targets for drug therapies may be suggested. Alternatively, psychotherapies with proven efficacy for certain anxiety disorders such as panic disorder may work by enhancing PFC-based inhibition or extinction of amygdala-mediated anxiety responses, and neuro-imaging experiments demonstrating brain changes induced by such psychotherapies are now possible. Indeed, elucidation of the neurocircuitry involved in anxiety disorders promises to allow development of a vast array of more specific, efficacious, and tolerable treatments.

MODES OF INFLUENCE OF THE AMYGDALA ON BRAIN RESPONSE TO THREAT

The general implication of much of the work reviewed here is that detection of danger is dependent on the amygdala through inputs it receives from the thalamus and cortex. The connectivity of the amygdala suggests three major modes of influence on brain activity. First, not only may direct connections to cortical areas modulate cortical processing of stimuli, but connections to areas such as the PFC may deliver information on the quantity of fear to be incorporated into working memory for a given experience (LeDoux 1996). The lateral PFC and the ACC have strong interconnections, and both have been implicated in working memory. Although the amygdala has relatively sparse connections with the lateral PFC, it has rather dense connections with the ACC. The orbitofrontal cortex (OFC), which is central to reward pathways, is also a region of the PFC that is closely connected with the amygdala and ACC. Although this is a speculative leap, such connections between fear pathways and areas implicated in attention, perception, and working memory may soon make it possible to put conscious feeling of fear back on the neuroanatomical map in considering subjective fear in the human.

Second, the amygdala's connections to serotonergic, noradrenergic, dopaminergic, and cholinergic neuronal areas in the brainstem may modulate the level of arousal as well as the more specific actions of these areas. And amygdala connections with thalamus and brainstem areas such as the nucleus tractus solitarius may serve a gating function in which the amygdala permits greater transmission from external and visceral sensory input sources, thereby heightening reception of sensory stimuli during a

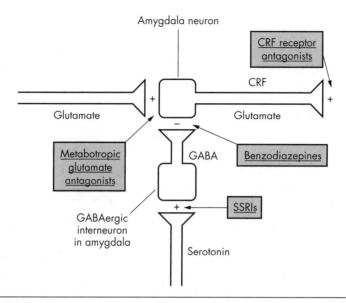

FIGURE 1–3   Theoretical amygdala-dependent synaptic effects of medicinal agents (*underlined*) in clinical use or under development for treatment of anxiety.

The signs + and – indicate that the presynaptic neuron is excitatory or inhibitory, respectively. Neurotransmitters released are indicated next to the axons of the four neurons represented. CRF = corticotropin-releasing factor, GABA = gamma-aminobutyric acid, SSRIs = selective serotonin reuptake inhibitors.

period of potential or real adversity. From this perspective, the brain could be conceived to be upping the gain and tuning in to particular stimuli for the purpose of protection from threat.

Third, well-described amygdalofugal pathways to the hypothalamus, brainstem nuclei, and striatum override tonic regulation of visceral and musculoskeletal systems for survival needs during real or perceived adversity. This results in the described hormonal, autonomic, and behavioral activation that make up a fear response. Once the process is set in motion, information about the visceral and hormonal activation states is transmitted back to the brain, resulting in further alteration of information processing and conscious perception. These three functions serve to place emotional valence on a situation, selectively heighten assessment of the situation, and engage systems appropriate for response to the situation. They also ultimately play a role in the emotional memory of the situation that is encoded through synaptic plasticity. Recent experiments suggest that consolidated implicit memories become labile upon reactivation, and that new protein synthesis is required for the memory to remain intact (Nader et al. 2000). Therefore, consolidation of implicit memory may not be a one-time event, but may be a process that is reiterated with subsequent activation of the memories and that depends on further synaptic plasticity.

CONCLUSIONS

In this review we have focused on the neuroscience of fear conditioning with particular emphasis on the plastic changes that occur at the level of the synapse. The fear system is but one of several implicit memory systems, and our personalities and behaviors depend on interactions between multiple systems involving memory, perception, and emotion that are beyond the scope of the current knowledge base. Yet research has moved beyond the notion that consciousness must be explained before we can address the neural substrates of emotions, including fear and anxiety. Analysis of the fear system may help explain many of the stereotyped fear-related behaviors common to the anxiety disorders. Synaptic microanatomy and activity in fear system structures such as the amygdala depend not only on genetics but also on learning. Synaptic plasticity is currently being revealed at a molecular level, and such plasticity depends on neuronal activity, receptor activation, second-messenger systems, new protein synthesis, and synaptic remodeling involving neurotrophic and other factors. The multitude of advances in neuroscience and translational efforts to understand psychiatric disorders promise to elucidate pathological anxiety in the short term, and in the long term may help us understand what makes up what we call the self.

REFERENCES

Adolphs R, Tranel D, Damasio H, et al: Fear and the human amygdala. J Neurosci 15:5879–5891, 1995

Adolphs R, Tranel D, Damasio AR: The human amygdala in social judgment. Nature 393:470–474, 1998

Amaral DG, Price JL, Pitkänen A, et al: Anatomical organization of the primate amygdaloid complex, in The Amygdala: Neurobiological Aspects of Emotion, Memory, and Mental Dysfunction. Edited by Aggleton JP. New York, Wiley-Liss, 1992, pp 1–66

Amorapanth P, Nader K, LeDoux JE: Lesions of periaqueductal gray dissociate conditioned freezing from conditioned suppression behavior in rats. Learn Mem 6:491–499, 1999

Amorapanth P, LeDoux JE, Nader K: Different lateral amygdala outputs mediate reactions and actions elicited by a fear-arousing stimulus. Nat Neurosci 3:74–79, 2000

Bechara A, Tranel D, Damasio H, et al: Double dissociation of conditioning and declarative knowledge relative to the amygdala and hippocampus in humans. Science 269:1115–1118, 1995

Blanchard RJ, Blanchard DC, Fial RA: Hippocampal lesions in rats and their effect on activity, avoidance, and aggression. J Comp Physiol Psychol 71:92–102, 1970

Braun K, Lange E, Metzger M, et al: Maternal separation followed by early social deprivation affects the development of monoaminergic fiber systems in the medial prefrontal cortex of *Octodon degus*. Neuroscience 95:309–318, 2000

Buchel C, Morris J, Dolan RJ, et al: Brain systems mediating aversive conditioning: an event-related fMRI study. Neuron 20:947–957, 1998

Calder AJ, Young AW, Rowland D, et al: Facial emotion recognition after bilateral amygdala damage: differentially severe impairment of fear. Cognitive Neuropsychology 13:699–745, 1996

Caldji C, Tannenbaum B, Sharma S, et al: Maternal care during infancy regulates the development of neural systems mediating the expression of fearfulness in the rat. Proc Natl Acad Sci U S A 95:5335–5340, 1998

Caldji C, Francis D, Sharma S, et al: The effects of early rearing environment on the development of GABAA and central benzodiazepine receptor levels and novelty-induced fearfulness in the rat. Neuropsychopharmacology 22:219–229, 2000

Cannon WB: Emergency function of the adrenal medulla in pain and major emotions. Am J Physiol 3:356–372, 1914

Canteras NS, Swanson LW: Projections of the ventral subiculum to the amygdala, septum, and hypothalamus: a PHAL anterograde tract-tracing study in the rat. J Comp Neurol 324:180–194, 1992

Cassell MD, Freedman LJ, Shi C: The intrinsic organization of the central extended amygdala. Ann N Y Acad Sci 877:217–241, 1999

Conrad CD, LeDoux JE, Magarinos AM, et al: Repeated restraint stress facilitates fear conditioning independently of causing hippocampal CA3 dendritic atrophy. Behav Neurosci 113:902–913, 1999

Coplan JD, Andrews MW, Rosenblum LA, et al: Persistent elevations of cerebrospinal fluid concentrations of corticotropin-releasing factor in adult nonhuman primates exposed to early life stressors: implications for the pathophysiology of mood and anxiety disorders. Proc Natl Acad Sci U S A 93:1619–1623, 1996

Coplan JD, Trost RC, Owens MJ, et al: Cerebrospinal fluid concentrations of somatostatin and biogenic amines in grown primates reared by mothers exposed to manipulated foraging conditions. Arch Gen Psychiatry 55:473–477, 1998

Corodimas KP, LeDoux JE, Gold PW, et al: Corticosterone potentiation of conditioned fear in rats. Ann N Y Acad Sci 746:392–393, 1994

Davis M: The role of the amygdala in conditioned fear, in The Amygdala: Neurobiological Aspects of Emotion, Memory, and Mental Dysfunction. Edited by Aggleton JP. New York, Wiley-Liss, 1992, pp 255–306

Fanselow MS: Neural organization of the defensive behavior system responsible for fear. Psychonomic Bulletin and Review 1:429–438, 1994

Frankland PW, Cestari V, Filipkowski RK, et al: The dorsal hippocampus is essential for context discrimination but not for contextual conditioning. Behav Neurosci 112:863–874, 1998

Garcia R, Vouimba RM, Baudry M, et al: The amygdala modulates prefrontal cortex activity relative to conditioned fear. Nature 402:294–296, 1999

Halgren E: The amygdala contribution to emotion and memory: current studies in humans, in The Amygdaloid Complex. Edited by Ben-Aris Y. Amsterdam, Elsevier, 1981, pp 395–408

Hirshfeld DR, Rosenbaum JF, Biederman J, et al: Stable behavioral inhibition and its association with anxiety disorder. J Am Acad Child Adolesc Psychiatry 31:103–111, 1992

Holland PC: "Occasion-setting" in conditional discriminations, in Quantitative Analyses of Behavior, Vol 4: Discrimination Processes. Edited by Commons ML, Herrnstein RJ, Wagners AR. New York, Ballinger, 1983, pp 183–206

Huang YY, Kandel ER: Postsynaptic induction and PKA-dependent expression of LTP in the lateral amygdala. Neuron 21:169–178, 1998

Huang YY, Nguyen PV, Abel T, et al: Long-lasting forms of synaptic potentiation in the mammalian hippocampus. Learn Mem 3:74–85, 1996

Huang YY, Martin KC, Kandel ER: Both protein kinase A and mitogen-activated protein kinase are required in the amygdala for the macromolecular synthesis-dependent late phase of long-term potentiation. J Neurosci 20:6317–6325, 2000

Huot RL, Thrivikraman KV, Meaney MJ, et al: Development of adult ethanol preference and anxiety as a consequence of neonatal maternal separation in Long Evans rats and reversal with antidepressant treatment. Psychopharmacology (Berl) 158:366–373, 2001

Kagan J, Reznick JS, Snidman N: The physiology and psychology of behavioral inhibition in children. Child Dev 58:1459–1473, 1987

Kagan J, Snidman N, Arcus D: Childhood derivatives of high and low reactivity in infancy. Child Dev 69:1483–1493, 1998

Kapp BS, Whalen PJ, Supple WF, et al: Amygdaloid contributions to conditioned arousal and sensory information processing, in The Amygdala: Neurobiological Aspects of Emotion, Memory, and Mental Dysfunction. Edited by Aggleton JP. New York, Wiley-Liss, 1992, pp 229–254

Kim JJ, Fanselow MS: Modality-specific retrograde amnesia of fear. Science 256:675–677, 1992

LaBar KS, LeDoux JE, Spencer DD, et al: Impaired fear conditioning following unilateral temporal lobectomy in humans. J Neurosci 15:6846–6855, 1995

LaBar KS, Gatenby JC, Gore JC, et al: Human amygdala activation during conditioned fear acquisition and extinction: a mixed-trial fMRI study. Neuron 20:937–945, 1998

LeDoux JE: Emotion, in Handbook of Physiology: The Nervous System, Vol V: Higher Functions of the Brain. Edited by Plums F. Bethesda, MD, American Physiological Society, 1987, pp 419–460

LeDoux JE: Emotion and the Amygdala, in The Amygdala: Neurobiological Aspects of Emotion, Memory, and Mental Dysfunction. Edited by Aggleton JP. New York, Wiley-Liss, 1992, pp 339–351

LeDoux JE: The Emotional Brain. New York, Simon & Schuster, 1996

LeDoux JE, Iwata J, Cicchetti P, et al: Different projections of the central amygdaloid nucleus mediate autonomic and behavioral correlates of conditioned fear. J Neurosci 8:2517–2529, 1988

LeDoux JE, Cicchetti P, Xagoraris A, et al: The lateral amygdaloid nucleus: sensory interface of the amygdala in fear conditioning. J Neurosci 10:1062–1069, 1990a

LeDoux JE, Farb CF, Ruggiero DA: Topographic organization of neurons in the acoustic thalamus that project to the amygdala. J Neurosci 10:1043–1054, 1990b

Liu D, Diorio J, Tannenbaum B, et al: Maternal care, hippocampal glucocorticoid receptors, and hypothalamic-pituitary-adrenal responses to stress. Science 277:1659–1662, 1997

Liu D, Caldji C, Sharma S, et al: Influence of neonatal rearing conditions on stress-induced adrenocorticotropin responses and norepinephrine release in the hypothalamic paraventricular nucleus. J Neuroendocrinol 12:5–12, 2000

Majidishad P, Pelli DG, LeDoux JE: Disruption of fear conditioning to contextual stimuli but not to a tone by lesions of the accessory basal nucleus of the amygdala (abstract). Abstr Soc Neurosci 22:1116, 1996

Manning BH: A lateralized deficit in morphine antinociception after unilateral inactivation of the central amygdala. J Neurosci 18:9453–9470, 1998

Maren S, Fanselow MS: Synaptic plasticity in the basolateral amygdala induced by hippocampal formation stimulation in vivo. J Neurosci 15:7548–7564, 1995

Maren S, Fanselow MS: The amygdala and fear conditioning: has the nut been cracked? Neuron 16:237–240, 1996

Maren S, Aharonov G, Fanselow MS: Neurotoxic lesions of the dorsal hippocampus and Pavlovian fear conditioning in rats. Behav Brain Res 88:261–274, 1997

Mascagni F, McDonald AJ, Coleman JR: Corticoamygdaloid and corticocortical projections of the rat temporal cortex: a phaseolus vulgaris leucoagglutinin study. Neuroscience 57:697–715, 1993

McDonald AJ: Cortical pathways to the mammalian amygdala. Prog Neurobiol 55:257–332, 1998

McEwen BS, Sapolsky RM: Stress and cognitive function. Curr Opin Neurobiol 5:205–216, 1995

Morgan MA, LeDoux JE: Differential contribution of dorsal and ventral medial prefrontal cortex to the acquisition and extinction of conditioned fear in rats. Behav Neurosci 109:681–688, 1995

Morgan MA, LeDoux JE: Contribution of ventrolateral prefrontal cortex to the acquisition and extinction of conditioned fear in rats. Neurobiol Learn Mem 72:244–251, 1999

Morgan MA, Romanski LM, LeDoux JE: Extinction of emotional learning: contribution of medial prefrontal cortex. Neurosci Lett 163:109–113, 1993

Morris JS, Ohman A, Dolan RJ: Conscious and unconscious emotional learning in the human amygdala. Nature 393:467–470, 1998

Morris JS, Ohman A, Dolan RJ: A subcortical pathway to the right amygdala mediating "unseen" fear. Proc Natl Acad Sci U S A 96:1680–1685, 1999

Nader K, Schafe GE, LeDoux JE: The labile nature of consolidation theory. Nat Rev Neurosci 1:216–219, 2000

Pare D, Smith Y, Pare JF: Intra-amygdaloid projections of the basolateral and basomedial nuclei in the cat: phaseolus vulgaris–leucoagglutinin anterograde tracing at the light and electron microscopic level. Neuroscience 69:567–583, 1995

Pavlov IP: Conditioned Reflexes. New York, Dover, 1927

Phillips RG, LeDoux JE: Differential contribution of amygdala and hippocampus to cued and contextual fear conditioning. Behav Neurosci 106:274–285, 1992

Pitkänen A, Savander V, LeDoux JL: Organization of intra-amygdaloid circuitries: an emerging framework for understanding functions of the amygdala. Trends Neurosci 20:517–523, 1997

Repa JC, Muller J, Apergis J, et al: Two different lateral amygdala cell populations contribute to the initiation and storage of memory. Nat Neurosci 4:724–731, 2001

Rescorla RA: Behavioral studies of Pavlovian conditioning. Annu Rev Neurosci 11:329–352, 1988

Rodrigues SM, Schafe GE, LeDoux JE: Intra-amygdala blockade of the NR2B subunit of the NMDA receptor disrupts the acquisition but not the expression of fear conditioning. J Neurosci 21:6889–6896, 2001

Romanski LM, LeDoux JE: Information cascade from primary auditory cortex to the amygdala: corticocortical and corticoamygdaloid projections of temporal cortex in the rat. Cereb Cortex 3:515–532, 1993

Rosenblum LA, Paully GS: The effects of varying environmental demands on maternal and infant behavior. Child Dev 55:305–314, 1984

Rosenblum LA, Coplan JD, Friedman S, et al: Adverse early experiences affect noradrenergic and serotonergic functioning in adult primates. Biol Psychiatry 35:221–227, 1994

Rudy JW: Postconditioning isolation disrupts contextual conditioning: an experimental analysis. Behav Neurosci 110:238–246, 1996

Rudy JW, Pugh CR: A comparison of contextual and generalized auditory-cue fear conditioning: evidence for similar memory processes. Behav Neurosci 110:1299–1308, 1996

Sapolsky RM: Stress, glucocorticoids, and damage to the nervous system: the current state of confusion. Stress 1:1–19, 1996

Schafe GE, LeDoux JE: Memory consolidation of auditory Pavlovian fear conditioning requires protein synthesis and protein kinase A in the amygdala. J Neurosci 20:RC96, 2000

Schafe GE, Nadel NV, Sullivan GM, et al: Memory consolidation for contextual and auditory fear conditioning is dependent on protein synthesis, PKA, and MAP kinase. Learn Mem 6:97–110, 1999

Schafe GE, Atkins CM, Swank MW, et al: Activation of ERK/MAP kinase in the amygdala is required for memory consolidation of Pavlovian fear conditioning. J Neurosci 20:8177–8187, 2000

Scott SK, Young AW, Calder AJ, et al: Impaired auditory recognition of fear and anger following bilateral amygdala lesions. Nature 385:254–257, 1997

Shepard JD, Barron KW, Myers DA: Corticosterone delivery to the amygdala increases corticotropin-releasing factor mRNA in the central amygdaloid nucleus and anxiety-like behavior. Brain Res 861:288–295, 2000

Squire LR, Knowlton B, Musen G: The structure and organization of memory. Annu Rev Psychol 44:453–495, 1993

Swanson LW, Petrovich GD: What is the amygdala? Trends Neurosci 21:323–331, 1998

Takahashi LK, Rubin WW: Corticosteroid induction of threat-induced behavioral inhibition in preweanling rats. Behav Neurosci 107:860–866, 1993

van de Kar LD, Piechowski RA, Rittenhouse PA, et al: Amygdaloid lesions: differential effect on conditioned stress and immobilization-induced increases in corticosterone and renin secretion. Neuroendocrinology 54:89–95, 1991

Weisskopf MG, Bauer EP, LeDoux JE: L-type voltage-gated calcium channels mediate NMDA-independent associative long-term potentiation at thalamic input synapses to the amygdala. J Neurosci 19:10512–10519, 1999

Welberg LA, Seckl JR, Holmes MC: Inhibition of 11beta-hydroxysteroid dehydrogenase, the foeto-placental barrier to maternal glucocorticoids, permanently programs amygdala GR mRNA expression and anxiety-like behaviour in the offspring. Eur J Neurosci 12:1047–1054, 2000

Whalen PJ, Rauch SL, Etcoff NL, et al: Masked presentations of emotional facial expressions modulate amygdala activity without explicit knowledge. J Neurosci 18:411–418, 1998

Yaniv D, Schafe GE, LeDoux JE, et al: A gradient of plasticity in the amygdala revealed by cortical and subcortical stimulation, in vivo. Neuroscience 106:613–620, 2001

2

Does Stress Damage the Brain?

Bruce S. McEwen, Ph.D.
Ana Maria Magarinos, Ph.D.

What is the capacity of the brain to withstand the ravages of stress? The answer to this question is evolving as our knowledge of the brain increases and as we better understand the complex interactions between the hormonal and tissue mediators of the response to stressors and their protective, as well as damaging, effects. The first major step was the recognition that the brain regulates the hormonal and neural response to stressful challenges through the hypothalamic outputs to the pituitary gland and the autonomic nervous system (Dallman et al. 1987; Harris 1970; Sawchenko et al. 1993; Spiess et al. 1981). Another major breakthrough was the realization that psychological stressors have a major influence in activating the hormonal and autonomic responses of the stress hormone axis (Mason 1968). Thus, the brain is the interpreter of what is "stressful" and the regulator of the behavioral, as well as physiological, responses to the perceived or actual stressor.

Another important revelation was the demonstration that the brain is a target for the actions of stress hormones (McEwen et al. 1968, 1986). This led first to the recognition of conditions in which stress hormones participate in some forms of brain damage (Landfield 1987; Sapolsky 1992) and then, somewhat later, to the realization that there are many protective and adaptive actions of stress mediators (McEwen 1998). Among these actions is their influence on the structural plasticity of brain regions involved in cognition and emotion. Although interpreted at first as signs of incipient brain damage, stress-induced structural plasticity of the adult brain appears to be largely adaptive and reversible, at least over the time span of weeks. This chapter summarizes the current status of this story in the context of its historical progression. We also discuss the implications for human disorders such as Cushing's disease and depressive illness in which cognitive deficits and atrophy of brain structures have been reported.

ADRENAL STEROID RECEPTORS IN THE HIPPOCAMPUS

Intracellular receptors for adrenal steroid hormones are found in the hippocampal formation and other regions of the adult brain such as the amygdala and hypothalamus (McEwen et al. 1968, 1986). There are two types of receptors: type I, or mineralocorticoid receptors, and type II, or glucocorticoid receptors (Reul and DeKloet 1986). They form a two-level recognition system for adrenal steroids: Type I receptors are occupied by adrenal steroid fluctuations during the diurnal cycle of sleep and activity, whereas type II receptors have a fivefold lower affinity for cortisol and corticosterone than type I receptors and are occupied by stress-induced levels of cortisol and corticosterone. Type I receptors are more discretely concentrated in brain regions such as the hippocampus, parts of the amygdala, septum, regions of the thalamus, and brainstem (Ahima et al. 1991), whereas type II receptors are more uniformly distributed throughout the brain (Ahima and Harlan 1990).

ROLE OF THE HIPPOCAMPUS, PREFRONTAL CORTEX, AND AMYGDALA IN COGNITION AND EMOTION

The hippocampus, prefrontal cortex, and amygdala play important roles in memory and emotional regulation. Whereas the prefrontal cortex has an important role in working memory (Goldman-Rakic 1999), the amygdala is a key structure in processing negative and positive emotions (LeDoux 2000; Roozendaal et al. 1996). The hippocampus is a way station for the processing of spatial and episodic memory (Eichenbaum and Otto 1992).

The hippocampus is important for contextual fear conditioning, but it is not as important in fear conditioning associated with specific stimuli such as tone (Anagnostaras et al. 2001; Phillips and LeDoux 1992).

DAMAGE IN HIPPOCAMPUS MADE WORSE BY ADRENAL STEROIDS

The hippocampus is vulnerable to damage by strokes, head trauma, and seizures, and it also shows early structural changes in the onset of Alzheimer's disease (Sapolsky 1992). The trisynaptic structure of the hippocampus is key to its vulnerability. Entorhinal cortex input to the hippocampus is the first area to show atrophy in the onset of Alzheimer's disease (Bobinski et al. 1999). The perforant pathway input from the entorhinal cortex to the dentate gyrus and CA3 region is the main entry point of information that is processed by the hippocampus. The organization of the CA3 region, with reciprocal connections to the dentate gyrus and collateral connections between CA3 pyramidal neurons (Li et al. 1994; Sik et al. 1994, 1995), is the basis of the synchronized firing of the CA3 that is postulated to play an important role in memory of sequences of events (Lisman 1999). This organization is also the basis for the susceptibility of the hippocampus to kindled seizures and to kainic acid, both of which cause damage and neuron loss that is heaviest in the CA3 region (Nadler et al. 1978; Roozendaal et al. 2001). The feedforward actions of glutamate on presynaptic kainate receptors cause further glutamate release and enhance the feedforward nature of the CA3 response to stimulation (Lauri et al. 2001; Schmitz et al. 2001).

Because of this anatomical organization, it is perhaps not surprising that kainate-induced damage to the CA3 region is exacerbated by adrenal steroids and can be reduced by blocking adrenal steroid synthesis in animals receiving kainic acid (Roozendaal et al. 2001). The CA1 region of the hippocampus is also susceptible to damage from ischemia, and these effects are also enhanced by adrenal steroids (Sapolsky and Pulsinelli 1985). This discovery has been the basis of efforts to avoid the use of glucocorticoids to treat brain edema in stroke and head trauma.

AGING, PREMATURE AGING, AND GLUCOCORTICOIDS

Prior to the aforementioned discoveries, the hippocampus was shown to be sensitive to high levels of adrenal steroids. Darkly stained cells were found in the guinea pig hippocampus after the administration of high doses of cortisone (AusDerMuhlen and Ockenfels 1969). More recent studies have reported darkly staining neurons after a cold swim stress in rats (Mizoguchi et al. 1992). Although the exact nature of these darkly staining neurons remains a mystery, the aging rat brain was found to undergo structural changes that could be prevented by adrenalectomy in midlife (Landfield et al. 1978). These changes include decreased neuronal density and increased numbers of astrocytes, as well as impairment of maze learning and performance (Landfield et al. 1986).

Robert Sapolsky mimicked some of the anatomical effects attributed to adrenal steroids in younger animals by treatment with high doses of glucocorticoids (Sapolsky et al. 1985). He also provided evidence for a role of the hippocampus in the shutoff of stress-induced elevations of glucocorticoids (for review, see Jacobson and Sapolsky 1991) and proposed the glucocorticoid cascade hypothesis of aging, in which the feedforward actions of adrenal steroids on the hippocampus during aging progressively impair hippocampal function and lead to progressively higher levels of glucocorticoids as the brain ages (Sapolsky 1992; Sapolsky et al. 1986). Individual differences in brain aging may therefore be tied to an increased "area under the curve" for the cumulative exposure of the brain to glucocorticoids, and some evidence for this has come from animal and human studies (Meaney et al. 1988; Star et al. 2002). One test of this notion has been the finding that the handling of young rats to produce a less reactive stress hormone axis leads to fewer rats showing age-related cognitive impairment (Meaney et al. 1988).

Both Landfield and Sapolsky have suggested that age-related cognitive impairment is related to loss of neurons in the hippocampus (Landfield and Eldridge 1994; Stein-Behrens et al. 1992). However, a number of studies have not found neuronal loss, although some form of functional, neurochemical impairment is evident in individual animals that show greater loss of cognitive function (Nicolle et al. 2001; Rapp and Gallagher 1996). Moreover, there are decreases in synapse density in the aging brain (Geinisman et al. 1992, 1995; Rapp et al. 1999; Smith et al. 2000).

Stress also produces impairment of cognitive functions that depend on the hippocampus, and some of these effects can be mimicked by exogenous glucocorticoid administration. One study of animals subjected to subordination as a chronic stressor for 1 month to several years found that there was shrinkage of neurons and apparent neuron loss in the hippocampus, particularly in the CA3 region (Rozovsky et al. 2002). Another study on rats showed that a cold-water swim stress produced dark-stained nerve cells in the hippocampus (Mizoguchi et al. 1992). Another study treated middle-aged rats with corticosterone for three cycles of 21 days each and found that previously nonimpaired rats became cognitively impaired as a result of the glucocorticoid treatment; impaired rats showed increased number of neurons that were darkly stained with cresyl violet (Arbel et al. 1994). Another study treated young or middle-aged rats for 1 or 3 months with corticosterone pellets; only the middle-aged rats treated for 3 months were impaired in a Morris water maze and in studies of long-term potentiation, but there was no decrease in neuronal density (Bodnoff et al. 1995).

Yet another study used a chronic stress in a shuttle-box shock avoidance paradigm for 6 months to cause impaired excitability in the hippocampus; the effects were evaluated 3 weeks after cessation of stress and were found

only in the stressed young animals; middle-aged and aging rats had reduced excitability that was not further reduced by stress (Kerr et al. 1991).
However, middle-aged and aging rats showed impaired stress-induced
downregulation of type II receptors in the hippocampus (Eldridge et al.
1989). It is possible that the failure to downregulate glucocorticoid receptors represents the failure of a protective mechanism, namely, reduction of
the sensitivity of the hippocampus to glucocorticoids that can exacerbate
excitotoxic damage. These findings raise the interesting possibility that
stress can cause some form of brain damage, but new information has
come to light suggesting another side to the story—namely, that stress hormones play an important role in adaptation and that the brain is capable
of considerable structural plasticity that may enable it to withstand the effects of fairly prolonged stress.

ROLES OF STRESS-RELATED HORMONES IN ADAPTATION

The amygdala and hippocampus are both involved in contextual fear conditioning and in passive avoidance learning. In fear conditioning, glucocorticoids enhance learned fear (Corodimas et al. 1994). They also play an
important role in forming the memory of context in contextual fear conditioning, but not of the actual effect of foot shock in rats that are already
familiar with the context where the shock is administered (Pugh et al.
1997a, 1997b). This suggests that the hippocampal role in contextual fear
conditioning is enhanced by moderate levels of glucocorticoids, but the
fear conditioning either is not heavily dependent on glucocorticoids or is
so strong that glucocorticoid influence is hard to demonstrate. Yet there is
evidence for an influence of glucocorticoids on the flow of information
within the amygdala.

   Glucocorticoids potentiate serotonin inhibition of the processing of excitatory input to the lateral amygdala from the thalamus, which suggests
that there is a mechanism for containing, or limiting, the sensory input that
is important for fear conditioning (Stutzmann et al. 1998). Thus, adrenal
steroids may regulate the nature of the signals that reach the amygdala and
allow for greater discrimination of the most salient cues for learning.

   Moreover, in passive avoidance, both catecholamines and glucocorticoids play a role in facilitating the learning (Cahill et al. 1994; Roozendaal
2000). Catecholamines work outside of the blood-brain barrier, and their
effects can be blocked by beta-adrenergic blocking agents that do not cross
the blood-brain barrier (Cahill et al. 1994). Glucocorticoids enter the
brain, and local implants of exogenous corticosterone into the hippocampus,

amygdala, and nucleus tractus solitarii (NTS) enhance passive avoidance learning (Roozendaal 2000).

Adrenal steroids also play a supporting role in the learning of a spatial navigation task in mice (Oitzl et al. 2001). Adrenalectomy impairs the acquisition of the memory of hidden platform location in the Morris water maze, and glucocorticoid administration restores the normal learning curve; however, in mice in which the glucocorticoid receptor was deleted and replaced with a glucocorticoid receptor that lacks the DNA binding domain, glucocorticoids have no effect in improving task acquisition (Oitzl et al. 2001). This finding illustrates a role for glucocorticoid receptors in acting on the genome in a task that is known to depend on the hippocampus. Interestingly, other actions of glucocorticoids via glucocorticoid receptors are known to involve the protein-protein interactions that are not prevented in mice carrying the glucocorticoid receptor defective in the DNA binding domain (Reichardt and Schutz 1998).

Other evidence for glucocorticoid actions supports an inverted U-shaped dose-response curve in which low to moderate levels of adrenal steroids enhance acquisition of tasks that involve the hippocampus, whereas high levels of glucocorticoids disrupt task acquisition (Conrad et al. 1999; Diamond et al. 1992, 1999; Pugh et al. 1997b). Adrenal steroids have biphasic effects on the excitability of hippocampal neurons that may underlie their biphasic actions on memory and recall (Diamond et al. 1992; Joels 1997; Pavlides and McEwen 1999; Pavlides et al. 1994, 1995).

The actions of adrenal steroids on behavior involve biphasic effects on conditioning and extinction of behaviors involving fear and anxiety that are mediated by type I and type II receptors (Korte 2001). Both unconditioned and conditioned fear show an inverted-U dose-response curve, with type I receptors facilitating acute fear and type II receptors promoting fear conditioning. However, both type I and type II receptors play a role in facilitating the extinction of learned fear during forced exposure to an inescapable stressor (Korte 2001). There are indications that extinction of learned fear is an active learning process not unlike the learning of the fear (Santini et al. 2001).

STRUCTURAL PLASTICITY OF THE HIPPOCAMPUS

One of the remarkable discoveries in modern neurobiology concerns the capacity of the adult brain to undergo structural remodeling as a result of experience. This was first shown in enriched-environment studies (Bennett et al. 1964) and later in response to brain lesions (Parnavelas et al.

1974). Patterns of synaptic activity reorganize synaptic connectivity and promote dendritic branching and sprouting of new synaptic connections (Das and Gilbert 1995; Jones et al. 1999; Wallace et al. 1992).

The adult hippocampus undergoes a number of types of structural remodeling. Estrogens and androgens regulate the formation of excitatory spine synapses on hippocampal pyramidal neurons, whereas glucocorticoids and repeated stress cause the remodeling of dendrites of CA3 pyramidal neurons and dentate gyrus granule neurons and the increased branching of neurons in the amygdala (McEwen 2000). In the dentate gyrus, there is ongoing neurogenesis in adult life that is enhanced by exercise and by an enriched environment and suppressed by certain acute and chronic stressors (Gould et al. 1997c, 1998; Kempermann et al. 1997; van Praag et al. 1999).

Role of Stress Mediators in Structural Plasticity

Chronic stress causes structural remodeling of the hippocampus and amygdala. These actions appear to be largely reversible and to occur in situations where the amount of stress or stress hormone secretion is not a major factor. Moreover, although glucocorticoid administration can "drive" aspects of this remodeling process, the major mediators are the excitatory amino acids aided by other neurotransmitter systems and by circulating glucocorticoids. As a result, we refer to these changes as adaptive plasticity and remodeling and avoid using the term *atrophy*. We postulate that this plasticity may not only help the brain adapt to new situations but may also help to protect it from actual damage. Following is a brief summary of the status of work concerning the stress effects on dentate gyrus cell proliferation and remodeling of dendrites.

Dentate Gyrus Neurogenesis
Cell proliferation and neurogenesis in the dentate gyrus of adult rodents has been reported (Altman and Bayer 1975; Kaplan and Bell 1984; Kaplan and Hinds 1977) but was never fully appreciated until recently. The rediscovery of this topic occurred in an unusual manner. First, bilateral adrenalectomy (ADX) of an adult rat was shown to increase granule neuron death by apoptosis (Gould et al. 1990; Sloviter et al. 1989). Subsequently, cell proliferation was also found to increase following ADX in adults rats (Cameron and Gould 1994), as well as in the perinatal dentate gyrus (Cameron and Gould 1996a). In adult rats, very low levels of adrenal steroids, sufficient to occupy type I adrenal steroid receptors, completely block dentate gyrus neuronal loss (Woolley et al. 1991). Con-

versely, in newborn rats, type II receptor agonists protect against neuronal apoptosis (Gould et al. 1997b). This is consistent with the fact that dentate gyrus neuronal loss in the developing rat occurs at much higher circulating steroid levels than in the adult, and it represents another example of the different ways that the two adrenal steroid receptor types are involved in hippocampal function (Lupien and McEwen 1997).

In adult rats, newly formed neurons arise in the hilus, very close to the granule cell layer, and then migrate into the granule cell layer, presumably along a vimentin-staining radial glial network that is also enhanced by ADX (Cameron et al. 1993). Most neuroblasts labeled with [^{3}H]thymidine lack both type I and type II adrenal steroid receptors (Cameron et al. 1993), indicating that steroidal regulation occurs via messengers from an unidentified steroid-sensitive cell that may involve a signaling role for transforming growth factor (TGF)–alpha and the epidermal growth factor (EGF) receptor system (Tanapat and Gould 1997) or possibly insulin-like growth factor–1 (IGF-1) (discussed later). The precursor cells for the new neurons use a glial fibrillary acidic protein (GFAP) promotor and may be a modified type of astrocyte (Seri et al. 2001).

It has been reported that dentate gyrus cell proliferation declines in the aging rodent (Kempermann et al. 1998) and rhesus monkey (Gould et al. 1999b). Recent studies of aging rats show that adrenalectomy could reverse the decline in dentate gyrus cell proliferation (Cameron and McKay 1999), suggesting that such decline is the result of age-related increases in hypothalamic-pituitary-adrenal (HPA) activity and glucocorticoid levels that have been reported (Landfield and Eldridge 1994; McEwen 1992; Sapolsky 1992; Sapolsky et al. 1986). The question of whether dentate gyrus cell neurogenesis is a widespread phenomenon among mammals was addressed recently by studies showing that it occurs in the marmoset (Gould et al. 1998), a New World primate, as well as in an Old World primate species, the rhesus monkey (Gould et al 1999b), and in the adult human dentate gyrus (Eriksson et al. 1998). Thus, changes in size of the human hippocampus, described earlier in relation to depressive illness, may include changes in neuron number in the dentate gyrus. In this connection, antidepressant treatments have been reported to increase cell proliferation in the otherwise untreated rat brain (Malberg et al. 2000) and in the tree shrew undergoing chronic psychosocial stress (Czeh et al. 2001).

Besides antidepressant treatments, granule neuron birth is accelerated by seizurelike activity (Parent et al. 1997), and the stimulus for this cell proliferation is likely to be apoptotic cell death because seizures kill granule neurons (Bengzon et al. 1997) and local increases in apoptosis simulate local neurogenesis (Cameron and Gould 1996b). Granule neuron birth is also accelerated by blocking N-methyl-D-aspartate (NMDA) receptors or lesioning the excitatory perforant pathway input from the entorhinal cortex (Cameron et al. 1995). Unlike ADX, these treatments do not increase granule neuron apoptosis, and a single dose of an NMDA blocking drug results in a 20% increase in dentate gyrus neuron number several weeks later (Cameron et al. 1995). Thus, although increased apoptosis leads to increased cell proliferation (Gould and Tanapat 1997), the two processes occur in different regions of the granule cell layer and can be uncoupled. Nevertheless, the adrenal steroid suppression of dentate gyrus cell proliferation is through an NMDA receptor mechanism (Gould et al. 1997a; Noguchi et al. 1990).

Very recently it was reported that serotonin may be a positive signal for cell proliferation and neurogenesis in the adult dentate gyrus. Treatment with the serotonin-releasing drug d-fenfluramine increased cell division (Gould 1999). Likewise, the 5-HT$_{1A}$ agonist 8-hydroxy-DPAT stimulated cell proliferation, whereas blockade of 5-HT$_{1A}$ receptors had the opposite effect and prevented the effect of d-fenfluramine treatment (Gould 1999), as well as preventing increased cell division caused by pilocarpine-induced seizures (Radley et al. 1998).

Circulating IGF-1 is another stimulator of dentate gyrus cell division (Aberg et al. 2000; O'Kusky et al. 2000). IGF-1 is a 7.5 kDa protein and yet is taken up into cerebrospinal fluid by a process that is independent of IGF receptors or binding proteins (Pulford and Ishii 2001). In rats, voluntary running in a running wheel has been reported to increase cell proliferation in the dentate gyrus (van Praag et al. 1999). Such exercise increases the uptake of IGF-1 from the blood and activates c-fos expression in dentate gyrus and other brain regions in a manner that is mimicked by IGF-1 administration into the circulation (Carro et al. 2000). Moreover, immunoneutralization of IGF-1 blocks the effects of exercise to enhance cell division (Trejo et al. 2001). Receptors for IGF-1, IGF-2, and insulin are expressed in the hippocampus (Dore et al. 1997b), with IGF-1 receptors undergoing a decrease after adrenalectomy (Islam et al. 1998). Although IGF-1, IGF-2, and insulin binding does not decrease with age in the rat hippocampus (Dore et al. 1997b), the level of IGF-1 mRNA undergoes a small but selective decrease in some hippocampal fields (Lai et al. 2000). Exogenous IGF-1 ameliorates memory deficits in aging rats (Markowska et al. 1998) and enhances glucose uptake in the aging hippocampus (Lynch et al. 2001), as well as having neuroprotective actions (Dore et al. 1997a; Gleichmann et al. 2000; Takadera et al. 1999).

Other important, albeit negative, regulators of cell proliferation are certain types of acute and chronic stress. Acute stress involving the odor of a natural predator, the fox, inhibits cell division and neurogenesis in the adult rat (Galea et al. 1996). Acute psychosocial stress in the adult tree shrew, involving largely visual cues, inhibits cell proliferation (Gould et al. 1997c), an effect that is reversed by treatment with an antidepressant (Czeh et al. 2001). Inhibition of cell division is also seen in the dentate gyrus of the marmoset after acute psychosocial stress (Gould et al. 1998).

Chronic psychosocial stress in the tree shrew results in a more substantial inhibition of cell proliferation than after a single acute stressful encounter. Moreover, the dentate gyrus is 30% smaller in the chronically stressed tree shrew, although granule neuron number shows only a trend for reduction (Gould et al. 1997c; E. Gould and E. Fuchs, unpublished observations, 2000). This finding suggests that there may be other changes such as remodeling of dendritic branching to account for the decrease in dentate gyrus volume. Recent studies on dendritic remodeling caused by glucocorticoids and also by repeated stress indicate that dentate gyrus dendrites undergo dendritic remodeling along with dendrites in CA3 and CA1 pyramidal neurons (Sousa et al. 2000).

One reason for turnover of dentate gyrus granule neurons in adult life is to adjust needs for hippocampal function in spatial learning and memory to environmental demands (Sherry et al. 1992). Birds that use space around them to hide and locate food, and voles as well as deer mice that traverse large distances to find mates, have larger hippocampal volumes than closely related species that do not (Sherry et al. 1992). Moreover, there are indications that hippocampal volume may change during the breeding season (Galea et al. 1994; Sherry et al. 1992). Indeed, the rate of neurogenesis in the male and female prairie vole varies according to the breeding season (Galea and McEwen 1999). In contrast, an enriched environment increases dentate gyrus volume in mice by increasing neuronal survival without altering the rate of neurogenesis (Kempermann et al. 1997). Thus, there are several ways to maintain the balance between neuronal apoptosis and neurogenesis.

Learning that involves the hippocampus also appears to affect the survival of newly formed dentate granule neurons. When rats were trained in a task involving the hippocampus, the survival of previously labeled granule neurons was prolonged (Gould et al. 1999a). Changes in dentate gyrus volume appear to have consequences for cognitive functions subserved by the hippocampus. In the enriched-environment studies (Kempermann et al. 1997), increased dentate gyrus volume was accompanied by better performance on spatial learning tasks. In contrast, decreased dentate gyrus volume in chronically stressed tree shrews is paralleled by impaired spatial learning and memory (Ohl and Fuchs 1999), although this might be as much due to remodeling of dendrites of CA3 pyramidal neurons and dentate granule neurons as to reduced dentate gyrus cell proliferation and neurogenesis.

Remodeling of Dendrites in Hippocampal Neurons

Remodeling of dendrites in hippocampal neurons was first described after treatment of adult male rats for 21 days with exogenous glucocorticoids (Woolley et al. 1990) (reviewed in McEwen 1999; McEwen et al. 1995). Subsequently, chronic restraint stress for 21 days in rats caused apical dendrites of CA3 pyramidal neurons to remodel (Watanabe et al. 1992b). A recent study using a multiple-stress paradigm, lasting 4 weeks, demonstrated that the remodeling of dendrites found in CA3 also occurs in the dentate gyrus and in CA1, although the effects in CA3 tend to be the greatest (Sousa et al. 2000). This important finding provides the basis for the hypothesis that remodeling of dendrites could be a factor in the shrinkage of the hippocampus reported in a number of disorders, such as recurrent major depression and aging with mild cognitive impairment (for reviews, see McEwen 1999; Sapolsky 1996).

Stress- and glucocorticoid-induced remodeling were prevented by the anti-epileptic drug phenytoin (Dilantin); this implicates the release and actions of excitatory amino acids, because phenytoin blocks glutamate release and antagonizes sodium channels and possibly also T-type calcium channels that are activated during glutamate-induced excitation (McEwen 1999). This result is consistent with evidence that stress induces the release of glutamate in the hippocampus and other brain regions (see Lowy et al. 1993; Moghaddam et al. 1994). Moreover, glucocorticoids increase extracellular levels of glutamate and aspartate in the hippocampus (Venero and Borrell 1999). The connection with excitatory amino acids is consistent with the finding that NMDA receptor blockade is also effective in preventing stress-induced dendritic remodeling (for reviews, see McEwen 1999; McEwen et al. 1995).

Besides glutamate, other participating neurotransmitters include GABA and serotonin. As for GABA, inhibitory interneurons have a significant role in controlling hippocampal neuronal excitability (Freund and Buzsaki 1996), and the involvement of the GABA-benzodiazepine receptor system is revealed by the ability of a benzodiazepine, adinazolam, to block dendritic remodeling (Magarinos et al. 1999). Serotonin is released by stressors, and tianeptine, an atypical tricyclic antidepressant, enhances serotonin reuptake and thus reduces extracellular 5-HT levels. Tianeptine prevented both stress- and corticosterone-induced dendritic remodeling of CA3 pyramidal neurons (Watanabe et al. 1992a), whereas fluoxetine and fluvoxamine, inhibitors of serotonin reuptake, and desipramine, an inhibitor of noradrenaline uptake, failed to block remodeling (Magarinos et al. 1999). Further evidence for serotonin involvement in dendritic remodeling comes from studies of psychosocial stress in rats (McKittrick et al. 2000).

Because both phenytoin and tianeptine block corticosterone- and stress-induced remodeling of CA3 pyramidal neurons (see McEwen et al. 1995), it is possible that serotonin released by stress or by corticosterone interacts pre- or postsynaptically with glutamate released by stress or by corticosterone. As a result of this interaction, the final common path may involve interactive effects between serotonin and glutamate receptors on the dendrites of CA3 neurons innervated by mossy fibers from the dentate gyrus. There is evidence for interactions between serotonin and NMDA receptors, indicating that serotonin potentiates NMDA receptor binding as well as activity of NMDA receptors, and may do so via $5\text{-}HT_2$ receptors (Mennini and Miari 1991; Rahmann and Neumann 1993).

Glucocorticoid treatment causes dendritic remodeling, and stress-induced remodeling is blocked by treatment with an adrenal steroid synthesis blocker, cyanoketone (see McEwen 1999; McEwen et al. 1995), indicating a role played by endogenous glucocorticoids in stress-induced dendritic remodeling. There appear to be several ways in which glucocorticoids affect the excitatory amino acid system:

- Adrenal steroids increase extracellular levels of glutamate in hippocampus by a mechanism that does not appear to be sensitive to mineralocorticoid and glucocorticoid receptor blockers (Venero and Borrell 1999). Moreover, adrenalectomy markedly reduces the magnitude of the excitatory amino acid release evoked by restraint stress (Lowy et al. 1993). Mossy fiber terminals in the stratum lucidum contain presynaptic kainate receptors that positively regulate glutamate release (Chittajallu et al. 1996); these presynaptic kainate receptors are decreased in density by ADX and restored to normal by corticosterone replacement (Watanabe et al. 1995). Moreover, repeated stress causes a reorganization of synaptic vesicles within mossy fiber terminals (MFTs), as reported recently in a study using electron microscopy (Magarinos et al. 1997). Whereas MFTs from control rats were packed with small, clear synaptic vesicles, those from rats receiving 21 days of restraint stress showed a marked rearrangement of vesicles, with more densely packed clusters localized in the vicinity of active synaptic zones. Moreover, compared with controls, restraint stress increased the area of the MFT occupied by mitochondrial profiles, which implies a greater, localized energy-generating capacity. A single stress session did not produce these changes either immediately after or the next day following the restraint session (Magarinos et al. 1997).

- Adrenal steroids modulate the expression of NMDA receptors in the hippocampus (Bartanusz et al. 1995; Weiland et al. 1995), with chronic glucocorticoid exposure leading to increased expression of NMDA receptor binding and both NR2A and NR2B subunit mRNA levels (Weiland et al. 1997).

- There are glucocorticoid effects on the expression of mRNA levels for specific subunits of $GABA_A$ receptors in CA3 and the dentate gyrus; low and high glucocorticoid levels have different effects on $GABA_A$ receptor subunit mRNA levels and receptor binding (Orchinik et al. 1994, 2001), suggesting that corticosterone may alter the excitability of hippocampal neurons through regulation of $GABA_A$ receptor expression. However, it remains to be seen if the corticosteroid effects on neuronal morphology involve changes in the number or pharmacological properties of $GABA_A$ receptors.

Translation of Anatomical Findings in Animal Models to the Human Brain

Studies with structural magnetic resonance imaging (MRI) and magnetic resonance spectroscopy (MRS) indicate that the hippocampus, amygdala, and prefrontal cortex undergo remodeling and reduced levels of neuronal markers such as N-acetyl aspartate (NAA) in disorders such as Cushing's disease, major depression, and posttraumatic stress disorder (Schuff et al. 2001; Winsberg et al. 2000) (for reviews, see McEwen 1997; Sapolsky 2001a, 2001c; Stoll et al. 2000). So far, only in the case of Cushing's disease is there some evidence that these changes are reversible after correction of the hypercortisolemia (Bourdeau et al. 2002; Starkman et al. 1999). In major depression, there is some evidence that is suggestive of brain lesions (Sheline et al. 1996). Yet there is almost no postmortem neuroanatomy that would support a permanent cell loss. Indeed, there is some recent research that fails to show evidence of neuronal loss in major depression (Lucassen et al. 2001; Muller et al. 2001). Yet there are indications from postmortem studies of brains from patients with mood disorders of a loss of glial cells in the prefrontal cortex (Rajkowska 2000).

How does one relate these findings to the animal studies described earlier? A recent study of the tree shrew model combined in vivo imaging with studies of the hippocampus with regard to neurogenesis and dentate gyrus volume (Czeh et al. 2001). Chronic psychosocial stress over 28 days leads to remodeling of dendrites in the CA3 region of the hippocampus and reduction in neurogenesis (Gould et al. 1997c; Magarinos et al. 1996), as well as reductions in levels of NAA, creatine, phosphocreatine, and choline-containing compounds determined by MRS (Czeh et al. 2001). Treatment with tianeptine starting 7 days into the psychosocial stress paradigm prevented the decrease in neurogenesis seen after 28 days and also prevented the decrease in NAA; it also increased overall hippocampal volume to levels seen in unstressed control animals (Czeh et al. 2001). Thus, for the first time, it is possible to see how changes at the cellular level in hippocampal structure may be related to the types of in vivo measurements that are possible in the human brain in relation to psychiatric illnesses.

PROTECTIVE AND DAMAGING EFFECTS OF STRESS MEDIATORS

We have seen for the brain that the response of hormonal and other tissue mediators to changes in the environment and unexpected challenges are largely adaptive, at least in the short run. Over the longer term, when these adaptive responses are either overused or dysregulated, there is a wear and tear that can contribute to pathophysiology. A similar situation applies to other systems (McEwen 1998). For the cardiovascular system, acute activation of heart rate and blood pressure is an important aspect of the "fight or flight" response and escape from danger, but repeated surges of blood pressure may damage the coronary arteries and accelerate atherosclerosis. For the metabolic system, catecholamines and glucocorticoids are important agents in mobilizing and replenishing energy in the aftermath of strenuous exercise; but these same hormones can become activated in situations in which there is an ample supply of energy in the body, possibly leading to obesity and diabetes. For the immune system, the acute secretion of glucocorticoids and catecholamines promote the movement of immune cells to places in the body where they are needed to fight an infection; yet these same agents can suppress immune function when secreted in excess or repeatedly over long periods of chronic stress.

Finally, although we pay the most attention to glucocorticoids and catecholamines as the mediators responsible for the acute and chronic aspects described previously, many other hormones and tissue mediators are affected by these hormones. The excitatory amino acid neurotransmitters are a prime example, but there are other mediators, such as the inflammatory cytokines and the *Nf-kB* transcriptional regulator (Bierhaus et al. 2001), as well as other hormones, such as prolactin (Torner et al. 2001). Moreover, there are intricate feedforward and feedback loops that govern interactions between circulating hormones and tissue mediators (McEwen and Gould 1990; Sapolsky 2001b). For example, defenses against excitotoxic insult involve decreases in neuronal excitability, extracellular glutamate accumulation, cytosolic calcium mobilization, a calcium-dependent degenerative event, and increased neuronal energy production (Sapolsky 2001b). In the case of *Nf-kB*, although it is linked to chronic inflammatory cytokine elevation, for example, in Type II diabetes and cell damage and death (Bierhaus et al. 2001), there are also indications that *Nf-kB* is involved in protecting cells against death under some circumstances (Bierhaus et al. 2001; Lezoualc'h and Behl 1998).

CONCLUSIONS

Does stress damage the brain? Although it is clear that stress hormones are able to make damage worse and that certain stress-related conditions may eventually cause brain damage, it is also increasingly clear that the mediators of the physiological response to challenge and change in an organism are largely working to promote protection and adaptation, at least in the short run. The complex networks of feedback and feedforward interactions that characterize every mediator from excitatory amino acids to glucocorticoids to the inflammatory-oxidative stress cascade, and the interactions between them, appear to have many ways of keeping themselves under control. Yet when the delicate balance of these systems is disrupted, the dysregulation that results can lead to pathophysiological changes that can in turn lead to damage and disease.

REFERENCES

Aberg MAI, Aberg ND, Hedbacker H, et al: Peripheral infusion of IGF-1 selectively induces neurogenesis in the adult rat hippocampus. J Neurosci 20:2896–2903, 2000

Ahima RS, Harlan RE: Charting of type II glucocorticoid receptor–like immunoreactivity in the rat central nervous system. Neuroscience 39:579–604, 1990

Ahima R, Krozowski Z, Harlan R: Type I corticosteroid receptor–like immunoreactivity in the rat CNS: distribution and regulation by corticosteroids. J Comp Neurol 313:522–538, 1991

Altman A, Bayer S: Postnatal development of the hippocampal dentate gyrus under experimental conditions, in The Hippocampus. Edited by Isaacson R, Pribram K. New York, Plenum, 1975, pp 95–122

Anagnostaras SG, Gale GD, Fanselow MS: Hippocampus and contextual fear conditioning: recent controversies and advances. Hippocampus 11:8–17, 2001

Arbel I, Kadar T, Silbermann M, et al: The effects of long-term corticosterone administration on hippocampal morphology and cognitive performance of middle-age rats. Brain Res 657:227–235, 1994

AusDerMuhlen K, Ockenfels H: Morphologische veranderungen im diencephalon und telencephalon: storungen des regelkreises adenohypophysenebennierenrinde. Mikrosck Anat 93:126–141, 1969

Bartanusz V, Aubry JM, Pagliusi S, et al: Stress-induced changes in messenger RNA levels of N-methyl-D-aspartate and Ampa receptor subunits in selected regions of the rat hippocampus and hypothalamus. Neuroscience 66:247–252, 1995

Bengzon J, Kokaia Z, Elmer E, et al: Apoptosis and proliferation of dentate gyrus neurons after single and intermittent limbic seizures. Proc Natl Acad Sci U S A 94:10432–10437, 1997

Bennett E, Diamond M, Krech D, et al: Chemical and anatomical plasticity of brain. Science 146:610–619, 1964

Bierhaus A, Schiekofer S, Schwaninger M, et al: Diabetes-associated sustained activation of the transcription factor nuclear factor-kB. Diabetes 50:2792–2808, 2001

Bobinski M, de Leon JJ, Convit A, et al: MRI of entorhinal cortex in mild Alzheimer's disease. Lancet 353:38–40, 1999

Bodnoff SR, Humphreys AG, Lehman JC, et al: Enduring effects of chronic corticosterone treatment on spatial learning, synaptic plasticity, and hippocampal neuropathology in young and mid-aged rats. J Neurosci 15:61–69, 1995

Bourdeau I, Bard C, Noel B, et al: Loss of brain volume in endogenous Cushing's syndrome and its reversibility after correction of hypercortisolism. J Clin Endocrinol Metab 87:1949–1954, 2002

Cahill L, Prins B, Weber M, et al: Beta-adrenergic activation and memory for emotional events. Nature 371:702–704, 1994

Cameron HA, Gould E: Adult neurogenesis is regulated by adrenal steroids in the dentate gyrus. Neuroscience 61:203–209, 1994

Cameron HA, Gould E: The control of neuronal birth and survival, in Receptor Dynamics in Neural Development. Edited by Shaw CA. New York, CRC Press, 1996a, pp 141–157

Cameron HA, Gould E: Distinct populations of cells in the adult dentate gyrus undergo mitosis or apoptosis in response to adrenalectomy. J Comp Neurol 369:56–63, 1996b

Cameron HA, McKay DG: Restoring production of hippocampal neurons in old age. Nat Neurosci 2:894–897, 1999

Cameron H, Woolley C, McEwen BS, et al: Differentiation of newly born neurons and glia in the dentate gyrus of the adult rat. Neuroscience 56:337–344, 1993

Cameron HA, McEwen BS, Gould E: Regulation of adult neurogenesis by excitatory input and NMDA receptor activation in the dentate gyrus. J Neurosci 15:4687–4692, 1995

Carro E, Nunez A, Busiguina S, et al: Circulating insulin-like growth factor I mediates effects of exercise on the brain. J Neurosci 20:2926–2933, 2000

Chittajallu R, Vignes M, Dev KK, et al: Regulation of glutamate release by presynaptic kainate receptors in the hippocampus. Nature 379:78–81, 1996

Conrad CD, Lupien SJ, McEwen BS: Support for a bimodal role for type II adrenal steroid receptors in spatial memory. Neurobiol Learn Mem 72:39–46, 1999

Corodimas KP, LeDoux JE, Gold PW, et al: Corticosterone potentiation of conditioned fear in rats. Ann N Y Acad Sci 746:392–393, 1994

Czeh B, Michaelis T, Watanabe T, et al: Stress-induced changes in cerebral metabolites, hippocampal volume and cell proliferation are prevented by antidepressant treatment with tianeptine. Proc Natl Acad Sci U S A 98:12796–12801, 2001

Dallman M, Akana S, Cascio C, et al: Regulation of ACTH secretion: variations on a theme of B. Recent Prog Horm Res 43:113–172, 1987

Das A, Gilbert C: Long-range horizontal connections and their role in cortical reorganization revealed by optical recording of cat primary visual cortex. Nature 375:780–784, 1995

Diamond DM, Bennett MC, Fleshner M, et al: Inverted-U relationship between the level of peripheral corticosterone and the magnitude of hippocampal primed burst potentiation. Hippocampus 2:421–430, 1992

Diamond DM, Park CR, Heman KL, et al: Exposing rats to a predator impairs spatial working memory in the radial arm water maze. Hippocampus 9:542–552, 1999

Dore S, Kar S, Quirion R: Insulin-like growth factor I protects and rescues hippocampal neurons against β-amyloid and human amylin-induced toxicity. Proc Natl Acad Sci U S A 94:4772–4777, 1997a

Dore S, Kar S, Rowe W, et al: Distribution and levels of [^{125}I]IGF-I, [^{125}I]IGF-II and [^{125}I]insulin receptor binding sites in the hippocampus of aged memory-unimpaired and -impaired rats. Neuroscience 80:1033–1040, 1997b

Eichenbaum H, Otto T: The hippocampus—what does it do? Behav Neural Biol 57:2–36, 1992

Eldridge JC, Brodish A, Kute TE, et al: Apparent age-related resistance of type II hippocampal corticosteroid receptors to down-regulation during chronic escape training. J Neurosci 9:3237–3242, 1989

Eriksson P S, Permlieva E, Bjork-Eriksson T, et al: Neurogenesis in the adult human hippocampus. Nat Med 4:1313–1317, 1998

Freund TF, Buzsaki G: Interneurons of the hippocampus. Hippocampus 6:345–470, 1996

Galea LAM, McEwen BS: Sex and seasonal differences in the rate of cell proliferation in the dentate gyrus of adult wild meadow voles. Neuroscience 89:955–964, 1999

Galea LAM, Kavaliers M, Ossenkopp K-P, et al: Sexually dimorphic spatial learning varies seasonally in two populations of deer mice. Brain Res 635:18–26, 1994

Galea LAM, Tanapat P, Gould E: Exposure to predator odor suppresses cell proliferation in the dentate gyrus of adult rats via a cholinergic mechanism. Abstr Soc Neurosci 22:1196, 1996

Geinisman Y, deToledo-Morrell L, Morrell F, et al: Age-related loss of axospinous synapses formed by two afferent systems in the rat dentate gyrus as revealed by the unbiased stereological dissector technique. Hippocampus 2:437–444, 1992

Geinisman Y, deToledo-Morrell L, Morrell F, et al: Hippocampal markers of age-related memory dysfunction: behavioral, electrophysiological and morphological perspectives. Prog Neurobiol 45:223–252, 1995

Gleichmann M, Weller M, Schulz JB: Insulin-like growth factor–1 mediated protection from neuronal apoptosis is linked to phosphorylation of the pro-apoptotic protein BAD but not to inhibition of cytochrome c translocation in rat cerebellar neurons. Neurosci Lett 282:69–72, 2000

Goldman-Rakic PS: The physiological approach: functional architecture of working memory and disordered cognition in schizophrenia. Biol Psychiatry 46:650–661, 1999

Gould E: Serotonin and hippocampal neurogenesis. Neuropsychopharmacology 21 (suppl 1): 46S–51S, 1999

Gould E, Tanapat P: Lesion-induced proliferation of neuronal progenitors in the dentate gyrus of the adult rat. Neuroscience 80:427–436, 1997

Gould E, Woolley C, McEwen BS: Short-term glucocorticoid manipulations affect neuronal morphology and survival in the adult dentate gyrus. Neuroscience 37:367–375, 1990

Gould E, Tanapat P, Cameron HA: Adrenal steroids suppress granule cell death in the developing dentate gyrus through an NMDA receptor-dependent mechanism. Brain Res Dev Brain Res 103:91–93, 1997a

Gould E, Tanapat P, McEwen BS: Activation of the type 2 adrenal steroid receptor can rescue granule cells from death during development. Brain Res Dev Brain Res 101:265–268, 1997b

Gould E, McEwen BS, Tanapat P, et al: Neurogenesis in the dentate gyrus of the adult tree shrew is regulated by psychosocial stress and NMDA receptor activation. J Neurosci 17:2492–2498, 1997c

Gould E, Tanapat P, McEwen BS, et al: Proliferation of granule cell precursors in the dentate gyrus of adult monkeys is diminished by stress. Proc Natl Acad Sci U S A 95:3168–3171, 1998

Gould E, Beylin A, Tanapat P, et al: Learning enhances adult neurogenesis in the hippo-campal formation. Nat Neurosci 2:260–265, 1999a

Gould E, Reeves AJ, Fallah M, et al: Hippocampal neurogenesis in adult Old World pri-mates. Proc Natl Acad Sci U S A 96:5263–5267, 1999b

Harris GW: Effects of the nervous system on the pituitary-adrenal activity. Prog Brain Res 32:86–88, 1970

Islam A, Ayer-LeLievre C, Heigenskold C, et al: Changes in IGF-1 receptors in the hippo-campal of adult rats after long-term adrenalectomy: receptor autoradiography and in situ hybridization histochemistry. Brain Res 797:342–346, 1998

Jacobson L, Sapolsky R: The role of the hippocampus in feedback regulation of the hypo-thalamic-pituitary-adrenocortical axis. Endocr Rev 12:118–134, 1991

Joels M: Steroid hormones and excitability in the mammalian brain. Front Neuroendocrinol 18:2–48, 1997

Jones TA, Chu CJ, Grande LA, et al: Motor skills training enhances lesion-induced struc-tural plasticity in the motor cortex of adult rats. J Neurosci 19:10153–10163, 1999

Kaplan MS, Bell DH: Mitotic neuroblasts in the 9 day old and 11 month old rodent hippo-campal. J Neurosci 4:1429–1441, 1984

Kaplan MS, Hinds JW: Neurogenesis in the adult rat: electron microscopic analysis of light radioautographs. Science 197:1092–1094, 1977

Kempermann G, Kuhn HG, Gage FH: More hippocampal neurons in adult mice living in an enriched environment. Nature 586:493–495, 1997

Kempermann G, Kuhn HG, Gage FH: Experience-induced neurogenesis in the senescent dentate gyrus. J Neurosci 18:3206–3212, 1998

Kerr S, Campbell L, Applegate M, et al: Chronic stress-induced acceleration of electrophys-iologic and morphometric biomarkers of hippocampal aging. J Neurosci 11:1316–1324, 1991

Korte SM: Corticosteroids in relation to fear, anxiety and psychopathology. Neurosci Biobe-hav Rev 25:117–142, 2001

Lai M, Hibberd CJ, Gluckman PD, et al: Reduced expression of insulin-like growth factor 1 messenger RNA in the hippocampus of aged rats. Neurosci Lett 288:66–70, 2000

Landfield P: Modulation of brain aging correlates by long-term alterations of adrenal ste-roids and neurally active peptides. Prog Brain Res 72:279–300, 1987

Landfield PW, Eldridge JC: Evolving aspects of the glucocorticoid hypothesis of brain aging: hormonal modulation of neuronal calcium homeostasis. Neurobiol Aging 15:579–588, 1994

Landfield PW, Waymire JC, Lynch G: Hippocampal aging and adrenocorticoids: quantita-tive correlations. Science 202:1098–1102, 1978

Landfield PW, Pitler TA, Applegate MD: The aged hippocampus: a model system for studies on mechanisms of behavioral plasticity and brain aging. Hippocampus 3:323–367, 1986

Lauri SE, Bortolotto ZA, Bleakman D, et al: A critical role of a facilitatory presynaptic kain-ate receptor in mossy fiber LTP. Neuron 32:697–709, 2001

LeDoux JE: Emotion circuits in the brain. Annu Rev Neurosci 23:155–184, 2000

Lezoualc'h F, Behl C: Transcription factor NF-kB: friend or foe of neurons? Mol Psychiatry 3:15–20, 1998

Li XG, Somogyi P, Ylinen A, et al: The hippocampal CA3 network: an in vivo intracellular labeling study. J Comp Neurol 339:181–208, 1994

Lisman J E: Relating hippocampal circuitry to function: recall of memory sequences by re-ciprocal dentate-CA3 interactions. Neuron 22:233–242, 1999

Lowy MT, Gault L, Yamamoto BK: Adrenalectomy attenuates stress-induced elevations in extracellular glutamate concentrations in the hippocampus. J Neurochem 61:1957–1960, 1993

Lucassen PJ, Muller MB, Holsboer F, et al: Hippocampal apoptosis in major depression is a minor event and absent from subareas at risk for glucocorticoid overexposure. Am J Pathol 158:453–468, 2001

Lupien SJ, McEwen BS: The acute effects of corticosteroids on cognition: integration of animal and human model studies. Brain Res Brain Res Rev 24:1–27, 1997

Lynch CD, Lyons D, Khan A, et al: Insulin-like growth factor–1 selectively increases glucose utilization in brains of aged animals. Endocrinology 142:506–509, 2001

Magarinos AM, McEwen BS, Flugge G, et al: Chronic psychosocial stress causes apical dendritic atrophy of hippocampal CA3 pyramidal neurons in subordinate tree shrews. J Neurosci 16:3534–3540, 1996

Magarinos AM, Verdugo Garcia JM, McEwen BS: Chronic restraint stress alters synaptic terminal structure in hippocampus. Proc Natl Acad Sci U S A 94:14002–14008, 1997

Magarinos AM, Deslandes A, McEwen BS: Effects of antidepressants and benzodiazepine treatments on the dendritic structure of CA3 pyramidal neurons after chronic stress. Eur J Pharmacol 371:113–122, 1999

Malberg JE, Eisch AJ, Nestler EJ, et al: Chronic antidepressant treatment increases neurogenesis in adult rat hippocampus. J Neurosci 20:9104–9110, 2000

Markowska AL, Mooney M, Sonntag WE: Insulin-like growth factor–1 ameliorates age-related behavioral deficits. Neuroscience 87:559–569, 1998

Mason JW: Organization of psychoendocrine mechanisms: the scope of psychoendocrine research. J Am Psychosom Soc 30:565–808, 1968

McEwen BS: Re-examination of the glucocorticoid cascade hypothesis of stress and aging, in Progress in Brain Research. Edited by Swaab D, Hoffman M, Mirmiran R, et al. Amsterdam, Elsevier, 1992, pp 365–383

McEwen BS: Possible mechanisms for atrophy of the human hippocampus. Mol Psychiatry 2:255–262, 1997

McEwen BS: Protective and damaging effects of stress mediators. N Engl J Med 338:171–179, 1998

McEwen BS: Stress and hippocampal plasticity. Annu Rev Neurosci 22:105–122, 1999

McEwen BS: Stress, sex, and the structural and functional plasticity of the hippocampus, in The New Cognitive Neurosciences, 2nd Edition. Edited by Gazzaniga MS. Cambridge, MA, MIT Press, 2000, pp 171–197

McEwen BS, Gould E: Adrenal steroid influences on the survival of hippocampal neurons. Biochem Pharmacol 40:2393–2402, 1990

McEwen BS, Weiss J, Schwartz L: Selective retention of corticosterone by limbic structures in rat brain. Nature 220:911–912, 1968

McEwen BS, DeKloet ER, Rostene W: Adrenal steroid receptors and actions in the nervous system. Physiol Rev 66:1121–1188, 1986

McEwen BS, Albeck D, Cameron H, et al: Stress and the brain: a paradoxical role for adrenal steroids, in Vitamins and Hormones, Vol 51. Edited by Litwack GD. San Diego, CA, Academic Press, 1995, pp 371–402

McKittrick CR, Magarinos AM, Blanchard DC, et al: Chronic social stress reduces dendritic arbors in CA3 of hippocampus and decreases binding to serotonin transporter sites. Synapse 36:85–94, 2000

Meaney M, Aitken D, Berkel H, et al: Effect of neonatal handling of age-related impairments associated with the hippocampus. Science 239:766–768, 1988

Mennini T, Miari A: Modulation of 3H glutamate binding by serotonin in rat hippocampus: an autoradiographic study. Life Sci 49:283–292, 1991

Mizoguchi K, Kunishita T, Chui DH, et al: Stress induces neuronal death in the hippocampus of castrated rats. Neurosci Lett 138:157–160, 1992

Moghaddam B, Boliano ML, Stein-Behrens B, et al: Glucocorticoids mediate the stress-induced extracellular accumulation of glutamate. Brain Res 655:251–254, 1994

Muller MB, Lucassen PJ, Yassouridis A, et al: Neither major depression nor glucocorticoid treatment affects the cellular integrity of the human hippocampus. Eur J Neurosci 14:1603–1612, 2001

Nadler JV, Perry BW, Cotman CW: Intraventricular kainic acid preferentially destroys hippocampal pyramidal cells. Nature 271:676–677, 1978

Nicolle MM, Gonzalez J, Sugaya K, et al: Signatures of hippocampal oxidative stress in aged spatial learning–impaired rodents. Neuroscience 107:415–431, 2001

Noguchi S, Higashi K, Kawamura M: A possible role of the b-subunit of (Na,K)-ATPase in facilitating correct assembly of the a-subunit into the membrane. J Biol Chem 265:5991–5995, 1990

Ohl F, Fuchs E: Differential effects of chronic stress on memory processes in the tree shrew. Brain Res Cogn Brain Res 7:379–387, 1999

Oitzl MS, Reichardt HM, Joels M, et al: Point mutation in the mouse glucocorticoid receptor preventing DNA binding impairs spatial memory. Proc Natl Acad Sci U S A 98:12790–12795, 2001

O'Kusky JR, Ye P, D'Ercole AJ: Insulin-like growth factor–1 promotes neurogenesis and synaptogenesis in the hippocampal dentate gyrus during postnatal development. J Neurosci 20:8435–8442, 2000

Orchinik M, Weiland NG, McEwen BS: Adrenalectomy selectively regulates GABA$_A$ receptor subunit expression in the hippocampus. Mol Cell Neurosci 5:451–458, 1994

Orchinik M, Carroll SS, Li Y-H, et al: Heterogeneity of hippocampal GABA$_A$ receptors: regulation by corticosterone. J Neurosci 21:330–339, 2001

Parent JM, Yu TW, Leibowitz RT, et al: Dentate granule cell neurogenesis is increased by seizures and contributes to aberrant network reorganization in the adult rat hippocampus. J Neurosci 17:3727–3738, 1997

Parnavelas J, Lynch G, Brecha N, et al: Spine loss and regrowth in hippocampus following deafferentation. Nature 248:71–73, 1974

Pavlides C, McEwen BS: Effects of mineralocorticoid and glucocorticoid receptors on long-term potentiation in the CA3 hippocampal field. Brain Res 851:204–214, 1999

Pavlides C, Kimura A, Magarinos AM, et al: Type I adrenal steroid receptors prolong hippocampal long-term potentiation. Neuroreport 5:2673–2677, 1994

Pavlides C, Watanabe Y, Magarinos AM, et al: Opposing role of adrenal steroid Type I and Type II receptors in hippocampal long-term potentiation. Neuroscience 68:387–394, 1995

Phillips RG, LeDoux JE: Differential contribution of amygdala and hippocampus to cued and contextual fear conditioning. Behav Neurosci 106:274–285, 1992

Pugh CR, Fleshner M, Rudy JW: Type II glucocorticoid receptor antagonists impair contextual but not auditory-cue fear conditioning in juvenile rats. Neurobiol Learn Mem 67:75–79, 1997a

Pugh CR, Tremblay D, Fleshner M, et al: A selective role for corticosterone in contextual-fear conditioning. Behav Neurosci 111:503–511, 1997b

Pulford BE, Ishii DN: Uptake of circulating insulin-like growth factors (IGFs) into cerebrospinal fluid appears to be independent of the IGF receptors as well as IGF-binding proteins. Endocrinology 142:213–220, 2001

Radley JJ, Jacobs BL, Tanapat P, et al: Blockade of 5HT$_{1A}$ receptors prevents hippocampal granule cell genesis during and after pilocarpine-induced status epilepticus. Abstr Soc Neurosci 24:1992, 1998

Rahmann S, Neumann RS: Activation of 5-HT$_2$ receptors facilitates depolarization of neocortical neurons by N-methyl-D-aspartate. Eur J Pharmacol 231:347–354, 1993

Rajkowska G: Postmortem studies in mood disorders indicate altered numbers of neurons and glial cells. Biol Psychiatry 48:766–777, 2000

Rapp PR, Gallagher M: Preserved neuron number in the hippocampus of aged rats with spatial learning deficits. Proc Natl Acad Sci U S A 93:9926–9930, 1996

Rapp PR, Stack EC, Gallagher M: Morphometric studies of the aged hippocampus, I: volumetric analysis in behaviorally characterized rats. J Comp Neurol 403:459–470, 1999

Reichardt HM, Schutz G: Glucocorticoid signalling—multiple variations of a common theme. Mol Cell Endocrinol 146:1–6, 1998

Reul J, DeKloet ER: Anatomical resolution of two types of corticosterone receptor sites in rat brain with in vitro autoradiography and computerized image analysis. J Steroid Biochem 24:269–272, 1986

Roozendaal B: Glucocorticoids and the regulation of memory consolidation. Psychoneuroendocrinology 25:213–238, 2000

Roozendaal B, Cahill L, McGaugh JL: Interaction of emotionally activated neuromodulatory systems in regulating memory storage, in Brain Process and Memory. Edited by Ishikawa K, McGaugh JL, Sakata H. Amsterdam, Elsevier, 1996, pp 39–54

Roozendaal B, Phillips RG, Power AE, et al: Memory retrieval impairment induced by hippocampal CA3 lesions is blocked by adrenocortical suppression. Nat Neurosci 4:1169–1171, 2001

Rozovsky I, Wei M, Stone DJ, et al: Estradiol (E2) enhances neurite outgrowth by repressing glial fibrillary acidic protein expression and reorganizing laminin. Endocrinology 143:636–646, 2002

Santini E, Muller RU, Quirk GJ: Consolidation of extinction learning involves transfer from NMDA-independent to NMDA-dependent memory. J Neurosci 21:9009–9017, 2001

Sapolsky R: Stress, the Aging Brain and the Mechanisms of Neuron Death, Vol 1. Cambridge, MA, MIT Press, 1992

Sapolsky RM: Why stress is bad for your brain. Science 273:749–750, 1996

Sapolsky RM: Atrophy of the hippocampus in posttraumatic stress disorder: how and when? Hippocampus 11:90–91, 2001a

Sapolsky RM: Cellular defenses against excitotoxic results. J Neurochem 76:1601–1611, 2001b

Sapolsky RM: Depression, antidepressants, and the shrinking hippocampus. Proc Natl Acad Sci U S A 98:12320–12322, 2001c

Sapolsky R, Pulsinelli W: Glucocorticoids potentiate ischemic injury to neurons: therapeutic implications. Science 229:1397–1399, 1985

Sapolsky R, Krey L, McEwen BS: Prolonged glucocorticoid exposure reduces hippocampal neuron number: implications for aging. J Neurosci 5:1222–1227, 1985

Sapolsky RM, Krey LC, McEwen BS: The neuroendocrinology of stress and aging: the glucocorticoid cascade hypothesis. Endocr Rev 7:284–301, 1986

Sawchenko PE, Imaki T, Potter E, et al: The functional neuroanatomy of corticotropin-releasing factor. Ciba Found Symp 172:5–21, 1993

Schmitz D, Mellor J, Nicoll RA: Presynaptic kainate receptor mediation of frequency facilitation at hippocampal mossy fiber synapses. Science 291:1972–1976, 2001

Schuff N, Neylan TC, Lenoci MA, et al: Decreased hippocampal N-acetyl aspartate in the absence of atrophy in posttraumatic stress disorder. Biol Psychiatry 50:952–959, 2001

Seri B, Garcia-Verdugo JM, McEwen BS, et al: Astrocytes give rise to new neurons in the adult mammalian hippocampus. J Neurosci 21:7153–7160, 2001

Sheline YI, Wang PW, Gado MH, et al: Hippocampal atrophy in recurrent major depression. Proc Natl Acad Sci U S A 93:3908–3913, 1996

Sherry DF, Jacobs LF, Gaulin SJ: Spatial memory and adaptive specialization of the hippocampus. Trends Neurosci 15:298–303, 1992

Sik A, Ylinen A, Penttonen M, et al: Inhibitory CA1-CA3-Hilar region feedback in the hippocampus. Science 265:1722–1724, 1994

Sik A, Penttonen M, Ylinen A, et al: Hippocampal CA1 interneurons: an in vivo intracellular labelling study. J Neurosci 15:6651–6665, 1995

Sloviter R, Valiquette G, Abrams G, et al: Selective loss of hippocampal granule cells in the mature rat brain after adrenalectomy. Science 243:535–538, 1989

Smith TD, Adams MM, Gallagher M, et al: Circuit-specific alterations in hippocampal synaptophysin immunoreactivity predict spatial learning impairment in aged rats. J Neurosci 20:6587–6593, 2000

Sousa N, Lukoyanov NV, Madeira MD, et al: Reorganization of the morphology of hippocampal neurites and synapses after stress-induced damage correlates with behavioral improvement. Neuroscience 97:253–266, 2000

Spiess J, Rivier J, Rivier C, et al: Primary structure of corticotropin-releasing factor from ovine hypothalamus. Proc Natl Acad Sci U S A 78:6517–6521, 1981

Star EN, Kwiatkowski DJ, Murthy VN: Rapid turnover of actin in dendritic spines and its regulation by activity. Nat Neurosci 5:239–246, 2002

Starkman MN, Giordani B, Gebrski SS, et al: Decrease in cortisol reverses human hippocampal atrophy following treatment of Cushing's disease. Biol Psychiatry 46:1595–1602, 1999

Stein-Behrens B, Elliot EM, Miller CA, et al: Glucocorticoids exacerbate kainic acid–induced extracellular accumulation of excitatory amino acids in the rat hippocampus. J Neurochem 58:1730–1735, 1992

Stoll AL, Renshaw PF, Yurgelun-Todd DA, et al: Neuroimaging in bipolar disorder: what have we learned? Biol Psychiatry 48:505–517, 2000

Stutzmann GE, McEwen BS, LeDoux JE: Serotonin modulation of sensory inputs to the lateral amygdala: dependency on corticosterone. J Neurosci 18:9529–9538, 1998

Takadera T, Matsuda I, Ohyashiki T: Apoptotic cell death and caspase-3 activation induced by N-methyl-D-aspartate receptor antagonists and their prevention by insulin-like growth factor I. J Neurochem 73:548–556, 1999

Tanapat P, Gould E: EGF stimulates proliferation of granule cell precursors in the dentate gyrus of adult rats. Abstr Soc Neurosci 23:317, 1997

Torner L, Toschi N, Pohlinger A, et al: Anxiolytic and anti-stress effects of brain prolactin: improved efficacy of antisense targeting of the prolactin receptor by molecular modeling. J Neurosci 21:3207–3214, 2001

Trejo JL, Carro E, Torres-Aleman I: Circulating insulin-like growth factor I mediates exercise-induced increases in the number of new neurons in the adult hippocampus. J Neurosci 21:1628–1634, 2001

van Praag H, Kempermann G, Gage FH: Running increases cell proliferation and neurogenesis in the adult mouse dentate gyrus. Nat Neurosci 2:266–270, 1999

Venero C, Borrell J: Rapid glucocorticoid effects on excitatory amino acid levels in the hippocampus: a microdialysis study in freely moving rats. Eur J Neurosci 1:2465–2473, 1999

Wallace CS, Kilman VL, Withers GS, et al: Increases in dendritic length in occipital cortex after 4 days of differential housing in weanling rats. Behav Neural Biol 58:64–68, 1992

Watanabe Y, Gould E, Cameron H, et al: Stress and antidepressant effects on hippocampus. Eur J Pharmacol 222:157–162, 1992a

Watanabe Y, Gould E, McEwen BS: Stress induces atrophy of apical dendrites of hippocampus CA3 pyramidal neurons. Brain Res 588:341–344, 1992b

Watanabe Y, Weiland NG, McEwen BS: Effects of adrenal steroid manipulations and repeated restraint stress on dynorphin mRNA levels and excitatory amino acid receptor binding in hippocampus. Brain Res 680:217–225, 1995

Weiland NG, Orchinik M, McEwen BS: Corticosterone regulates mRNA levels of specific subunits of the NMDA receptor in the hippocampus but not in cortex of rats. Abstr Soc Neurosci 21:502, 1995

Weiland NG, Orchinik M, Tanapat P: Chronic corticosterone treatment induces parallel changes in N-methyl-D-aspartate receptor subunit messenger RNA levels and antagonist binding sites in the hippocampus. Neuroscience 78:653–662, 1997

Winsberg ME, Sachs N, Tate DL, et al: Decreased dorsolateral prefrontal *N*-acetyl aspartate in bipolar disorder. Biol Psychiatry 47:475–481, 2000

Woolley CS, Gould E, McEwen BS: Exposure to excess glucocorticoids alters dendritic morphology of adult hippocampal pyramidal neurons. Brain Res 531:225–231 1990

Woolley C, Gould E, Sakai R, et al: Effects of aldosterone or RU28362 treatment on adrenalectomy-induced cell death in the dentate gyrus of the adult rat. Brain Res 554:312–315, 1991

3

Neuropsychobiology of the Variable Foraging Demand Paradigm in Nonhuman Primates

Jeremy D. Coplan, M.D.
Anca D. Paunica, M.D.
Leonard A. Rosenblum, Ph.D.

PSYCHIATRIC AND MEDICAL SEQUELAE OF ADVERSE EARLY REARING

Extensive preclinical and clinical data point to the vitally important role adverse early rearing plays in the etiology of human clinical conditions across the life span. Modern theories of depression and anxiety explicitly postulate the existence of a vulnerable biological diathesis resulting from the interaction of a genetic predisposition and untoward early life events (Nemeroff 1998, 1999).

Early life stress is increasingly recognized as an etiological factor in other adult conditions as well. These conditions include obesity, hypertension (Bjorntorp et al. 2000), Type II diabetes (the preceding three conditions comprise features of metabolic syndrome X [Bjorntorp and Rosmond 1999]), short physical stature, retarded intellectual development (Trickett and McBride-Chang 1995), atherosclerosis (Felitti et al. 1998), fibromyalgia (Anderberg et al. 2000), irritable bowel syndrome, and migraine, as well as other somatoform conditions (Romans et al. 2002).

With its advantages of environmental control and random genetic assignment, translational research using a primate model of adverse early rearing facilitates understanding of the subtle interactions of nature and

Financial support was provided by National Institute of Mental Health grants MH59990 and MH58911 and by a National Alliance for Research on Schizophrenia and Depression Independent Investigator Award (J.D.C.).

nurture at very early stages of development and the affective consequences of these interactions. The relatively unconfounded data derived
from such an animal model make it feasible to relate affective behavioral
outcomes to specific neurobiological findings.

THE VARIABLE FORAGING DEMAND PARADIGM

The early life stress paradigm used in our primate laboratory was designed
by Rosenblum and Paully (1984) to study the impact of disruption of
mother–infant attachment. In the variable foraging demand (VFD) rearing
paradigm, the offspring of mothers confronted with unpredictability and
lack of consistency in the time and work necessary to find their daily food
are compared with offspring of mothers exposed to consistent and predictable foraging requirements. For both groups adequate daily rations are always available. The VFD maternal food procurement schedule consists of
alternating blocks of 2 weeks in which food is easy to find (low foraging
demand [LFD]) with a 2-week period in which food procurement is difficult, involving more work and effort (high foraging demand [HFD]). We
have usually used 12 to 16 weeks of these conditions, with six to eight alternating 2-week periods of HFD and LFD, always starting with the LFD
component.

A simple device referred to as a foraging cart is constructed in such a
way that food is either buried in wood chips or sawdust or left freely exposed in containers within the cart. During the HFD component, animals
are required to manually search for and retrieve the apportioned buried
food through multiple apertures visible on the side of the cart. The procedure and the biological data discussed here all involve animals exposed to
the VFD or control conditions during the first 6 months of life.

The VFD procedure involves repeated, abrupt, and evidently unpredictable shifts from easy to difficult and then back to easy foraging. The repeated
shifting of foraging demand appears to overwhelm maternal coping capacities and, to varying degrees, appears to induce a form of functional emotional separation between mother and infant. As a consequence, we have
hypothesized that the affected mother becomes "psychologically unavail-
able" toward her infant. Even when maternal response to the infant's initiation for bodily contact and comfort is present, a qualitative disruption of
focus and execution of maternal interactive repertoire occurs and the critical
process of "affective reciprocity" between mother and infant is hampered.
The VFD mothers appear unable to respond contingently to their infants'
attempts to elicit affection, huddling, and ventral contact. Additionally,

VFD mothers fail to engage in the intense compensatory patterns toward their infants typically seen in control conditions following normal acute disturbances of the dyadic relationship (Andrews and Rosenblum 1991).

EFFECTS ON THE OFFSPRING OF MOTHERS EXPOSED TO VFD

One advantage of the VFD paradigm resides in its ability to permit the detailed study of patterns of dysregulation in several key central nervous system (CNS) components induced on a persistent basis by the VFD form of early life stress. These components include the noradrenergic (Rosenblum et al. 1994), serotonin, and dopamine systems (Coplan et al. 1998; Rosenblum et al. 1994); the hypothalamic-pituitary-adrenal (HPA) axis/corticotropin-releasing factor (CRF) system (Coplan et al. 1996, 2001; Mathew et al. 2002; Smith et al. 2002); somatotropic systems (Coplan et al. 1998, 2000); and cytokine elements (Smith et al. 2002). Finally, indirect evidence for hyperactivity of the excitatory and potentially neurotoxic glutamatergic neurotransmitter system is suggested by magnetic resonance spectroscopic studies of fully grown male VFD offspring (Mathew et al. 2002; see Chapter 8, "Neuroimaging Studies in Nonhuman Primates Reared Under Early Stressful Conditions").

CORTISOL AND CORTICOTROPIN-RELEASING FACTOR IN VFD OFFSPRING

It is clear that VFD rearing produces a mosaic of disturbances in CRF/cortisol regulatory systems (Mathew et al., in press). Coplan et al. (1996) found increased cerebrospinal fluid (CSF) CRF and decreased CSF cortisol in VFD offspring compared with either LFD- or HFD-reared groups. An increase in CSF CRF concentrations was found to persist into young adulthood, according to studies using an ad lib–reared age-matched control group (Coplan et al. 2001). In this same VFD cohort, an elevation in CSF concentrations of somatostatin, a neuropeptide with known inhibitory influence over the somatotropic axis (Coplan et al. 1998), prompted additional growth hormone secretion studies. Parallel clinical studies in panic disorder patients, using basal plasma cortisol measures as an indicator of HPA-axis/CRF hypersecretion, revealed an inverse relationship toward the growth hormone (GH) response to the adrenergic GH-secretagogue adrenoreceptor agonist clonidine (Coplan et al. 1997). In corollary primate studies, an inverse relationship between mean serial CSF CRF concentrations and the GH response to clonidine was noted, suggesting an antitrophic effect of CRF hypersecretion (Coplan et al. 2000). Collectively, the data suggest a diffusely antitrophic effect of adverse early rearing, potentially mediated proximally by CRF hypersecretion, although the data can be interpreted only in the correlative domain. A neuroendocrine profile of reduced GH response to GH secretagogues has long been noted as a reliable biological marker in psychiatric conditions such as major depression (Charney et al. 1982) and other anxiety disorders, such as panic disorder (Coplan et al. 1997). Thus, in both primate models of adverse early rearing and panic disorder, somatotropic activity is inversely related to CRF/HPA-axis activity. The full neural consequences or "signal" value of peripheral GH responsivity requires further characterization.

RELATIONSHIP BETWEEN CEREBROSPINAL FLUID CRF AND BIOGENIC AMINES

In VFD offspring, but not normal control subjects, CSF CRF was highly correlated with other CSF neurochemicals, including the metabolites of serotonin (5-hydroxyindoleacetic acid [5-HIAA]) and dopamine (homovanillic acid [HVA]) but not norepinephrine (3-methoxy-4-hydroxyphenethyleneglycol [MHPG]). The levels of both dopamine and serotonin amine turnover, including the anti-somatotropic neuropeptide somatostatin, were generally higher in VFD subjects (Coplan et al. 1998). Within the correlation matrix analysis, CSF CRF appears to be a point of confluence for multiple correlations specifically within VFD subjects, suggesting a key modulatory effect of this neuropeptide over a range of biological systems, evident following stressful rearing conditions but otherwise latent (Coplan et al. 1998).

CRF SECRETION AND NEUROPATHOLOGICAL CONSEQUENCES

The supposition that early increases in CSF CRF may be neurotoxic, independent of glucocorticoid effect, remains understudied. Hypersensitivity of central glucocorticoid negative-feedback systems has been invoked to account for the hippocampal volume loss and/or compromised functional integrity of the hippocampus, as reflected by magnetic resonance spectroscopy (MRS), in clinical posttraumatic stress disorder (PTSD) subjects (Schuff et al. 2001). It is curious that compromise of hippocampal neuronal viability occurs within the context of low to normal basal cortisol levels reported in PTSD (Yehuda et al. 1995). The facilitatory effect of amygdaloid CRF on enhancement of potentially neurotoxic glutamatergic neurotransmission has clearly been identified in the locus ceruleus region (Valentino et al. 2001) and may well occur at other central sites.

To address the long-term impact of excessive CRF exposure early in life, Brunson et al. (2001) examined adult rodents following repeated central CRF injections during early development. Administration of the neuropeptide to rats early in life and followed into adulthood caused a series of effects: progressive loss of hippocampal CA3 pyramidal layer cells, upregulated CRF receptors in the CA3 region, and exuberant growth or "sprouting" of mossy fibers from the dentate gyrus to the CA3 region. The synapses of the hippocampal CA3 region are glutamatergic, and the alterations resulting from the heightened CRF levels may promote a hyperglutamatergic state and excitotoxicity in this region. Studies of hippocampal CA3 neuronal cell loss in rodents developmentally exposed to CRF may be of key significance in understanding the neurobiological impact of adverse early rearing (Brunson et al. 2001). Additional corroborative studies are still needed to fully characterize the role of exuberant "mossy fiber sprouting" as a purported source of hyperglutamatergic activity, and therefore a proximal causative factor in hippocampal cell loss. The full impact of enhanced CRF secretion has yet to be fully integrated within the context of one of the most challenging scientific observations of the last decade—namely, that the neurons in the dentate gyrus of the hippocampus are capable of neurogenesis (Gould et al. 1999a). It is of striking note that the granular zone of the dentate gyrus is a primary site of neurogenesis across mammalian phylogeny, as has been demonstrated in postmortem studies by introduction of the thymidine analogue bromodioxyuridine (BRDU) in live primates (Gould et al. 1999a) or in terminal human cancer patients (Eriksson et al. 1998).

Several factors are now suggested to impede hippocampal neurogenesis, including stress, inflammation, CRF and glucocorticoids, glutamate and N-methyl-D-aspartate (NMDA) receptor agonists, as well as opiates. Other factors that stimulate and enhance neurogenesis include electroconvulsive shock (ECS), lithium and anticonvulsants, antidepressants and other 5-hydroxytryptamine (serotonin) type 1A (5-HT_{1A}) receptor agonists, and brain-derived neurotrophic factor (BDNF) (Czeh et al. 2001; Gould et al. 1999a). The VFD model of adverse early rearing conceivably offers the opportunity to examine the long-term impact of early life stress on adult patterns of neurogenesis.

Gould (1999b) demonstrated that learning and exercise in rats and primates stimulate neurogenesis, a finding that has extraordinary conceptual implications for humans. It shows that the brain has plastic capacities beyond synaptic plasticity. Learning and psychotherapy that imply the reframing and rethinking of the memories of early traumatic events involve emotional reprocessing and hence, as these current concepts imply, may ultimately involve certain forms of neuronal restructuring in order to provide amnestic reactions to adverse early events.

In the 1930s, Papez proposed a limbic substrate for emotional regulation, represented by a circuit that involves the anterior thalamus, anterior cingulate gyrus, parahippocampal gyrus, hippocampus, fornix, mammillary bodies, back to the thalamus (Allman et al. 2001). Although all these structures play important roles, the anterior cingulate has emerged as being central to normal and abnormal affective and emotional regulation (Allman et al. 2001). Untoward early life events seem to negatively affect regions of the limbic system. Among the most documented changes are those in the dentate gyrus (Liu et al. 2000), and rats exposed to adverse early rearing have different expression of the gamma subunits of the gamma-aminobutyric acid (GABA) receptors in the amygdala and the frontal cortex (Caldji et al. 2000). The anterior cingulate cortex seems to have certain specialized cells called spindle cells that appeared in the very late phases of primate evolution (Nimchinsky et al. 1995). In human infants, these cells cannot be discerned at birth, and their emergence at the age of 4 months coincides with the infant's capacity to hold the head steady, smile spontaneously, track an object visually, and reach for an object (Eisenberg et al. 1996).

Given the centrality of the abovementioned structures in affect and stress regulation, it is conceivable that in the offspring of VFD mothers these regions would be affected. MRS is a noninvasive neuroimaging methodology that permits assessment of the quantitative neurochemistry of regions of interest within the brain. An MRS study of the brains of VFD offspring compared with control subjects by Mathew et al. (see Chapter 8, "Neuroimaging Studies in Nonhuman Primates Reared Under Early Stressful Conditions") demonstrated significant differences in the quantitative neurochemistry of the hippocampus and anterior cingulate gyrus. In the hippocampus, the choline/creatine ratio was found to be higher in the VFD offspring compared with non-VFD. The choline/creatine ratio is indicative of neuronal membrane turnover and, along with the high CRF levels observed in these same subjects as juveniles (Coplan et al. 1996), could suggest increased mossy fiber sprouting, although histological confirmation is required. In the anterior cingulate the Glx/creatine (Glx is an indicator of glutamate/glutamine/GABA resonance [see Mathew et al., in press]) ratio was significantly greater in the VFD offspring. In accordance with current concepts of postnatal anterior cingulate neuronal vulnerability, the *N*-acetyl-aspartate/creatine ratio was significantly decreased, suggesting that increased glutamatergic tone was associated with decreased indices of neuronal viability. These studies are addressed in greater detail in Chapter 8, "Neuroimaging Studies in Nonhuman Primates Reared Under Early Stressful Conditions."

MATERNAL BIOBEHAVIORAL CHARACTERISTICS ACROSS THE VFD PERIOD

It has become clear that the VFD paradigm imposed on primate mothers critically affects the capacity to provide "good mothering" toward their infants. The biological mechanism by which this process is mediated has yet to be explored. In an effort to understand the nature of the effects of VFD stress on mothers, a study was undertaken to look at a range of biological measures, including plasma cortisol levels, prior to and at the cessation of the VFD experience. We focus on maternal plasma cortisol levels in relation to a number of maternal characteristics, including age, weight, and position within the social hierarchy of her cohort. Cortisol is a primary indicator of HPA axis activity and is therefore a physiological indicator of level of stress.

Twenty-three mother–infant dyads were the subjects of the study. They were distributed in four pens of five to seven dyads each. Mothers were assessed for hierarchical status during the final HFD phase of a 16-week (four-LFD, four-HFD) VFD cycle. In this study venous blood and cisternal CSF measures were performed prior to the onset of the 16-week VFD period and were repeated in the last week of the fourth HFD component. All biological measures were performed between 11:00 A.M. and 12:30 P.M., to avoid diurnal confounds. No intermediate measures were performed, so as to minimally perturb the VFD experimental process and concomitant behavioral measures. This novel biobehavioral database was intended to allow examination of several aspects of those maternal features that may conceivably contribute to the pattern and expression of the life trajectory of VFD offspring.

A complex interplay of maternal characteristics, present prior to imposition of the VFD stress and dubbed "pre-VFD," appears to strongly determine patterns of both social behavior and neurobiological response to 16 weeks of VFD. As noted in Figure 3–1, maternal pre-VFD cortisol levels were strongly negatively correlated ($r=-0.85$) with HPA axis response to the VFD stressor, predicting both the degree and directionality of change in cortisol from pre-VFD to "post-VFD." Hence, maternal pre-VFD cortisol levels below the post hoc cutoff at the approximate median

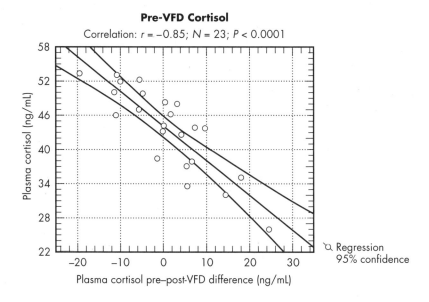

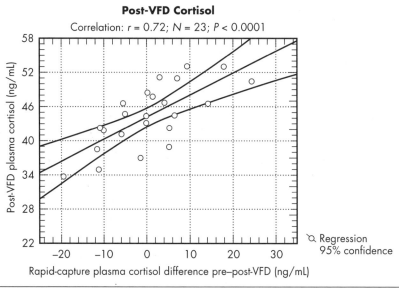

FIGURE 3–1 Variable foraging demand (VFD)–associated cortisol inversion. Mothers with high pre-VFD cortisol show lower cortisol levels after the stress (pre>post); mothers with low pre-VFD cortisol exhibit higher cortisol levels after the stress (post>pre).

of 45 ng/mL were associated with significant increases in plasma cortisol measures following VFD. Conversely, subjects whose values pre-VFD were above the 45 ng/mL mark demonstrated significant reductions in plasma cortisol. Essentially, mothers with low baseline cortisol showed increases in cortisol levels in response to VFD, whereas those with high baseline cortisol showed reductions. The drop in high pre-VFD maternal cortisol and the increase in low pre-VFD maternal cortisol accounts for what appears to be, to our knowledge, a novel social stress response that we have termed cortisol level inversion. It should be noted that the process exceeds the statistical phenomenon referred to as regression to the mean because the rank in cortisol level is also inverted: Animals that start out with the highest cortisol levels manifest the lowest cortisol levels following VFD exposure, and vice versa. Regression to the mean is not compatible with the observation of rank inversion.

It has been shown in wild social groups that relatively high cortisol levels are evident among dominant baboons in unstable hierarchies (Sapolsky 1992). On the contrary, in stable social hierarchies, the dominant animals have the lowest cortisol levels within the troop. In our studies, dominance emerges as a multidimensional characteristic. As reflected in Figure 3–2, within our dyadic groups the dominant animals are significantly older.

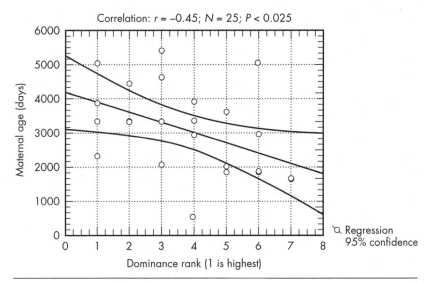

FIGURE 3–2   Relationship between maternal dominance and maternal age. Older mothers are more likely to be dominant.

Moreover, as Figure 3–3 suggests, regardless of hierarchical status, older mothers have lower pre-VFD baseline cortisol levels. Our observations are in accordance with work in humans (Rasheed 1993; Vleugels et al. 1986), where increased parity has also been associated with lower cortisol levels. Thus, older mothers generally started with lower cortisol levels in comparison with their younger and generally lower-parity counterparts.

As expected, weight and age were highly positively correlated. Thus, not surprisingly, as reflected in Figure 3–4, heavier mothers showed lower pre-VFD cortisol levels and were more likely to raise their cortisol levels after the VFD, whereas lighter and presumably younger mothers were mostly characterized by cortisol decrement effects observed in association with the VFD condition.

In keeping with these characteristics, social dominance rank correlated positively with change in cortisol in response to VFD. Higher-dominance animals had increases in cortisol whereas lower-dominance animals showed decrements in cortisol (see Figure 3–5). Dominance rank also significantly predicted post-VFD cortisol (see Figure 3–6). About 50% of maternal post-VFD cortisol variance was dependent on the magnitude and direction of the cortisol response to the VFD stressor. In turn, cortisol response was highly dependent on pre-VFD cortisol measures. However, there was no significant relationship between absolute pre- and post-VFD cortisol levels.

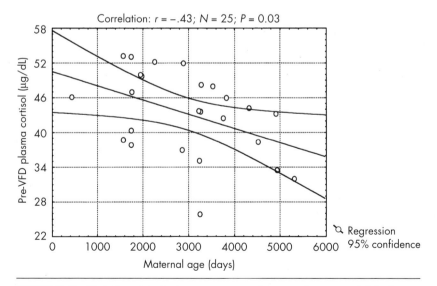

FIGURE 3–3   Relationship between maternal age and pre–variable foraging demand (VFD) cortisol.

Data suggest that older mothers tend to have lower baseline cortisol levels.

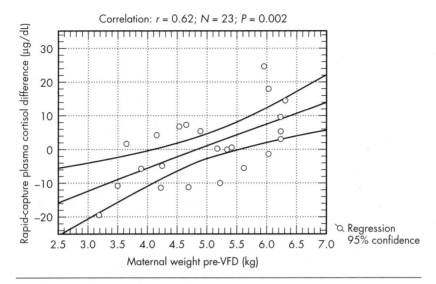

FIGURE 3–4   Relationship of maternal weight with pre/post–variable foraging demand (VFD) cortisol difference.

Heavier animals are more likely to have raised cortisol levels and lighter animals to have lowered cortisol levels after the VFD stressor.

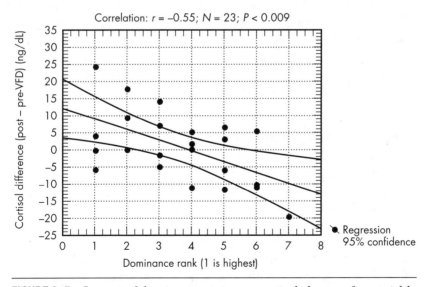

FIGURE 3–5   Impact of dominance status on cortisol change after variable foraging demand (VFD).

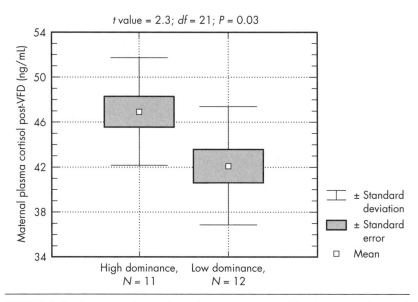

FIGURE 3–6   Impact of social rank on post–variable foraging demand (VFD) cortisol.

High-dominance animals have low pre-VFD cortisol and raise their cortisol after the VFD, whereas low-dominance animals have high pre-VFD cortisol and lower their cortisol after the VFD.

On regression analysis, both pre-VFD cortisol and social rank significantly predicted change in cortisol in response to the VFD imposition. Thus, the maternal plasma cortisol stress response to VFD appears to depend on social rank and related basal cortisol levels, but age and weight, in all likelihood mediated in part by their influence on dominance status, are also significantly related to this process (see Figure 3–7).

CONCLUSIONS AND DISCUSSION

The psychosocial stress induced by the VFD paradigm has a clear impact on the ability of primate mothers to provide consistent and adequate parenting toward their infants. The extensive data on the neuropsychobiology of the offspring demonstrates the powerful influence unpredictable rearing wields over the future development of the primate CNS. However, intimate knowledge regarding the mechanisms by which stress imposed on the mother is transmitted to the infant is lacking. This lack of knowledge originates in large part from the paucity of data on the neurobiology

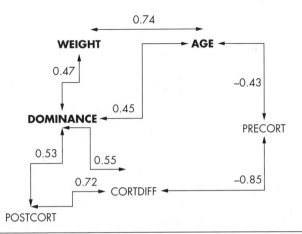

FIGURE 3–7   Variance relationship in maternal variable foraging demand (VFD): significant ($P < 0.05$; two tailed) Pearson correlations from 25 VFD-exposed mothers, as data set permitted.

Weight is positively correlated with age ($r = 0.74$) and dominance ($r = 0.47$). Age is correlated positively with dominance ($r = 0.45$) and negatively with pre-VFD cortisol (PRECORT) ($r = -0.43$). Dominance is positively correlated with post-VFD cortisol (POSTCORT) ($r = 0.53$) and with post–pre-VFD cortisol difference (CORTDIFF) ($r = 0.55$). Post–pre-VFD cortisol difference is strongly negatively correlated with pre-VFD cortisol and positively with post-VFD cortisol.

of VFD stress on primate mothers. Most of the subsequent data in this chapter deals with factors affecting the nature of the VFD stress on the mothers. In an attempt to decipher what may emerge as the most important and relevant factors in the transmission of the stress from the mothers to the infants, a central feature of the social dimension of the mothers' groups was studied in relation to cortisol, a biological indicator of HPA axis activation.

Social instability seems to constitute a major source of stress for all individuals within cohesive groups. Sapolsky (1992) reviewed a range of animal studies investigating the relationship between social rank and glucocorticoid secretion. In general, subordinate animals of many species (baboons, squirrel monkeys, rats, tree shrews, and others) have elevated basal corticoid levels whereas dominant animals, at least when groups are stable, have lower baseline glucocorticoid levels.

Our data are generally consistent with previous studies (Sapolsky 1992). The groups of mothers before imposition of the VFD condition essentially represent stable social hierarchies in which the dominant animals (who tend to be older, heavier, and multiparous) had relatively low cortisol levels and the subordinate animals (who are generally younger and slimmer and have a lower parity) had higher cortisol levels. When VFD is imposed, the social group seems to maintain the previous hierarchical structure, which nonetheless becomes more apparent with progressive perception of food insecurity. What is not clear, however, is the degree to which this type of stress affects the relative stability of the social hierarchy.

Sachser et al. (1998) described two major types of social relationships in mammalian social systems: dominance relationships established and maintained by agonistic behaviors, and social bonding relationships (mother–infant, female–male). Sachser et al. argued that both forms of social relationships are important for stress management. The established dominance status in a stable social hierarchy results in predictable behavior. Therefore, low positions in the hierarchy do not necessarily lead to intense HPA activation. According to Sachser et al. (1998), predictability seems to be the key factor that determines the stress response in a social group. Each individual's stress level is somewhat determined by the uncertainty of the social interactions. If the group is maintained undisturbed, we expect that hierarchical stratification will ultimately be established and the stress level of all individuals diminished.

In our experiments, VFD is a stress imposed on subjects within what appear to be relatively stable social hierarchies. Nonetheless, under the evidently stressful VFD condition, the dominants and the subordinates showed strikingly divergent patterns of HPA axis response; dominants started with relatively low cortisol and showed increases during VFD, whereas the subordinates started with higher levels and lowered their cortisol after the VFD. At the behavioral level, the dominants seemed to spend more time patrolling the resource cart, were more likely to display aggressive behavior, and seemed to neglect ventral contact with their infants. The subordinates, on the other hand, seemed to restrict their movement in the pen, and they looked more fearful and submissive, while clinging to their infants. Systematic analysis of the behavioral data is pending.

One possible hypothesis is that at baseline, particularly if the newly formed maternal-infant groups have not fully stabilized, dominants control and predict all significant features of the environment. On the other hand, subordinates may predict (but not control) food procurement but are less able to predict or control their interactions with the other members of the social group. The subordinates at baseline are stressed by the unpredictability of the dominants' reaction toward them. Hence, at baseline dominants' cortisol is low and subordinates' cortisol levels are higher. With the imposition of VFD, the hierarchy becomes progressively "crystallized" and hence social interactions become more predictable for the subordi-nates. Thus, in VFD the dominant animals may be more affected by the unpredictability of the foraging than the subordinates, who may ironically experience a more adverse yet more predictable social environment. We therefore present one possible explanation as to why over the course of the VFD, dominants show increases and subordinates show decreases in cor-tisol levels. Somewhat contrary to the assumption of Sachser et al. (1998) that the hierarchical structure increases the predictability of social interac-tion and thereby tends to reduce the stress of the individuals, the VFD condition seemed to crystallize the social hierarchy and differentially af-fected individuals at different strata in the hierarchy.

A recent study of army recruits undergoing boot camp produced results consistent with our data (Hellhammer et al. 1997). That study assessed the effects of stress (boot camp training) and social rank on adrenocortical ac-tivity and reactivity. Sixty-three recruits were randomly distributed to nine groups, and weekly measurements of social hierarchy within each group were determined. Baseline salivary cortisol measures were obtained throughout the training period and showed increases during the first few weeks of training irrespective of social status. Under experimental psycho-logical and physical stress a differentiated pattern of cortisol response was demonstrated between the dominants and subordinates. The socially dominant subjects markedly increased their salivary cortisol across the training period whereas only very modest increases were found in subor-dinate men. These findings are consistent with the increases in cortisol lev-els observed in our dominant mothers but nevertheless fail to account for the down-modulation of the cortisol response to the VFD of our subordi-nate mothers.

Another explanation is that reductions of cortisol levels in response to stress may represent an alternative yet equally valid and relevant modifi-cation of the HPA axis. Certainly many human clinical conditions inti-mately related to stress are characterized by low rather than high cortisol levels (Heim et al. 2000). These include PTSD, chronic fatigue syndrome, fibromyalgia, headache and migraine, and irritable bowel syndrome. Mechanisms for the induction of low cortisol states remain unclear, and the reductions of cortisol observed in subordinate mothers exposed to VFD represents a viable future animal model for studying this clinically pertinent but poorly understood and rarely documented transition from relatively high to relatively low HPA axis activity in adult animals without direct injury to the adrenal glands, as occurs in Addison's disease.

Many questions remain to be answered regarding the factors that influ-ence the rearing of the infants by mothers exposed to VFD and other forms of stress. The work presented here is an initial attempt to look at several sociobiological factors affecting the mothers of the infants reared under VFD, infants that show significant and enduring neurobiobehavioral effects following the VFD experience. For now, although we have identified several factors shaping maternal response, we have yet to decipher how these maternal effects mediate the apparently permanent biobehavioral effects observed in their offspring. Nonetheless, these data point to the tremendous importance of social factors in determining stress reactivity and response of the mothers and thus their ability to provide adequate mothering to their developing infants.

REFERENCES

Allman JM, Hakeem A, Erwin JM, et al: The anterior cingulate cortex: the evolution of an interface between emotion and cognition (review). Ann N Y Acad Sci 935:107–117, 2001

Anderberg UM, Marteinsdottir I, Theorell T, et al: The impact of life events in female patients with fibromyalgia and in female healthy controls. Eur Psychiatry 15:295–301, 2000

Andrews MW, Rosenblum LA: Attachment in monkey infants rose in variable- and low-demand. Child Dev 62:686–693, 1991

Bjorntorp P, Rosmond R: Hypothalamic origin of the metabolic syndrome X. Ann N Y Acad Sci 892:297–307, 1999

Bjorntorp P, Holm G, Rosmond R, et al: Hypertension and the metabolic syndrome: closely related central origin? Blood Press 9:71–82, 2000

Brunson KL, Eghbal-Ahmadi M, Bender R, et al: Long-term, progressive hippocampal cell loss and dysfunction induced by early life administration of corticotropin-releasing hormone reproduce the effects of early life stress. Proc Natl Acad Sci U S A. 98:8856–8861, 2001

Caldji C, Francis D, Sharma S, et al: The effects of early rearing environment on the development of GABAA and central benzodiazepine receptor levels and novelty-induced fearfulness in the rat. Neuropsychopharmacology 22:219–229, 2000

Charney DS, Henniger GR, Steinberg DE, et al: Adrenergic receptor sensitivity in depression: effects of clonidine in depressed patients and healthy subjects. Arch Gen Psychiatry 39:290–294, 1982

Coplan JD, Andrews MW, Rosenblum LA, et al: Persistent elevations of cerebrospinal fluid concentrations of corticotropin-releasing factor in adult nonhuman primates exposed to early life stressors: implications for the pathophysiology of mood and anxiety disorders. Proc Natl Acad Sci U S A. 93:1619–1623, 1996

Coplan JD, Pine D, Papp L, et al: A window on noradrenergic, hypothalamic-pituitary-adrenal axis and corticotropin-releasing factor function in anxiety and affective disorders: the growth hormone response to clonidine. Psychopharmacol Bull 33: 193–204, 1997

Coplan JD, Trost RC, Owens MJ, et al: Cerebrospinal fluid concentrations of somatostatin and biogenic amines in grown primates reared by mothers exposed to manipulated foraging conditions. Arch Gen Psychiatry 55:473–477, 1998

Coplan JD, Smith EL, Trost RC, et al: Growth hormone response to clonidine in adversely reared young adult primates: relationship to serial cerebrospinal fluid corticotropin-releasing factor concentrations. Psychiatry Res 95:93–102, 2000

Coplan JD, Smith EL, Altemus M, et al: Variable foraging demand rearing: sustained elevations in cisternal cerebrospinal fluid corticotropin-releasing factor concentrations in adult primates. Biol Psychiatry 50:200–204, 2001

Czeh B, Michaelis T, Watanabe T, et al: Stress-induced changes in cerebral metabolites, hippocampal volume, and cell proliferation are prevented by antidepressant treatment with tianeptine. Proc Natl Acad Sci U S A 98:12796–12801, 2001

Eisenberg N, Fabes RA, Murphy BC: Parents' reactions to children's negative emotions: relations to children's social competence and comforting behavior. Child Dev 67:2227–2247, 1996

Eriksson PS, Perfilieva E, Bjork-Eriksson T, et al: Neurogenesis in the adult human hippocampus. Nat Med 4:1313–1317, 1998

Felitti VJ, Anda RF, Nordenberg D, et al: Relationship of childhood abuse and household dysfunction to many of the leading causes of death in adults: the Adverse Childhood Experiences (ACE) study. Am J Prev Med 14:245–258, 1998

Gould E, Reeves AJ, Fallah M, et al: Hippocampal neurogenesis in adult Old World primates. Proc Natl Acad Sci U S A 96:5263–5267, 1999a

Gould E, Beylin A, Tanapat P, et al: Learning enhances adult neurogenesis in the hippocampal formation. Nat Neurosci 2:260–265, 1999b

Heim C, Ehlert U, Hellhammer DH: The potential role of hypocortisolism in the pathophysiology of stress-related bodily disorders. Psychoneuroendocrinology 25:1–35, 2000

Hellhammer DH, Buchtal J, Gutberlet I, et al: Social hierarchy and adrenocortical stress reactivity in men. Psychoneuroendocrinology 22:643–650, 1997

Liu D, Diorio J, Day JC, et al: Maternal care, hippocampal synaptogenesis and cognitive development in rats. Nat Neurosci 3:799–806, 2000

Mathew SJ, Coplan JD, Smith ELP, et al: Cerebrospinal fluid concentrations of biogenic amines and corticotropin-releasing factor in adolescent nonhuman primates as a function of the timing of adverse early rearing. Stress 5:185–193, 2002

Mathew SJ, Shungu DC, Mao X, Perera GM, Kegeles LS, Smith EL, Perera T, Lisanby SH, Rosenblum LA, Gorman JM, Coplan JD: A magnetic resonance spectroscopic imaging study of hippocampus and anterior cingulate in adult nonhuman primates reared under variable foraging demand conditions. Biol Psychiatry, in press

Nemeroff CB: The neurobiology of depression. Sci Am 278:42–49, 1998

Nemeroff CB: The preeminent role of early untoward experience on vulnerability to major psychiatric disorders: the nature-nurture controversy revisited and soon to be resolved. Mol Psychiatry 4:106–108, 1999

Nimchinsky EA, Vogt BA, Morrison JH, et al: Spindle neurons of the human anterior cingulate cortex. J Comp Neurol 355:27–37, 1995

Rasheed, JN: Parity, birthweight and cortisol. Lancet 339:828, 1993

Romans S, Belaise C, Martin J, et al: Childhood abuse and later medical disorders in women: an epidemiological study. Psychother Psychosom 71:141–150, 2002

Rosenblum LA, Paully GS: The effects of varying environmental demands on maternal and infant behavior. Child Dev 55:305–314, 1984

Rosenblum LA, Coplan JD, Friedman S, et al: Adverse early experiences affect noradrenergic and serotonergic functioning in adult primates. Biol Psychiatry 35:221–227, 1994

Sachser N, Durschlag M, Hirzel D: Social relationships and the management of stress. Psychoneuroendocrinology 23:891–904, 1998

Sapolsky R: Stress, the Aging Brain, and the Mechanisms of Neuron Death. Cambridge, MA, MIT Press, 1992

Schuff N, Neylan TC, Lenoci MA, et al: Decreased hippocampal N-acetyl-aspartate in the absence of atrophy in posttraumatic stress disorder. Biol Psychiatry 50:952–959, 2001

Smith EL, Batuman OA, Trost RC, et al: Transforming growth factor–beta 1 and cortisol in differentially reared primates. Brain Behav Immun 16:140–149, 2002

Trickett PK, Noll JG, Reiffman A, et al: Variants of intrafamilial sexual abuse experience: implications for short- and long-term development. Dev Psychopathol 13:1001–1019, 2001

Valentino RJ, Rudoy C, Saunders A, et al: Corticotropin-releasing factor is preferentially colocalized with excitatory rather than inhibitory amino acids in axon terminals in the peri-locus coeruleus region. Neuroscience 106:375–384, 2001

Vleugels MP, Eling WM, Rolland R, et al: Cortisol levels in pregnancy in relation to parity and age. Am J Obstet Gynecol 155:118–121, 1986

Yehuda R, Boisoneau D, Lowy MT, et al: Dose-response changes in plasma cortisol and lymphocyte glucocorticoid receptors following dexamethasone administration in combat veterans with and without posttraumatic stress disorder. Arch Gen Psychiatry 52:583–593, 1995

4

Offspring at High Risk for Anxiety and Depression

Preliminary Findings From a Three-Generation Study

Myrna M. Weissman, Ph.D.
Virginia Warner, M.P.H.
Priya Wickramaratne, Ph.D.
Yoko Nomura, Ph.D.
Kathleen R. Merikangas, Ph.D.
Gerard E. Bruder, Ph.D.
Craig E. Tenke, Ph.D.
Christian Grillon, Ph.D.

Numerous studies have demonstrated the familial transmission of major depressive disorder (MDD) in adult first-degree relatives of depressed patients (Gershon et al. 1982; Klein et al. 2001; Taylor et al. 1980; Weissman et al. 1982; Winokur 1982). Recent comprehensive reviews of controlled family studies of depression reveal that the average risk ratio (RR) for major depression among relatives of probands with major depression compared with control subjects was 2.0, indicating a moderate influence of familial aggregation on nonbipolar mood disorders (Sullivan et al. 2000). A recent meta-analysis of community-based twin studies of major depression yielded a heritability estimate of 0.37 (95% confidence interval [CI] 0.28 to 0.42). These estimates are in the range of estimates for other complex genetic disorders such as diabetes and breast cancer and

This research was funded by National Institute of Mental Health grant MH036197 (M.M.W., Principal Investigator).

suggest that environmental risk factors also make a substantial contribution (Sullivan et al. 2000). Retrospective data on onset and course from existing family studies indicate that early age of onset and recurrence are associated with increased familial clustering of depression (Wickramaratne et al. 2000). In parallel, studies of offspring of parents with affective disorders reveal an approximately threefold increased risk of depression among child and adolescent offspring (Downey and Coyne 1990; Hammen et al. 1990; Keller et al. 1986; Kovacs et al. 1997; Kutcher and Marton 1991; Lieb et al. 2002; Orvaschel et al. 1988; Puig-Antich et al. 1989; Weissman et al. 1984, 1987; Williamson et al. 1995). However, the results of recent family and twin studies of youth suggest that prepubertal depression may be less heritable than postpubertal depression (Harrington et al. 1997; Kaufman et al. 2001; Merikangas and Angst 1995; Rende and Weissman 1999; Rende et al. 1999; Silberg et al. 1999, 2001). The discrepancy in these findings may be attributable to anxiety as a prodromal form of depression or that prepubertal MDD is diagnostically heterogeneous into adulthood (Avenevoli et al. 2001; Breslau et al. 1995; Cole et al. 1998; Kovacs et al. 1989; Lewinsohn et al. 1994; Pine et al. 1998; Reinherz et al. 1993; Rende et al. 1999; Rohde et al. 1991; Thapar and McGuffin 1997; Weissman 2002; Weissman et al. 1999). There also appear to be differences in both the specificity and risk factors for preadolescent and adolescent-onset depression that will be examined in future analyses of the present study.

The overall aim of this research is to examine the familial aggregation of mood disorders and other psychiatric disorders across the generations. By following the second and third generations of a cohort with well-characterized mood disorders (generation 1) compared with non–psychiatrically ill control subjects, we aimed to understand the stability of risk across the generations, to identify premorbid vulnerability factors (biological markers, early signs), and to apply this information to the development of appropriate and targeted preventive interventions.

This study incorporates a combined family study–high-risk design with a prospective longitudinal follow-up of three generations of families that were initially identified more than 17 years ago. Table 4–1 and Figure 4–1 present a summary of the study design. There are numerous advantages to the combined high-risk and longitudinal design. The potential case yield is increased as is the power to detect risk factor associations, as well as mediating and moderating effects on risk factors (e.g., children of depressed parents with vs. without a divorce). Other important benefits include the ability to identify early patterns and sequence of disease given

TABLE 4–1   Study design

High–risk	Comparison between individuals with and without risk of parental depression
Longitudinal	Four assessments over 17 years (baseline, 2, 10, and 17 years) from childhood to adulthood in the second generation
Three generations	

exposure to risk, which in this case is parental depression, and maximization of the reliability of estimates of specificity and stability of transmission (Merikangas et al. 1999).

The present study is unique in examining familial aggregation of mood and anxiety disorders across three generations. Other design features that differentiate the present study from the majority of prior family/high-risk studies include systematic interviewing of both parents regarding not only child psychopathology but also their own psychopathology; prospective follow-up of high- and low-risk groups; inclusion of a demographically comparable control group, which has rarely been incorporated in prior high-risk studies of depression; and measures of potential biological markers for mood and anxiety disorders (i.e., psychophysiological measures, described later).

We hypothesized that the grandchildren of depressed grandparents would have an increased risk of mood disorders. Further, we predicted that multigenerational MDD (i.e., the presence of MDD in both grandparent and parent) would be associated with a significantly greater risk of mood disorders among grandchildren. Finally, in light of the familial links between depression and anxiety disorders, we expected that offspring of parents in both generations would have an increased risk of anxiety disorders, irrespective of parental comorbidity for anxiety and depression. This chapter presents preliminary findings from this three-generation study to illustrate the potential advantages of the design for translational research.

METHODS

In the original study, probands with major depression were selected from outpatient clinical specialty settings for the treatment of mood disorders (generation 1). The nondepressed probands, who were required to show no lifetime history of psychiatric illness on the basis of several interviews, were selected from a community sample of adults from the same commu-

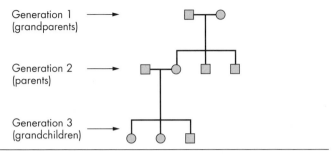

FIGURE 4–1   The three generations.

nity, New Haven, Connecticut (for more details see Weissman et al. 1982, 1992, 1997; Warner et al. 1999). The proband, spouse, offspring (generation 2) and grandchildren (generation 3) were interviewed independently. The six families in which either the control proband or spouse in the control group subsequently developed MDD were removed from the study.

The diagnostic interviews across all waves were conducted using a semistructured diagnostic assessment (the Schedule for Affective Disorders and Schizophrenia, Lifetime Version [SADS-L] for adults [Mannuzza et al. 1986], and for subjects between the ages of 6 and 17 the Schedule for Affective Disorders and Schizophrenia for School-Aged Children, Epidemiological Version [K-SADS-E] [Orvaschel et al. 1982] modified for DSM-IV [American Psychiatric Association 1994] at wave 4 by Kaufman). The diagnostic assessments were administered by highly trained clinical interviewers who were blind to the clinical status of the parents or grandparents. Multiple sources of information were obtained, including independent assessments of the subjects by direct interview, by parent report, and by direct assessment of both biological parents as often as possible. All final diagnoses (best estimates) were made blindly by experienced psychiatrists or psychologists based on all available information (Leckman et al. 1982). The data presented are based on extensive interviews concerning medical history, psychiatric diagnoses, and social functioning, as well as medical records when available at four waves over 17 years on grandparents and parents, and for grandchildren at the last two waves). The results presented here from the fourth wave are preliminary, based on about 80% of the sample and based on interviews and not best-estimate diagnoses. The response rate for probands, offspring, and grandchildren ranged from 76% to 86% over the previous three waves and did not differ by proband groups. The total sample available for interview and the data collected at wave 4 for these preliminary analyses are described in Figure 4–2.

Generation 1   ⟶ One or both grandparents had
(grandparents)   major depression *or* both were
              never mentally ill ($n = 133$)

Generation 2   ⟶ Offspring ages 6+ followed over
(parents)   15–17 years into adulthood
              ($n = 182$)

Generation 3   ⟶ Grandchildren ages 6+ ($n = 160$)
(grandchildren)

FIGURE 4–2   Descriptions of the three generations.

RESULTS

Sequence of Onset and Age-Specific Rates of Anxiety Disorder and MDD

Figures 4–3 and 4–4, respectively, show the age-specific rates of anxiety and MDD in the second generation stratified by the MDD status of the grandparents (generation 1). The peak incidence of an anxiety disorder, at ages 5 to 10 (Figure 4–3), is much earlier than that for MDD, which occurs between the ages of 15 and 20 (Figure 4–4).

The age-specific rates in the third generation follow a similar pattern as in the second generation, with the exception that the second generation had a longer period of follow-up (Figures 4–5 and 4–6). Not shown here is the finding that grandchildren with a diagnosis of anxiety (prior to the onset of MDD) had a 2.4-fold increase in risk for MDD compared with grandchildren without a prior diagnosis of anxiety. These findings are consistent with the hypothesis that anxiety may act either as a predisposition or temporal antecedent to recurrent, early-onset MDD. This form of MDD is characteristically the most severe and has the poorest treatment outcome. The observation that anxiety disorder also was a precursor of MDD in the second generation in wave 4 led us to examine psychophysiological indicators of anxiety in youth based on prior research demonstrating increased startle response among offspring of parents with anxiety disorders compared with those of probands with substance use disorders and control subjects (Grillon et al. 1997a, 1997b, 1998; Merikangas et al. 1999).

Effect of Parent and Grandparent MDD on Grandchildren

Grandparent MDD has a strong impact on the risk of mood disorders in the grandchildren. The grandchildren in the high-risk group (i.e., those with at least one depressed grandparent) have higher rates of mood disorders

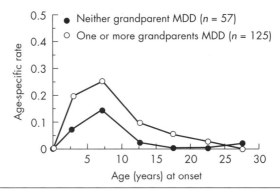

FIGURE 4–3 Age-specific rates of any anxiety disorder in parent (generation 2) by major depressive disorder (MDD) status of grandparent (generation 1).

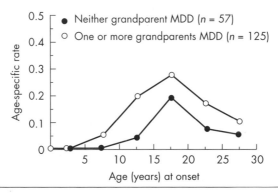

FIGURE 4–4 Age-specific rates of major depressive disorder (MDD) in parent (generation 2) by MDD status of grandparent (generation 1).

than those in the low-risk group (22.1% vs. 3.6%, RR 4.5 [95% CI 1.1 to 15.2]) after adjusting for age and gender of grandchild, using Cox proportional hazard regression models. These results support the use of the original high- and low-risk classification.

The following results are preliminary.

We further categorized the grandchildren by grandparent and parent depression status. Grandparents without MDD (groups 1 and 2) were defined as low risk and grandparents with MDD (groups 3 and 4) as high risk (Figure 4–7). We found that grandchildren with a depressed grandparent, regardless of their parents' depression status, were at increased risk for mood disorder. This may be because the majority of the depressed grandparents were originally selected through a depression treatment clinic.

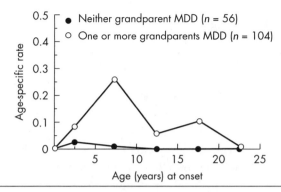

FIGURE 4–5 Age-specific rates of any anxiety disorder in grandchild (generation 3) by major depressive disorder (MDD) status of grandparent (generation 1).

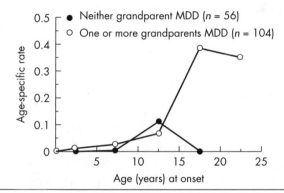

FIGURE 4–6 Age-specific rates of major depressive disorder (MDD) in grandchild (generation 3) by MDD status of grandparent (generation 1).

Their depression may have been of a more severe or chronic form, which also tends to be more familial. The grandchildren from groups 2 and 4 had the poorest overall functioning (not shown). These findings were independent of grandparent depression status, suggesting that parental MDD also has an impact on offspring.

Group 2 (grandparent not depressed, parent depressed) is of considerable interest. Our previous findings in the offspring (generation 2) of depressed grandparents showed, both cross-sectionally and over a 10-year follow-up, that these offspring were at a threefold increased risk for MDD. We also found that some of the offspring (generation 2) with nondepressed parents (generation 1) developed MDD (group 2). However, Fendrich et al. (1990), in an analysis of the second wave of these data, showed that they had a lower rate of MDD, a later age of onset, and more family environment risk factors (discord between parents and children, poor parental bonding, etc.) compared with control subjects. These findings were replicated by Nomura et al. (2002) in the same sample at 10-year follow-up (the third wave), when the second generation were all adults. These findings raised questions about the transmission of depression to the third generation (grandchildren in group 2). We hypothesized that cases of parental depression in group 2 may be nonfamilial phenocopies that will not result in transmission of MDD to the grandchildren. Our findings in the grandchildren (third generation in group 2) are consistent with this hypothesis (see Figure 4–7). The rate of MDD in grandchildren did not differ between low-risk groups (groups 1 and 2). When the full-sample and best-estimate diagnoses are completed, we will examine the nature, severity, and onset of the mood disorders in the grandchildren in the four groups. We will also assess the transmission of familial risk factors across the generations and the range of disorders in the grandchildren.

DISCUSSION

Summary of Findings

The preliminary data confirm our major hypotheses. First, there was a strong degree of familial aggregation across the three generations investigated in the present study. Mood disorders in the grandparents were associated with mood disorders in the grandchildren, irrespective of parental mood disorder. We also confirmed our second hypothesis, that multigenerational depression was associated with the greatest level of depression in offspring. In addition, we found that the third generation was at increased risk for anxiety disorders in childhood, followed by MDD in adolescence. This increased risk of MDD preceded by anxiety was stable across the three generations in high-risk samples. If confirmed in the full sample, this finding could provide a powerful index of genetic risk.

The findings illustrate the potential importance of collecting family history data beyond the first generation for research studies that involve children. Although the offspring of depressed parents without a grandparent history of depression may represent phenocopies, they did not appear to differ clinically from the offspring with both a depressed parent and a depressed grandparent. However, the risk for depression in the next generation of these groups may be quite different. Alternatively, depression-free adults with a depressed parent may confirm an increased risk of depression in the third generation.

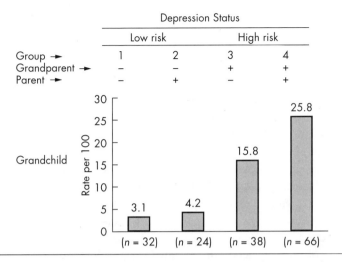

FIGURE 4–7   Mood disorder rates in grandchildren, by major depressive disorder (MDD) status of grandparents and parents.

Psychophysiological Measures

A convergence of evidence suggests that psychophysiological measures, which are noninvasive, cost-effective, and easily obtained in children, are good candidates for biological markers of vulnerability to depressive or anxiety disorders. This includes electroencephalogram (EEG) findings from 1) studies in infants or young children who are at risk for depressive or anxiety disorders by virtue of family history of depression (Dawson et al. 1997; Field et al. 1995), 2) studies of behaviorally inhibited and uninhibited children (Davidson and Fox 1989; Fox et al. 1992), and 3) studies in adults and adolescents with depressive or anxiety disorders (Bruder et al. 1997; Davidson 1992; Kentgen et al. 2000). Davidson (1992) reviewed evidence that frontal brain asymmetry, as measured by EEG alpha asymmetry, identifies a diathesis predisposing individuals to respond with predominantly negative or positive affect, which may relate to the risk for depression or anxiety. Reduced left frontal activation is hypothesized to be associated with a deficit in approach-related behaviors and right frontal activation with withdrawal-related behaviors. In several studies, infants of depressed mothers exhibited reduced left frontal activity compared with infants of nonsymptomatic mothers (Dawson et al. 1997; Field et al. 1995). Similarly, behaviorally inhibited children showed an EEG alpha asymmetry indicative of right frontal activation, whereas uninhibited children showed the opposite asymmetry (Davidson 1992). Depressed adults have been reported to show greater left than right frontal alpha asymmetry (Davidson et al. 1987; Gotlib et al. 1998; Henriques and Davidson 1991), but not all studies have found this frontal asymmetry (Reid et al. 1998).

Some studies have found the opposite alpha asymmetry at posterior sites in depressed adults, indicative of reduced right relative to left posterior activity (Davidson et al. 1987; Reid et al. 1998), but other studies have not found this asymmetry (Henriques and Davidson 1991). Heller et al. (1995) suggested that the failure of some studies to find evidence of reduced right posterior activation in depression may be due to the opposing effects of anxiety on parietotemporal activity. This is supported by EEG findings of less right than left posterior activation in adults and adolescents having MDD without an anxiety disorder, but not in those with a comorbid anxiety disorder (Bruder et al. 1997; Kentgen et al. 2000). Remitted depressed patients who were normothymic during EEG testing displayed evidence of both reduced left frontal and right posterior activity, which supports the hypothesis that these EEG alpha asymmetries may represent state-independent trait markers (Henriques and Davidson 1991).

Because of the preceding findings, an additional aim of this study was to evaluate the potential of EEG alpha asymmetry measures as biological markers of a phenotype of depression characterized by early onset of anxiety and familial loading for MDD. It was hypothesized that frontal alpha asymmetry will vary as a function of familial loading of MDD and will be associated with risk for MDD alone and MDD comorbid with anxiety. Resting EEG is measured in both parents (generation 2) and grandchildren (generation 3) who are at high or low risk for depression by virtue of their family history. Both grandchildren and parents who come from high-risk families in which a grandparent had MDD show EEG alpha asymmetries indicative of greater right than left frontal activation, whereas offspring from low-risk families do not show this pattern of alpha asymmetry. Moreover, based on findings of abnormal posterior alpha asymmetries in adult and adolescent depression, high-risk offspring are expected to differ from low-risk offspring in showing evidence of less right than left activation at posterior sites. Offspring with both parents depressed or who have both a parent and a grandparent who are depressed, show the greatest difference in the alpha asymmetries compared with low-risk offspring. Data collection and analysis are ongoing.

The startle reflex was also included in this study and is a relatively new approach to investigating emotions. Since the early 1990s, the startle reflex has provided unique and integrative ways of probing aversive states and psychopathology in adults and children. Startle presents several advantages that make it an ideal tool to identify vulnerability markers for mood and anxiety disorders. It is sensitive to aversive states. It is also a translational methodology that not only links neuroscience to psychological sciences, but also permits cross-generational research in humans.

The startle reflex is a cross-species response to an intense and surprising stimulus. In animals, startle is measured by assessing the whole-body reflex. In humans, the "startle pattern" consists of a forward thrusting of the head and a descending flexor wave reaction, extending through the trunk and knees (Landis and Hunt 1939). The amplitude and the latency of the startle reflex can be measured by recording the eyeblink reflex, the most consistent and persistent component of the startle pattern. Although a startle response can be elicited with visual and tactile stimuli as long as the stimuli are sufficiently intense and have a fast rise time, most startle studies use acoustic stimuli (e.g., brief bursts of white noise at 90 to 115 dBA).

One appealing characteristic of startle is its extreme sensitivity to aversive emotional states in both humans and animals. Brown et al. (1951) first reported that startle was increased or potentiated by conditioned fear in animals. Since this seminal study, the so-called fear-potentiated startle effect has been replicated many times using different procedures in different laboratories. Thus, startle is increased or sensitized following administration of shocks (Davis 1989). It is also increased upon reexposure to aversive contexts in which shocks have been previously administered (Gewirtz et al. 1998). Finally, it is facilitated by innately aversive stimuli such as bright lights. Despite the fact that Brown et al.'s (1951) initial study was prompted by the anecdotal clinical observations that anxious people show an exaggerated startle response to loud sounds, it is only recently that the startle reflex methodology has been used to study fear and anxiety in humans. Several studies have documented potentiated startle during aversive states in humans. Grillon et al. (1991) reported a robust and highly reliable increase in startle when subjects were verbally informed to expect unpleasant aversive stimuli such as shocks. Similar results were obtained for aversive expectation following learned fear (i.e., fear conditioning) (Grillon and Davis 1997; Hamm et al. 1993). Startle is also increased during the processing of unpleasant stimuli (e.g., aversive pictures) (Lang et al. 1990). Finally, anxiogenic situations such as darkness facilitate startle (Grillon et al. 1997b). Grillon et al. (1997b) suggested that the facilitation of startle in the dark in humans and the facilitation of startle in rodents exposed to bright light have similar evolutionary bases. Rodents are nocturnal animals and are vulnerable in bright spaces, whereas humans are diurnal and are more vulnerable in the dark. In general, threatening environments facilitate startle in both species. Experiments with changes in lighting conditions illustrate another advantage of startle as a translational tool of investigation. Because very similar experiments can be conducted in two species, human and animal research can inform each other.

Perhaps the most compelling feature of the startle reflex is the abundant basic research that informs its underlying anatomic and functional basis, thereby shedding light on the biological pathways involved in fear and anxiety states. Clinicians have long recognized that anxiety is not a unitary phenomenon but can take several forms (Barlow 2000). An accepted distinction is that between fear, a phasic response associated with an identifiable threat, and anxiety, a more sustained state of apprehension not obviously associated with a specific cue. Davis (1998) described two separate pathways mediating fear-potentiated startle that may be associated with these two aversive states (i.e., fear and anxiety). The first pathway is responsible for the phasic potentiation of startle during anticipation of an aversive event (e.g., a shock) signaled by a cue (e.g., a light). This pathway, which appears to activate cue-specific fear, is critically dependent on the central nucleus of the amygdala. Another structure, the bed nucleus of the stria terminalis (BNST), is involved in a second type of aversive response more indicative of generalized anxiety than fear. For example, under certain conditions, baseline startle reflex shows a gradual elevation over the course of aversive conditioning that may reflect a response to chronic stress (Gewirtz et al. 1998). This elevation is blocked by lesions of the BNST, but not by lesions of the amygdala (Gewirtz et al. 1998). Further evidence of a functional dissociation between the amygdala and the BNST is presented by the fact that lesions of the BNST, but not lesions of the amygdala, block the facilitation of startle by bright light (Walker and Davis 1997a, 1997b). Systemic injections of the stress hormone corticotropin-releasing hormone produce a sustained elevation in baseline startle that is blocked by lesions of the BNST, but not by lesions of the amygdala (Lee and Davis 1997). Based on this result, it has been suggested that the symptom of aversive anticipation that characterizes anxiety may be mediated by a sustained activation of the BNST via corticotropin-releasing hormone (Davis 1998).

There is an emerging literature suggesting that the latter pathway (i.e., BNST) may be implicated in the pathophysiology of anxiety disorders. Empirical evidence from startle studies suggests that anxious patients are overly sensitive to threatening contexts but show fairly normal response to cued fear. Grillon et al. (1994a) showed that patients with panic disorder and posttraumatic stress disorder (PTSD) exhibit increased baseline startle but normal fear-potentiated startle when anticipating signaled shocks. Similarly, Cuthbert et al. (1994) reported normal affective modulation of startle during aversive imagery procedures in patients with various anxiety disorders (simple and social phobia, PTSD, and panic disorders). However, startle stimuli presented during intertrial periods were significantly elevated in these patients. These elevated baseline levels seem specific to aversive contexts because patients with anxiety disorders do not show increased startle in nonthreatening environments (Grillon et al. 1994b). These results are consistent with the hypothesis of greater contextual fear in anxious patients. There is preliminary evidence that this sensitivity to threatening experimental contexts could constitute a marker for anxiety disorders. Grillon et al. (1997b, 1998) reported that children at high risk for anxiety disorders because of a parental history of these conditions exhibited increased baseline startle.

One important issue in high-risk research on anxiety is to ensure that experiments are developmentally appropriate and that they lead to comparable results across generations. Procedures in which electric shocks are anticipated are obviously unethical for research in children. Recently, Grillon and Ameli (1998) developed a procedure that substituted intense jets of air (air blasts) directed at the neck at the level of the larynx for electric shocks. Anticipation of air blasts activates the amygdala (Pine et al. 2001a, 2001b) and yields robust and reliable startle potentiation in children (Grillon et al. 1999) and in adults of all ages (C. Grillon, unpublished observations). Other procedures, such as testing subjects in the dark, also facilitate startle in children and adults (Grillon et al. 1999), providing additional ways of assessing startle potentiation as a vulnerability marker in high-risk studies.

Based on the preceding evidence, one would expect that the magnitude of startle in grandchildren and parents will increase as a function of familial loading for anxiety and will be associated with increased risk for anxiety alone and anxiety comorbid with MDD. In those high-risk families in which MDD is comorbid with an anxiety disorder, the magnitude of the startle response should be greater in grandchildren and parents compared with both high-risk families with MDD not comorbid with anxiety and low-risk families. Data collection and analyses are ongoing.

Implications for Prevention

The ultimate aim of this research is to develop appropriate and targeted preventive interventions based on familial and individual risk factors. At least two intervention studies are suggested by our findings. The finding that anxiety disorder is an early precursor of MDD across the generations suggests that treatment of primary anxiety may lead to the prevention of secondary depression (Kessler et al. 1996). Furthermore, these findings indicate that it may be fruitful to implement early intervention efforts to reduce the severity and recurrence of mood disorders in susceptible youth as they proceed through adolescence.

Finally, the application of prevention efforts among youth of parents with MDD, prior to its onset in the youth, may actually reduce the incidence of depression in a high-risk cohort. This could be accomplished by treatment of parental depression to reduce its impact on the familial environment of exposed youth. For example, Beardslee et al. (1993, 1997) developed a program for offspring of depressed parents. A psychoeducational approach was compared with a purely educational approach among 36 parents, largely middle-class and Caucasian, with a lifetime history of MDD and at least one child age 8 to 15 ($N=52$). These parents were randomly assigned to a psychoeducational intervention, consisting of 6 to 10 sessions, or a control condition, consisting of two 1-hour standardized group lectures on depression. Parental depression was not treated. Parents receiving psychoeducation reported better communication with their children than those in the control group. Their children, compared with children in the control condition, experienced higher levels of overall functioning, as measured by the Children's Global Assessment Scale (CGAS), and gained an increased understanding of their parents' illness. There were no group differences between children in the psychoeducational group and those in the control condition in the amount of change observed on various symptom scales (Beardslee et al. 1993, 1997). Future studies employing more aggressive treatment strategies of either the affected parent or child may address the relevance of this strategy in reducing the impact of depression in youth.

There are three ongoing studies of the impact of treatment of depressed mothers on their children that may inform future treatment efforts among high-risk youth. Garber and colleagues at Vanderbilt University are conducting a study focusing on the impact of treating parental MDD on children's (age 8 to 16) socioemotional adjustment. Their study includes three groups receiving 16 weekly sessions of cognitive-behavioral therapy (CBT), pharmacotherapy, or placebo, with approximately 60 patients per group, as well as a comparison group of 90 nondepressed mothers. Patients are recruited from psychiatric settings. Riley and colleagues at Johns Hopkins targeted 150 depressed women and their children (75 mothers receiving 16 weekly group CBT sessions and 75 receiving paroxetine) and a comparison group of 50 nondepressed mothers and their children, recruited from a family planning clinic.

A third study by Weissman and Pilowsky, ancillary to the multisite Sequential Treatment Alternatives to Relieve Depression (STAR*D) study, is examining the impact of remission of maternal MDD on the psychiatric and social functioning of children (N=320). The STAR*D study will compare the effectiveness of different treatment options for MDD, focusing on the common clinical question of what to do when patients fail to respond to standard treatment with an antidepressant medication. STAR*D will define which subsequent treatment strategies are acceptable to patients and provide the best clinical results. Children are being followed over the course of the depressed mother's treatment.

CONCLUSIONS

The major findings are the stability of depression across generations and the role of anxiety disorder as a precursor to the development of depression. These findings are consistent with those of numerous previous studies based on retrospective reports or investigations of only two generations. Our results, although preliminary, suggest the stability of the findings across generations. Whether biological markers can be found that can further strengthen the risk predictions awaits the final results. Regardless of these results, findings thus far suggest several opportunities for early intervention.

REFERENCES

American Psychiatric Association: Diagnostic and Statistical Manual of Mental Disorders, 4th Edition. Washington, DC, American Psychiatric Association, 1994

Avenevoli S, Stolar M, Li J, et al: Comorbidity of depression in children and adolescents: models and evidence from a prospective high-risk family study. Biol Psychiatry 49:1071–1081, 2001

Barlow DH: Unraveling the mysteries of anxiety and its disorders from the perspective of emotion theory. Am Psychol 55:1247–1263, 2000

Beardslee WR, Keller MB, Lavori PW, et al: The impact of parental affective disorder on depression in offspring: a longitudinal follow-up, in a non-referred sample. J Am Acad Child Adolesc Psychiatry 32:723–730, 1993

Beardslee WR, Wright EJ, Salt P, et al: Examination of children's responses to two preventive intervention strategies over time. J Am Acad Child Adolesc Psychiatry 36:196–204, 1997

Breslau N, Schultz L, Peterson E: Sex differences in depression: a role for preexisting anxiety. Psychiatry Res 58:1–12, 1995

Brown JS, Kalish HI, Farber IE: Conditioned fear as revealed by the magnitude of startle response to an auditory stimulus. J Exp Psychol 41:317–327, 1951

Bruder GE, Fong R, Tenke CE, et al: Regional brain asymmetries in major depression with or without an anxiety disorder: a quantitative electroencephalographic study. Biol Psychiatry 41:939–948, 1997

Cole DA, Peeke LG, Martin JM, et al: A longitudinal look at the relation between depression and anxiety in children and adolescents. J Consult Clin Psychol 66:451–460, 1998

Cuthbert BN, Drobes DJ, Patrick CJ, et al: Autonomic and startle responding during affective imagery among anxious patients. Psychophysiology 31:S37, 1994

Davidson RJ: Anterior cerebral asymmetry and the nature of emotion. Brain Cogn 20:125–151, 1992

Davidson RJ, Fox NA: Frontal brain asymmetry predicts infants' response to maternal separation. J Abnorm Psychol 98:127–131, 1989

Davidson RJ, Chapman JP, Chapman LJ: Task-dependent EEG asymmetry discriminates between depressed and non-depressed subjects. Psychophysiology 24:585, 1987

Davis M: Sensitization of the acoustic startle reflex by footshock. Behav Neurosci 103:495–503, 1989

Davis M: Are different parts of the extended amygdala involved in fear versus anxiety? Biol Psychiatry 44:1239–1247, 1998

Dawson G, Frey K, Panagiotides H, et al: Infants of depressed mothers exhibit atypical frontal brain activity: a replication and extension of previous findings. J Child Psychol Psychiatry 38:179–186, 1997

Downey G, Coyne JC: Children of depressed parents: an integrative review. Psychol Bull 108:50–76, 1990

Fendrich M, Warner V, Weissman MM: Family risk factors, parental depression and psychopathology in offspring. Dev Psychol 25:40–50, 1990

Field T, Fox NA, Pickens J, et al: Relative right frontal EEG activation in 3- to 6-month-old infants of "depressed" mothers. Dev Psychol 31:358–363, 1995

Fox NA, Bell MA, Jones NA: Individual differences in response to stress and cerebral asymmetry. Dev Neuropsychol 8:161–184, 1992

Gershon ES, Hamovit JA, Guroff JJ, et al: A family study of schizoaffective bipolar I, bipolar II, unipolar, and normal control probands. Arch Gen Psychiatry 39:1157–1167, 1982

Gewirtz JC, McNish KA, Davis M: Lesions of the bed nucleus of the stria terminalis block sensitization of acoustic startle reflex produced by repeated stress, but not fear-potentiated startle. Prog Neuropsychopharmacol Biol Psychiatry 22:625–648, 1998

Gotlib IH, Ranganath C, Rosenfeld JP: Frontal EEG alpha asymmetry, depression, and cognitive functioning. Cognition and Emotion 12:449–478, 1998

Grillon C, Ameli R: Effects of threat and safety signals on startle during anticipation of aversive shocks, sounds, or airblasts. Journal of Psychophysiology 12:329–337, 1998

Grillon C, Davis M: Fear-potentiated startle conditioning in humans: explicit and contextual cue conditioning following paired versus unpaired training. Psychophysiology 34:451–458, 1997

Grillon C, Ameli R, Woods SW, et al: Fear-potentiated startle in humans: effects of anticipatory anxiety on the acoustic blink reflex. Psychophysiology 28:588–595, 1991

Grillon C, Ameli R, Goddard A, et al: Baseline and fear-potentiated startle in panic disorder patients. Biol Psychiatry 35:431–439, 1994a

Grillon C, Morgan A, Charney D: Startle response and prepulse inhibition in Vietnam veterans with PTSD. Psychophysiology 31:S53, 1994b

Grillon C, Dierker L, Merikangas KR: Startle modulation in children at risk for anxiety disorders and/or alcoholism. J Am Acad Child Adolesc Psychiatry 36:925–932, 1997a

Grillon C, Pellowski M, Merikangas KR, et al: Darkness facilitates the acoustic startle in humans. Biol Psychiatry 42:453–460, 1997b

Grillon C, Dierker L, Merikangas KR: Fear-potentiated startle in adolescent offspring of Parents with Anxiety Disorders. Biol Psychiatry 44:990–997, 1998

Grillon C, Merikangas KR, Dierker L, et al: Startle potentiation by threat of aversive stimuli and darkness in adolescents: a multi-site study. Int J Psychophysiol 32:63–73, 1999

Hamm AO, Greenwald MK, Bradley MM, et al: Emotional learning, hedonic changes, and the startle probe. J Abnorm Psychol 102:453–465, 1993

Hammen C, Burge D, Burney E, et al: Longitudinal study of diagnoses in children of women with unipolar and bipolar affective disorder. Arch Gen Psychiatry 47:1112–1117, 1990

Harrington, R, Rutter M, Weissman MM, et al: Psychiatric disorders in the relatives of depressed probands, I: comparison of prepubertal, adolescent and early adult onset cases. J Affect Disord 42:9–22, 1997

Heller W, Etienne MA, Miller GA: Patterns of perceptual asymmetry in depression and anxiety: implications for neuropsychological models of emotion and psychopathology. J Abnorm Psychol 104:327–333, 1995

Henriques JB, Davidson RJ: Left frontal hypoactivation in depression. J Abnorm Psychol 100:535–545, 1991

Kaufman J, Martin A, King RA, et al: Are child-, adolescent-, and adult-onset depression one and the same disorder? Biol Psychiatry 49:980–1001, 2001

Keller MB, Beardslee WR, Dorer DJ, et al: Impact of severity and chronicity of parental affective illness on adaptive functioning and psychopathology in children. Arch Gen Psychiatry 43:930–937, 1986

Kentgen LM, Tenke CE, Pine DS, et al: Electroencephalographic asymmetries in adolescents with major depression: influence of comorbidity with anxiety disorders. J Abnorm Psychol 109:797–802, 2000

Kessler RC, Nelson CB, McGonagle KA, et al: The epidemiology of co-occurring addictive and mental disorders: implications for prevention and service utilization. Am J Orthopsychiatry 66:17–31, 1996

Klein DN, Lewinsohn PM, Seeley JR, et al: A family study of major depressive disorder in a community sample of adolescents. Arch Gen Psychiatry 58:13–20, 2001

Kovacs M, Gatsonis C, Paulauskas SL, et al: Depressive disorders in childhood, IV: a longitudinal study of comorbidity with and risk for anxiety disorders. Arch Gen Psychiatry 66:451–460, 1989

Kovacs M, Devlin B, Pollock M, et al: A controlled family history study of childhood-onset depressive disorder. Arch Gen Psychiatry 54:613–623, 1997

Kutcher S, Marton P: Affective disorders in first-degree relatives of adolescent onset bipolars, unipolars, and normal controls. J Am Acad Child Adolesc Psychiatry 30:75–78, 1991

Landis C, Hunt WA: The Startle Pattern. New York, Farrar & Rinehart, 1939

Lang PJ, Bradley MM, Cuthbert BN: Emotion, attention, and the startle reflex. Psychol Rev 97:1–19, 1990

Leckman JF, Sholomskas D, Thompson D, et al: Best estimate of lifetime psychiatric diagnosis: a methodological study. Arch Gen Psychiatry 39:879–883, 1982

Lee Y, Davis M: Role of the hippocampus, the bed nucleus of the stria terminalis, and the amygdala in the excitatory effect of corticotropin-releasing hormone on the acoustic startle reflex. J Neurosci 17:6434–6446, 1997

Lewinsohn PM, Clarke GN, Seeley JR, et al: Major depression in community adolescents: age at onset, episode duration, and time to recurrence. J Am Acad Child Adolesc Psychiatry 33:809–818, 1994

Lieb R, Isensee B, Hofler M, et al: Parental major depression and the risk of depression and other mental disorders in offspring. Arch Gen Psychiatry 59:365–374, 2002

Mannuzza S, Fyer AJ, Klein DF, et al: Schedule for Affective Disorders and Schizophrenia—Lifetime Version modified for the study of anxiety disorders (SADS-LA): rationale and conceptual development. J Psychiatr Res 20:317–325, 1986

Merikangas KR, Angst J: The challenge of depressive disorders in adolescence, in Psychosocial Disturbances in Young People: Challenges for Prevention. Edited by Rutter M. New York, Cambridge University Press, 1995, pp 131–165

Merikangas RK, Avenevoli S, Dierker L, et al: Vulnerability factors among children at risk for anxiety disorders. Biol Psychiatry 46:1523–1535, 1999

Nomura Y, Wickramaratne PJ, Warner V, et al: Family discord, parental depression and psychopathology in offspring: ten-year follow-up. J Am Acad Child Adolesc Psychiatry 41:402–409, 2002

Orvaschel H, Puig-Antich J, Chambers W, et al: Retrospective assessments of prepubertal major depression with Kiddie-SADS-E. J Am Acad Child Adolesc Psychiatry 21:392–397, 1982

Orvaschel H, Walsh-Allis G, Ye WJ: Psychopathology in children of parents with recurrent depression. J Abnorm Child Psychol 16:17–28, 1988

Pine DS, Cohen P, Gurley D, et al: The risk for early adulthood anxiety and depressive disorders in adolescents with anxiety and depressive disorders. Arch Gen Psychiatry 55:56–64, 1998

Pine DS, Cohen P, Gurley D, et al: Adolescent fear as predictors of depression. Biol Psychiatry 50:721–724, 2001a

Pine DS, Fyer A, Grun J, et al: Methods for developmental studies of fear conditioning circuitry. Biol Psychiatry 50:225–228, 2001b

Puig-Antich J, Goetz D, Davies M, et al: A controlled family history study of prepubertal major depressive disorder. Arch Gen Psychiatry 46:406–418, 1989

Reid SA, Duke LM, Allen JJ: Resting frontal electroencephalographic asymmetry in depression: inconsistencies suggest the need to identify mediating factors. Psychophysiology 35:389–404, 1998

Reinherz HZ, Giaconia RM, Pakiz B, et al: Psychosocial risks for major depression in late adolescence: a longitudinal community study. J Am Acad Child Adolesc Psychiatry 32:1155–1163, 1993

Rende R, Weissman MM: Sibling aggregation for psychopathology in offspring of opiate addicts: effects of parental comorbidity. J Clin Child Psychol 3:342–348, 1999

Rende R, Warner V, Wickramaratne P, et al: Sibling aggregation for psychiatric disorders in offspring at high and low risk for depression: 10-year follow-up. Psychol Med 6:1291–1298, 1999

Rohde P, Lewinsohn PM, Seeley JR. Comorbidity of unipolar depression, II: comorbidity with other mental disorders in adolescents and adults. J Abnorm Psychol 100:214–222, 1991

Silberg J, Pickles A, Rutter M, et. al: The influence of genetic factors and life stress on depression among adolescent girls. Arch Gen Psychiatry 56:225–232, 1999

Silberg JL, Rutter M, Eaves L: Genetic and environmental influences on the temporal association between earlier anxiety and later depression in girls. Biol Psychiatry 49:1040–1049, 2001

Sullivan PF, Neale MC, Kendler KS: Genetic epidemiology of major depression: review and meta-analysis. Am J Psychiatry 157:1552–1562, 2000

Taylor MA, Abrams R, Hayman MA: The classification of affective disorders: a reassessment of the bipolar-unipolar dichotomy. J Affect Disord 2:95–109, 1980

Thapar A, McGuffin P: Anxiety and depressive symptoms in childhood: a genetic study of comorbidity. J Child Psychol Psychiatry 38:651–656, 1997

Walker DL, Davis M: Double dissociation between the involvement of the bed nucleus of the stria terminalis and the central nucleus of the amygdala in startle increases produced by conditioned versus unconditioned fear. J Neurosci 17:9375–9383, 1997a

Walker DL, Davis M: Anxiogenic effects of high illumination levels assessed with the acoustic startle response in rats. Biol Psychiatry 42:461–471, 1997b

Warner V, Weissman MM, Mufson L, et al: Grandparents, parents, and grandchildren at high risk for depression: a three-generation study. J Am Acad Child Adolesc Psychiatry 38:289–296, 1999

Weissman MM: Juvenile-onset major depression includes childhood- and adolescent-onset depression and may be heterogeneous. Arch Gen Psychiatry 59:223–224, 2002

Weissman MM, Kidd KK, Prusoff BA: Variability in the rates of affective disorders in the relatives of depressed and normal probands. Arch Gen Psychiatry 39:1397–1403, 1982

Weissman MM, Wickramaratne P, Merikangas KR, et al: Onset of major depression in early adulthood: increased familial loading and specificity. Arch Gen Psychiatry 41:1136–1143, 1984

Weissman MM, Gammon GD, John K, et al: Children of depressed parents: increased psychopathology and early onset of major depression. Arch Gen Psychiatry 44:847–853, 1987

Weissman MM, Fendrich M, Warner V, et al: Incidence of psychiatric disorder in offspring at high and low risk for depression. J Am Acad Child Adolesc Psychiatry 31:640–648, 1992

Weissman MM, Warner V, Wickramaratne P, et al: Offspring of depressed parents. 10 years later. Arch Gen Psychiatry 54:932–940, 1997

Weissman MM, Wolk S, Wickramaratne PJ, et al: Children with prepubertal-onset major depressive disorder and anxiety grown up. Arch Gen Psychiatry 56:794–801, 1999

Wickramaratne PJ, Warner V, Weissman MM: Selecting early onset probands for genetic studies: results from a longitudinal high risk study. Am J Med Genet (Neuropsych Genet) 96:93–101, 2000

Williamson DE, Ryan ND, Birmaher B, et al: A case control family history study of depression in adolescents. J Am Acad Child Adolesc Psychiatry 34:1596–1607, 1995

Winokur G: The development and validity of familial subtypes in primary unipolar depression. Pharmacopsychiatria 15:142–146, 1982

5

Pathophysiology of Anxiety

A Developmental Psychobiological Perspective

Daniel S. Pine, M.D.

Recent studies in both clinical and basic science domains generate considerable enthusiasm for developmental approaches to the pathophysiology of anxiety disorders. From the clinical perspective, considerable research suggests that early signs of many chronic mental disorders manifest during childhood or adolescence. These include the anxiety disorders, the focus of the current review. From the basic science perspective, other research documents the impact of environmental factors during development on the long-term functioning of brain systems and behaviors related to threat perception and response. Because anxiety disorders can be viewed as disorders of aberrant threat perception (Ehlers and Clark 2000), such basic research appears relevant to the pathophysiology of clinical anxiety states. Advances in molecular genetics, cognitive neuroscience, and neuroimaging set the stage for research designed to integrate these insights from the clinical and basic domains. In support of this conclusion, this chapter summarizes a series of studies pertinent to the pathophysiology of anxiety.

The opinions and assertions contained in this chapter are the private views of the authors and are not to be construed as official or as reflecting the views of the National Institute of Mental Health or the U.S. Department of Health and Human Services.

In summarizing such research, the chapter focuses on four specific anxiety disorders: specific phobia, social anxiety disorder, separation anxiety disorder, and generalized anxiety disorder. However, current nosological categories of childhood anxiety disorders are based on descriptive phenomenology, as opposed to underlying pathophysiology. Consequently, current categories may change as understandings of pathophysiology advances (Costello et al. 2002). Accordingly, the chapter also focuses on the broader issue of anxiety symptoms among children, independent of any particular diagnosis.

This review proceeds in three stages, addressing a set of related phenomena that are hypothesized to bear increasingly specific relationships with functional aspects of brain circuits thought to engender anxiety disorders. Figure 5–1 illustrates the multiple levels of phenomena to be considered, referencing examples of the phenomena described throughout the chapter. At the most superficial layer, the first section of the chapter reviews data in developmental psychopathology, focusing on results from longitudinal and family-based studies of anxiety symptoms and disorders in children and their parents. The second section reviews data on physiological, neuroendocrine, and cognitive correlates of anxiety disorders, again referencing examples described later in the chapter. This section focuses on correlates that extend basic science research on brain systems engaged by threat perception and response. This section also focuses on correlates that can be measured in the laboratory and used to inform studies that more directly examine neural functions, through imaging approaches. The final section reviews data concerning the neural circuitry of anxiety based on neuroimaging studies. Data among adults are reviewed, along with the few available studies in children, with the goal of informing potential future studies in childhood anxiety disorders.

DEVELOPMENTAL PSYCHOPATHOLOGY

Three main observations support the conceptualization of anxiety disorders as developmental conditions. These include the observation that anxiety symptoms exhibit characteristic fluctuations across development, the observation that early signs emerge during childhood of chronic anxiety as well as affective disorders among adults followed prospectively over time, and the observation that children of parents with anxiety as well as affective disorders exhibit high rates of anxiety symptoms and disorders themselves.

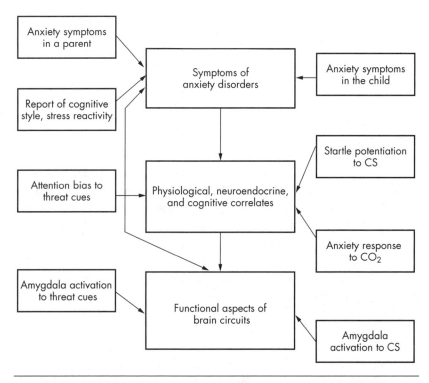

FIGURE 5–1 Multiple levels of phenomena examined in developmental psychopathology.

Cross-Sectional Associations With Developmental Stage

In terms of associations between anxiety and developmental stage, anxiety symptoms consistently exhibit characteristic fluctuations as children pass from toddlerhood into elementary school and then adolescence. Fluctuations in levels of anxiety are observed among most normally developing children and adolescents. These fluctuations exhibit relationships with clinically significant levels of anxiety. For example, separation anxiety typically emerges during toddlerhood as a normal aspect of early development. This type of anxiety typically is followed by fears of bodily harm or of dangerous objects during elementary school, which in turn are followed by fears or concerns about embarrassment or social competence (Klein and Pine 2002). Normal changes in levels of anxiety at adolescence are paralleled by changes in aspects of mood regulation, in which more profound, pervasive periods of unhappiness emerge during adolescence relative to preadolescence. This pattern of developmental fluctuations in anxiety and mood symptoms among typically developing children is accompanied by similar developmental fluctuations in rates of pathological anxiety disorders. Specifically, rates of separation anxiety disorder peak during the elementary school years, shortly after normal separation anxiety diminishes. This has led some to suggest that separation anxiety disorder represents a variant of normal anxiety that becomes pathological by persisting into developmental periods in which separation anxiety typically diminishes (Klein and Pine 2002). Other conditions, including major depression and social anxiety disorder, show marked increases in prevalence after puberty (Angold et al. 1998; Hayward et al. 1992; Pine et al. 1998). These changes show parallels with the previously noted changes in moodiness and social anxiety among typically developing adolescents, again suggesting that anxiety disorders might be conceptualized as aberrancies in normal developmental processes.

Given the relationship between developmental fluctuations in both normal and pathological fears, major questions emerge concerning factors that distinguish normal from pathological anxiety states. Such states can be distinguished clinically, in that only anxiety disorders are characterized by impairment and clinically significant distress. On the other hand, some forms of "normal" childhood fears exhibit stronger associations with later-life psychopathology than forms of "abnormal" childhood fears. For example, fear of the dark during childhood, even in the absence of clinically significant distress or impairment, exhibits a stronger association with later-life major depression than clinically significant phobias during childhood (Pine et al. 2001a). This suggests that some aspects of fear irrespective of clinical significance may indicate underlying long-term risk, possibly by indexing underlying dysfunction in fear-related brain systems. This finding emphasizes the need for studies of pathophysiology to develop measures that go beyond indices of clinical significance, distress, or impairment. Using modern neuroscience methods, it may be possible to identify underlying signs of brain dysfunction that predict risk for specific conditions, independent of their effect on impairment or distress.

Prospective Associations

In terms of prospective longitudinal research, various types of behaviors in children have been linked to risk for later anxiety disorders. Perhaps the earliest manifestation of risk for anxiety emerges in the form of specific temperament types. For example, the term *behavioral inhibition* refers to children who exhibit signs of wariness, caution, or minimal spontaneous communication and movement in response to novelty, particularly social novelty. This temperament type is hypothesized to reflect functional aspects of brain circuitry, reviewed later, that is engaged when humans process threats (Kagan and Snidman 1999; Kagan et al. 2001). Longitudinal studies find that children with behavioral inhibition face an elevated risk for a range of anxiety disorders during the elementary school years, as well as a particularly elevated risk for social anxiety disorder during adolescence (Schwartz et al. 1999).

Beyond temperamental constructs, longitudinal studies also establish associations between specific anxiety disorders present during childhood, adolescence, and adulthood. An expanding series of epidemiological studies examine longitudinal associations among anxiety disorders present during various stages of childhood and adolescence (Achenbach et al. 1995; Last et al. 1996; McGee et al. 1992; Pine et al. 1998; Stein et al. 2001). In general, these studies find that anxiety disorders during one stage of development predict an elevated risk for various anxiety as well as affective syndromes at other stages of development. The most recent studies in this area establish associations extending into the early adult years, such that childhood anxiety disorders represent a potent risk factor for adult anxiety disorders.

Two main questions emerge from the available prospective studies, both of which pertain to heterogeneity in clinical outcomes. First, more research is needed on specificity in outcomes, because many studies consider associations among a broad array of anxiety disorders and symptom categories. Some evidence does emerge for specificity in the outcome of phobias, with childhood specific phobia showing a strong association with adult specific phobia and childhood social phobia showing a strong association with adult social phobia (Pine et al. 1998; Stein et al. 2001). Similarly, childhood separation anxiety disorder shows some evidence of a specific association with panic disorder (Klein and Pine 2002), whereas childhood generalized anxiety disorder shows ties with a range of adult conditions, including major depression, generalized anxiety disorder, and social phobia. More research is needed to clarify the underlying causes of such heterogeneity in outcome. For example, nonspecificity in outcome of conditions such as generalized anxiety disorder may suggest the need for refinements in nosology. Alternatively, generalized anxiety disorder, as currently conceived, may represent a general risk factor for a range of other conditions. Answers to such questions require increasing understanding of the underlying causes of generalized anxiety disorder, as well as other anxiety disorders, so that nosology can be informed by knowledge of pathophysiology.

Second, although the presence of a childhood anxiety disorder does indicate an increased risk for a range of conditions, most children with an anxiety disorder will exhibit few if any signs of psychiatric impairment as adults (Klein and Pine 2002; Last et al. 1996). Hence, another major question concerns factors that distinguish those children with an anxiety disorder who will go on to develop chronic mood or anxiety symptoms from those who will exhibit relatively few such symptoms. Current data provide limited insights on this issue (Achenbach et al. 1995; Pine 1999). For example, there is some evidence that cognitive factors predict onset or persistence of mood and anxiety disorders (Hankin and Abramson 2001). However, most studies documenting such associations rely on self-reports of cognitive style or stress reactivity that appear conceptually similar to self-reports of psychiatric symptoms. Again, knowledge of the underlying causes of anxiety disorders in children and adolescents might address questions in this area. For example, if underlying abnormalities in brain function associated with persistent anxiety disorders could be identified, children with anxiety disorders might be classified with respect to such abnormalities, in the hopes of identifying children who face a high risk for chronic symptoms. Available cognitive neuroscience studies examining aspects of threat perception may provide an avenue for examining such abnormalities, possibly through ties with self-reports of cognitive styles or stress reactivity.

Familial Associations

Much like research on age-related fluctuations in prevalence and longitudinal outcome, family studies also suggest the utility of a developmental perspective on anxiety disorders. Perhaps the most consistent findings in this area document associations among diagnoses in parents and their children. Many studies find strong associations between childhood anxiety disorders and a range of adult mood and anxiety disorders, including major depression and panic disorder (Merikangas et al. 1999; Rosenbaum et al. 2000; Weissman et al. 1984, 1997; Wickramaratne and Weissman 1998). These studies also extend such associations to the preschool years, in which parental panic or depression exhibits an association with childhood behavioral inhibition (Rosenbaum et al. 2000).

Behavioral genetic studies have begun to examine the possible role of genetic and environmental factors in such familial associations, relying on studies in twins. Among adults, the available data implicate both environmental and genetic factors in anxiety disorders, with genetic factors typically accounting for less of the variance in risk than environmental factors (Kendler 2001). Fewer studies examine these issues among children, and complications arise in such studies. For example, divergent degrees of genetic contribution have been found for anxiety symptoms assessed by parent report as opposed to child report. This again illustrates limitations in current nosology and emphasizes the need to develop measures of anxiety firmly grounded in indices of brain function. Nevertheless, the available data do suggest that genetic factors make a significant contribution to childhood anxiety, as they do to adult anxiety. Moreover, environmental factors in children, as in adults, typically account for a greater proportion of the variance in risk than genetic factors (Klein and Pine 2002).

As in the area of longitudinal studies, major questions concerning specificity arise from research in familial aggregation. For example, major depression in parents appears to confer a strong risk for both anxiety and depression in children, with some evidence that early childhood anxiety in children of depressed parents may indicate particularly high risk for later-life major depression (Weissman et al. 1997). Consistent with these findings, available twin data suggest that common genetic factors may predispose to childhood anxiety and adolescent depression (Silberg et al. 2001). It remains unclear in light of such data if childhood anxiety should be considered an entirely distinct entity from major depression or if it should be considered a nosologically related disorder.

In summary, cross-sectional, prospective, and family-based studies document strong associations between anxiety during childhood and both anxiety and depression in adulthood. Considerable questions arise in this area, many related to aspects of heterogeneity. Research on developmental psychopathology suggests that anxiety disorders, like many mental illnesses, represent disorders whose initial signs manifest during childhood and persist to varying degrees into adulthood. Anxiety disorders are hypothesized to represent conditions that result from perturbations in underlying brain function. The key to answering questions pertaining to heterogeneity in outcome and familial aggregation may depend on refining our ability to examine brain function as it relates to symptoms of anxiety disorders. The remainder of the chapter provides an outline for methods that might lead to such refinements.

BEHAVIORAL AND PHYSIOLOGICAL CORRELATES

Efforts to study the pathophysiology of anxiety disorders benefit from research in basic science. Ample basic science research delineates brain systems that are engaged by various forms of threat. In these studies, the term *threat* refers to a stimulus that predicts a high likelihood of experiencing a punishment, whereas the term *punishment* refers to a stimulus that an animal will expend effort to avoid. Research examining aspects of threat response demonstrates considerable similarity in behavior, physiology, and underlying brain circuitry across various mammalian species, from rodents to humans. Such parallels presumably reflect the evolutionary advantages afforded by brain systems that facilitate adaptive responses to threats. Such parallels also provide an important opportunity on which to capitalize in an effort to refine understandings of pathophysiology. Given strong cross-species parallels in physiological, cognitive, and behavioral responses to threat presentation, knowledge concerning functional aspects of threat-responsive brain systems in animals might be used to inform understanding of human anxiety disorders. This section of the chapter provides a brief review of current basic science research on fear systems and integrates this review with a summary of parallel studies in humans.

Basic Science

Research on fear conditioning provides a basis for much of the ongoing research on fear states in rodents and nonhuman primates. In the fear conditioning experiment, a neutral conditioned stimulus (CS), such as a tone or a light, is repeatedly paired with a punishing unconditioned stimulus (US), such as a shock or a sudden air puff. Following such pairings, the CS comes to represent a threat or predictor of the aversive, punishing US. As a result, the CS comes to elicit behaviors formerly associated with the US. The significance of the fear conditioning paradigm derives from the precise delineation of neural structures engaged by distinct components of the paradigm and associated psychological processes. These include perceptual processing of threats, learning about the salience of threats, and organizing behavioral responses to threats. The amygdala, a collection of nuclei in the medial temporal lobe, makes a central contribution to each of these processes. Specifically, the amygdala is thought to be centrally involved in processes that allow an organism to associate mental representations of a punishment and a neutral stimulus. Moreover, aspects of threats are processed in two parallel pathways that converge on the amygdala. In one subcortical pathway, coarse sensory details pertaining to threat are rapidly channeled to the amygdala from the thalamus, facilitating rapid response to a broad range of stimuli that may indicate threat. In the second, cortically based pathway, more sensory details are processed, allowing a more precise evaluation of threat level. The availability of rapid and slow pathways allows an organism to rapidly avoid possible threats but also to counteract any tendencies to treat an overly abundant array of stimuli as threatening. As described in more detail later, research on attention bias among humans suggests that anxiety disorders may result from specific deficits in these two pathways.

Particularly among primates, some controversy remains on the precise role played by the amygdala in response to various forms of threat, beyond formerly neutral conditioned stimuli. For example, amygdala lesions appear to produce relatively subtle changes in fear-related behaviors among humans and monkeys (Amaral 2002). More substantial effects on threat response may emerge as a result of lesions in other brain regions, such as the ventral prefrontal cortex. Such regions may regulate activity in a distributed neural circuit encompassing the amygdala (Baxter et al. 2000; Bechara et al. 2001). Similarly, debate continues on the degree to which the amygdala plays a specific and selective role in the threat response, given ample evidence implicating the amygdala in perception and response to rewards.

Basic research delineating functional aspects of circuits engaged by threats may provide particularly relevant insights for developmental studies. Research suggests that environmental manipulations early in development can exert long-term organizational effects on a rodent's response to threat (Meaney 2001). For example, following brief handling manipulations, rat pups receive extensive maternal care. This maternal care in turn produces long-term reductions in anxiety-related behaviors in response to threat presentation. These behavioral changes are accompanied by parallel changes in functioning of the hypothalamic-pituitary-adrenal (HPA) axis and amygdala. Most of this research examines rodents, but studies in primates are beginning to note parallel findings. For example, a variable foraging demand manipulation in bonnet macaques produced long-term alterations in the HPA axis and increases in anxiety behaviors (Coplan et al. 2001).

Experimental Paradigms in Humans

Clinically oriented researchers face a major hurdle in trying to capitalize on insights from basic science research on threat response in an effort to enhance understandings on the pathophysiology of human anxiety. One of the keys to advancing research in this area may lie in the successful implementation of paradigms that generate comparable data across rodents, primates, and humans. The current section reviews two families of experimental paradigms designed to generate such data. Both sets of paradigms track changes in indirect measures of brain function during exposure to various forms of threat. These measures can be used to test the hypothesis that anxiety disorders in both children and adults are characterized by abnormal behavioral, physiological, and cognitive responses to threatening stimuli.

Psychophysiology and Neuroendocrinology

One set of paradigms attempts to assess functional aspects of underlying fear circuitry by examining changes in psychophysiological or endocrinological measures during exposure to threats. These data can be referenced against data documenting changes on such measures in rodents and non-human primates. Given the wealth of information on neural circuits underlying fear conditioning and associated physiological changes, considerable work is occurring in this area using variants of fear conditioning procedures employed among rodents (Gorman et al. 2000). The startle reflex can be modulated by changes in affective state, showing increases and decreases in magnitude under states of increasing or decreasing threat (Lang et al. 1998). Many studies in humans measure changes in startle levels to index levels of fear during exposure to threats, such as conditioned stimuli. This convention is based on strong cross-species parallels in mechanisms of startle modulation (Davis and Whalen 2001). In general, the weight of the evidence documents small or inconsistent relationships between clinical measures of anxiety and startle-based measures of fear acquisition during fear conditioning paradigms (Grillon 2002; Grillon and Morgan 1999). Many factors may contribute to such inconsistencies in subjective and physiological measures of threat response. For example, abnormalities in startle potentiation may relate more closely to underlying risk for anxiety disorders, as opposed to the presence of symptoms or disorders (Merikangas et al. 1999). Alternatively, other aspects of threat perception or response, beyond simple measures of fear acquisition, may show more consistent associations with clinical measures of anxiety. For example, humans and other mammals develop fear responses to the general context in which a conditioning experiment has been conducted. Some evidence suggests that high levels of subjective anxiety, as experienced by anxiety disorder patients, interferes with cognitive processing in stressful contexts (Grillon 2002). Patients with anxiety disorders also show signs of abnormal contextual conditioning (Grillon and Morgan 1999). Finally, much of the literature on fear conditioning in animals focuses on learning, whereby a neutral stimulus comes to acquire threat value through experience. Clinical levels of anxiety may show stronger relationships with innately threatening stimuli (Davis 1998). Consistent with this possibility, adult patients with snake or spider phobias do show enhanced startle while viewing pictures of such feared objects (Lang et al. 1998). Similarly, patients with posttraumatic stress disorder exhibit enhanced startle potentiation to darkness, which may relate to abnormalities in rodent brain systems that facilitate responses to threatening scenarios (Davis 1998). Given that corticotropin-releasing factor (CRF) influences such psychophysiological measures, these findings may also be relevant to research on childhood fear of the dark and its association with adult major depression (Pine et al. 2001a).

Research using other psychophysiological paradigms provides additional evidence of abnormal response to innate threats in clinical anxiety states. Probably the most extensive evidence of abnormalities in this area relies on respiratory stimulation paradigms to study panic disorder. Adult patients with panic disorder exhibit enhanced anxiety and enhanced respiratory physiology responses when exposed to various respiratory stimulants, such as carbon dioxide (CO_2), that signal potential respiratory compromise (Klein 1996). Moreover, these abnormalities appear independent of state-anxiety levels, in that non-ill first-degree relatives of panic patients also exhibit such abnormalities (Coryell 1997). These abnormalities have been conceptualized as reflecting a hypersensitivity to the threat of suffocation. Finally, children with various anxiety disorders, particularly separation anxiety disorder, exhibit many of the same subjective and physiological abnormalities when exposed to respiratory stimulants (Pine et al. 2000). Hence, some subset of childhood anxiety disorders, much like adult panic disorder, may result from a pathological perturbation in brain systems designed to assess and respond to a subset of innately threatening stimuli or scenarios.

Other forms of innately threatening stimuli also have been used to document parallel abnormalities among children and adults with panic disorder. For example, both adults with panic disorder and children with separation anxiety disorder exhibit abnormal responses to pharmacological challenges with yohimbine, a noradrenergic α_2-receptor antagonist that increases activity of the locus ceruleus (Sallee et al. 2000). Such findings, noting consistent abnormalities in response to innate threats, raise hopes of generating acceptable laboratory-based paradigms for research in pediatric anxiety disorders. Precise understanding of cross-species parallels in startle regulation provide one opportunity to generate such paradigms. However, studies relying on other psychophysiological or neuroendocrinological measures may be more difficult to integrate with research in the basic sciences. Cognitive paradigms may provide clearer avenues for such extensions.

Cognitive Paradigms

The second set of paradigms relies on behavioral measures to assess the degree to which select cognitive processes are engaged by threats. The most consistent findings in this area derive from studies employing attention paradigms. Mammals possess elaborate neural systems that allocate cognitive resources to prioritize perceptual stimuli in the environment for enhanced levels of processing. The need to prioritize stimuli derives from the fact that cognitive resources are limited, preventing full processing of all stimuli. The term *attention* has been applied to neural processes devoted to prioritizing one set of stimuli for further analysis, at the expense of other stimuli. As in the area of fear conditioning, considerable work in the basic sciences delineates basic brain systems involved in attention modulation (Miller and Cohen 2001). Threats represent one class of stimuli that receive enhanced attention. An enhanced tendency to direct attention toward threats is hypothesized to represent a key vulnerability factor in individuals with anxiety disorders (MacLeod et al. 2002; Williams et al. 1996).

Two main paradigms have been used to quantify levels of attention bias toward threats. In one paradigm, the emotional Stroop task, words printed in letters of various colors are presented to research participants, and participants are asked to name the colors of the letters as quickly as possible. The words vary systematically in the level of threat conveyed. For example, a patient with panic disorder might see the word *kill* printed in blue letters or the word *ball* printed in yellow letters. Attention bias for threat in this paradigm is manifest as a slowing of the reaction time when naming a threat word, such as a longer latency to identify "blue" as opposed to "yellow" in the previous example. In this paradigm, both children and adults with anxiety disorders exhibit evidence of enhanced attention bias to threat words, particularly words that appear highly relevant to their anxiety disorder (Williams et al. 1996). Despite the consistency of these findings, complications arise in the interpretation of the findings due to the complexity of the task, in which attention bias is indexed based on interference with color naming.

The second main cognitive paradigm attempts to provide a more direct measure of attention bias, using a dot-probe task. In this task, subjects must identify the location of a probe that appears in one of two locations on a computer screen. Cues appear in these locations immediately prior to probe presentation, and measures of attention bias are provided based on the effect of differential cue types on reaction times (see Figure 5–2). In general, a subject will exhibit a faster response to a probe that appears in an attended location, relative to a probe that appears in an unattended location. For example, a threat word (*kill*) may appear on the right location, and a neutral word (*ball*) may appear on the left. Here, attention bias for threat would manifest as a faster reaction time to the probe when it appears on the right or a slower reaction time when it appears on the left. As with the emotional Stroop task, patients with anxiety disorders consistently exhibit such signs of attention bias on the dot-probe task (Bradley et al. 1999; MacLeod et al. 2002). Moreover, these abnormalities emerge both among children and adults (Daleiden and Vasey 1997).

Two variations of the dot-probe task may facilitate research on developmental psychopathology. First, as with the emotional Stroop task, many of the early dot-probe tasks relied on verbal stimuli as threats. These methods may be problematic in children and adolescents, where some degree of verbal elaboration may be required as part of the threat assessment. That is, because verbal skills continue to mature through adolescence, studies relying on verbally based stimuli may confound the effects of linguistic and emotionally based processes. More recent studies elicit attention bias through ecologically valid stimuli less closely linked to verbal processes, such as evocative pictures or angry faces (Bradley et al. 1999; Mogg and Bradley 1998; Mogg et al. 2000). For example, adults with anxiety disorders have been shown to exhibit an enhanced attention bias for angry faces (see Figure 5–2). Such measures may be well suited for research in pediatric anxiety disorders. Second, as noted in reviewing circuitry underlying fear conditioning, threat stimuli are processed through two parallel streams: a rapid, coarse subcortical stream and a slow, detailed cortical stream. Through "masking" procedures, the dot-probe task has been adapted to separately engage each of these streams. For example, an "emotion threat" face, such as an angry face, can be briefly presented on one side of the display and then masked with a neutral face. Subjects will fail to notice such briefly presented angry faces, though they may exhibit an attention bias for such faces. These methods enable selective engagement of the rapid subcortical path. Patients with anxiety disorders may exhibit a specific abnormality in this path, manifested as an abnormal attention bias during masked-face presentations (Mogg and Bradley 1998).

The main advantage of the emotional Stroop and dot-probe tasks derives from the ease with which these tasks can be used in neuroimaging paradigms. Particularly for studies among children, functional magnetic resonance imaging (fMRI) provides a safe, tolerable means for acquiring data relating behavior to brain function with adequate temporal and spatial resolution. One of the keys to implementing fMRI research with patients involves developing a thorough knowledge concerning relationships between a diagnosis and a specific behavior, such as dot-probe performance. In the final section of this chapter, data from fMRI studies are reviewed.

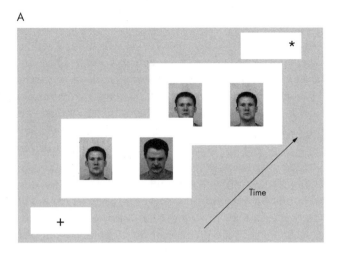

FIGURE 5–2   Example of dot-probe paradigm used to evaluate attention bias to rapidly presented threat cues.

A: Sequence of events in a dot-probe trial. Subject is told to monitor visual display for a dot-probe (*) and indicate the side of the display (right/left) on which it appears with a button press. Fixation is presented (500 ms), followed by brief "emotion-threat" photographs of neutral and angry faces (14–33 ms). The emotion-threat photographs are then masked with a photograph of neutral faces (486–467 ms). Finally, the subject indicates with a button- press the side of the probe when it appears subsequently (250 ms).

B: Measure of attention bias for threat. Attention bias toward or away from the "emotion-threat" photograph is indicated by the reaction time advantage when the dot-probe appears congruent with the "emotion-threat" face, minus when it appears incongruent with the "emotion-threat" face.

NEURAL CIRCUITRY

As of this writing, only one fMRI study has examined children with any mood or anxiety disorder (Thomas et al. 2001). This study found an enhanced amygdala response in patients with anxiety disorders during passive viewing of fear faces, one potential form of threatening stimulus. This chapter provides a more general review of fMRI paradigms relevant to future studies in this area. Two specific sets of paradigms will be reviewed.

Fear Conditioning Paradigms

One set of imaging studies, largely among adults, has used fear conditioning procedures to extend the considerable literature examining neural circuits involved in fear conditioning among rodents and primates. As reviewed elsewhere (Buchel and Dolan 2000), a series of fMRI studies consistently documents engagement of the amygdala during presentation of conditioned stimuli. Interestingly, amygdala engagement selectively occurs early in conditioning, consistent with a role in initial appraisals of stimuli showing changes in salience. Moreover, some evidence emerges for a stronger response to conditioned stimuli in adults with social phobia compared with healthy adults (Birbaumer et al. 1998).

A few questions do arise from the available studies in this area. First, fear conditioning clearly involves a distributed circuit. Whereas the initial studies focused most extensively on the amygdala, future studies might consider the role of prefrontal regions in moderating amygdala response. This interest might follow based on evidence of prefrontal involvement in human anxiety (Davidson 2002), coupled with evidence of strong prefrontal-amygdala interaction in nonhuman primates (Baxter et al. 2000). Second, as noted earlier, psychophysiological studies document inconsistent associations between clinical measures of anxiety and fear conditioning indices. Given preliminary evidence of abnormal amygdala response to conditioning paradigms in patients, the degree to which patients with anxiety disorders might exhibit underlying neural abnormalities in the absence of psychophysiological abnormalities remains unclear. Finally, because developmental data suggest that abnormalities in fear conditioning may represent premorbid risk factors for later anxiety disorders (Grillon et al. 1998), it is important to extend fMRI conditioning studies to child and adolescent populations. Following methods developed in the psychophysiology laboratory (Grillon et al. 1999), unconditioned stimuli more appropriate for use with children may be employed in such paradigms. For example, a mildly aversive air-puff US has been shown in psychophysiological studies to consistently potentiate the startle reflex and produce conditioning. This same US was recently shown to engage the amygdala in a conditioning paradigm (Pine et al. 2001b).

Face Processing Tasks

Probably more than for any other paradigm, imaging studies using face emotion-processing paradigms generate key insights on neural structures engaged during various emotion states. As noted previously, the only fMRI study in pediatric anxiety disorders documented increased amygdala activation to fear faces, conceived as threat cues (Thomas et al. 2001). Psychological processes engaged during face processing have been differentiated based on the degree to which a given process relates to evaluating features of faces in general, as opposed to evaluating features of one particular class of faces (Haxby et al. 2002). For example, processes related to threat evaluation ascertain differences among a collection of possible faces and facial expressions encountered in social relationships. Such faces convey different degrees of threat, depending on variation in emotional expressions or other relevant features, such as eye gaze. In patients with clinical disorders, abnormalities are thought to emerge in the latter set of processes, related to evaluating differences among faces. Prior imaging paradigms have manipulated two main parameters in an effort to map brain regions relevant to anxiety: the nature of emotions in face stimuli and the nature of attention sets during face viewing.

In terms of variations in the nature of face emotions, studies conducted over the past decade consistently document meaningful differences in the degree to which select brain regions are engaged by different types of emotional facial expressions. Hence, a wealth of studies document amygdala engagement during fear face viewing, consistent with lesion studies demonstrating impairment in appraisal of fear following amygdala damage (Haxby et al. 2002). Similarly, other studies document ventral prefrontal engagement during angry face viewing, consistent with another set of lesion studies. Thus, levels of various emotions in facial photographs reliably engage relevant brain structures.

The degree to which conscious processing of face emotion relates to engagement in these brain structures remains unclear. Some evidence documents amygdala engagement even to subliminally presented fear faces, as well as enhanced engagement to such faces in patients with major depression or posttraumatic stress disorder (Rauch et al. 2000; Sheline et al. 2001). This suggests that differential amygdala engagement in patients relates to measures that are independent of verbal reports pertaining to current anxiety state. One set of theories suggests that amygdala engagement relates to attention, in that the amygdala is involved in determining stimulus evaluation priorities, particularly in the face of changing or ambiguous stimuli (Davis and Whalen 2001). Increased engagement of the amygdala in patients to subliminally presented faces is consistent with evidence of attention bias to threats presented subliminally (Williams et al. 1996). These findings suggest directions for future imaging studies. Given that clinical anxiety is associated with enhanced amygdala response and enhanced attention bias to threat faces, abnormalities in attention bias are hypothesized to result from amygdala dysfunction.

In terms of variations in attention set, recent fMRI studies document relationships between attention set and specific activations. For example, attending to emotional aspects of stimuli tends to engage components of the prefrontal cortex, including the medial or ventral portions (Drevets 2000; Lane et al. 1997), whereas attending to other features, such as the identity of the individual, tends to engage association cortex of the temporal region (Haxby et al. 2002). As noted earlier, anxiety disorders are hypothesized to result from abnormal attention regulation in response to threat stimuli, as manifest in reaction time data. Thus, behavioral abnormalities in this area are hypothesized to relate to abnormalities detected with brain imaging paradigms. For example, anxiety disorders are hypothesized to be associated with abnormal activation of prefrontal regions during tasks that require attention to be directed toward or away from emotional aspects of stimuli.

CONCLUSIONS

Research with rodents, nonhuman primates, and humans suggests that developmental factors have an impact on lifetime anxiety-related behaviors. This finding provides potential major insights for pathophysiological models of clinical anxiety disorders. Clinical research among patients with anxiety disorders also has found evidence of abnormal attention regulation during presentation of threat stimuli, a process that is understood relatively well among rodents and nonhuman primates. In particular, studies have found enhanced threat-related bias using both the emotional Stroop and dot-probe paradigms, among both adults and children. Similarly, some abnormalities in fear conditioning have been noted among patients with anxiety disorders, though with less consistency. Given advances in fMRI research on mechanisms of fear conditioning and attention, these data may provide an avenue for future studies in children and adults with anxiety disorders.

REFERENCES

Achenbach TM, Howell CT, McConaughy SH, et al: Six-year predictors of problems in a national sample of children and youth, I: cross-informant syndromes. J Am Acad Child Adolesc Psychiatry 34:336–347, 1995

Amaral DG: The primate amygdala and the neurobiology of social behavior: implications for understanding social anxiety. Biol Psychiatry 51:11–17, 2002

Angold A, Costello EJ, Worthman CM: Puberty and depression: the roles of age, pubertal status and pubertal timing. Psychol Med 28:51–61, 1998

Baxter MG, Parker A, Lindner CC, et al: Control of response selection by reinforcer value requires interaction of amygdala and orbital prefrontal cortex. J Neurosci 20:4311–4319, 2000

Bechara A, Dolan S, Denburg N, et al: Decision-making deficits, linked to a dysfunctional ventromedial prefrontal cortex, revealed in alcohol and stimulant abusers. Neuropsychologia 39:376–389, 2001

Birbaumer N, Grodd W, Diedrich O, et al: fMRI reveals amygdala activation to human faces in social phobics. Neuroreport 9:1223–1226, 1998

Bradley BP, Mogg K, White J, et al: Attentional bias for emotional faces in generalized anxiety disorder. Br J Clin Psychol 38:267–278, 1999

Buchel C, Dolan RJ: Classical fear conditioning in functional neuroimaging. Curr Opin Neurobiol 10:219–223, 2000

Coplan JD, Smith EL, Altemus M, et al: Variable foraging demand rearing: sustained elevations in cisternal cerebrospinal fluid corticotropin-releasing factor concentrations in adult primates. Biol Psychiatry 50:200–204, 2001

Coryell W: Hypersensitivity to carbon dioxide as a disease-specific trait marker. Biol Psychiatry 41:259–263, 1997

Costello EJ, Pine DS, Hammen C, et al: Development and natural history of mood disorders. Biol Psychiatry 52:529–542, 2002

Daleiden EL, Vasey MW: An information-processing perspective on childhood anxiety. Clin Psychol Rev 17:407–429, 1997

Davidson RJ: Anxiety and affective style: role of prefrontal cortex and amygdala. Biol Psychiatry 51:68–80, 2002

Davis M: Are different parts of the extended amygdala involved in fear versus anxiety? Biol Psychiatry 44:1239–1247, 1998

Davis M, Whalen PJ: The amygdala: vigilance and emotion. Mol Psychiatry 6:13–34, 2001

Drevets WC: Neuroimaging studies of mood disorders. Biol Psychiatry 48:813–829, 2000

Ehlers A, Clark DM: A cognitive model of posttraumatic stress disorder. Behav Res Ther 38:319–345, 2000

Gorman JM, Kent JM, Sullivan GM, et al: Neuroanatomical hypothesis of panic disorder, revised. Am J Psychiatry 157:493–505, 2000

Grillon C: Associative learning deficits increase symptoms of anxiety in humans. Biol Psychiatry 51:851–858, 2002

Grillon C, Morgan CA III: Fear-potentiated startle conditioning to explicit and contextual cues in Gulf War veterans with posttraumatic stress disorder. J Abnorm Psychol 108:134–142, 1999

Grillon C, Dierker L, Merikangas KR: Fear-potentiated startle in adolescent offspring of parents with anxiety disorders. Biol Psychiatry 44:990–997, 1998

Grillon C, Merikangas KR, Dierker L, et al: Startle potentiation by threat of aversive stimuli and darkness in adolescents: a multi-site study. Int J Psychophysiol 32:63–73, 1999

Hankin BL, Abramson LY: Development of gender differences in depression: an elaborated cognitive vulnerability-transactional stress theory. Psychol Bull 127:773–796, 2001

Haxby JV, Hoffman EA, Gobbini MI: Human neural systems for face recognition and social communication. Biol Psychiatry 51:59–67, 2002

Hayward C, Killen JD, Hammer LD, et al: Pubertal stage and panic attack history in sixth- and seventh-grade girls. Am J Psychiatry 149:1239–1243, 1992

Kagan J, Snidman N: Early childhood predictors of adult anxiety disorders. Biol Psychiatry 46:1536–1541, 1999

Kagan J, Snidman N, McManis M, et al: Temperamental contributions to the affect family of anxiety. Psychiatr Clin North Am 24:677–688, 2001

Kendler KS: Twin studies of psychiatric illness: an update. Arch Gen Psychiatry 58:1005–1014, 2001

Klein DF: Panic disorder and agoraphobia: hypothesis hothouse. J Clin Psychiatry 57 (suppl)6:21–27, 1996

Klein RG, Pine DS: Anxiety disorders, in Child and Adolescent Psychiatry, 4th Edition. Edited by Rutter M, Taylor E, Hersov L. New York, Elsevier, 2002, pp 486–509

Lane RD, Fink GR, Chau PM, et al: Neural activation during selective attention to subjective emotional responses. Neuroreport 8:3969–3972, 1997

Lang PJ, Bradley MM, Cuthbert BN: Emotion, motivation, and anxiety: brain mechanisms and psychophysiology. Biol Psychiatry 44:1248–1263, 1998

Last CG, Perrin S, Hersen M, et al: A prospective study of childhood anxiety disorders. J Am Acad Child Adolesc Psychiatry 35:1502–1510, 1996

MacLeod C, Rutherford E, Campbell L, et al: Selective attention and emotional vulnerability: assessing the causal basis of their association through the experimental manipulation of attentional bias. J Abnorm Psychol 111:107–123, 2002

McGee R, Feehan M, Williams S, et al: DSM-III disorders from age 11 to age 15 years. J Am Acad Child Adolesc Psychiatry 31:50–59, 1992

Meaney MJ: Maternal care, gene expression, and the transmission of individual differences in stress reactivity across generations. Annu Rev Neurosci 24:1161–1192, 2001

Merikangas KR, Avenevoli S, Dierker L, et al: Vulnerability factors among children at risk for anxiety disorders. Biol Psychiatry 46:1523–1535, 1999

Miller EK, Cohen JD: An integrative theory of prefrontal cortex function. Annu Rev Neurosci 24:167–202, 2001

Mogg K, Bradley BP: A cognitive-motivational analysis of anxiety. Behav Res Ther 36:809–848, 1998

Mogg K, Millar N, Bradley BP: Biases in eye movements to threatening facial expressions in generalized anxiety disorder and depressive disorder. J Abnorm Psychol 109:695–704, 2000

Pine DS: Pathophysiology of childhood anxiety disorders. Biol Psychiatry 46:1555–1566, 1999

Pine DS, Cohen P, Gurley D, et al: The risk for early adulthood anxiety and depressive disorders in adolescents with anxiety and depressive disorders. Arch Gen Psychiatry 55:56–64, 1998

Pine DS, Klein RG, Coplan JD, et al: Differential carbon dioxide sensitivity in childhood anxiety disorders and nonill comparison group. Arch Gen Psychiatry 57:960–967, 2000

Pine DS, Cohen P, Brook J: Adolescent fears as predictors of depression. Biol Psychiatry 50:721–724, 2001a

Pine DS, Fyer A, Grun J, et al: Methods for developmental studies of fear conditioning circuitry. Biol Psychiatry 50:225–228, 2001b

Rauch SL, Whalen PJ, Shin LM, et al: Exaggerated amygdala response to masked facial stimuli in posttraumatic stress disorder: a functional MRI study. Biol Psychiatry 47:769–776, 2000

Rosenbaum JF, Biederman J, Hirshfeld-Becker DR, et al: A controlled study of behavioral inhibition in children of parents with panic disorder and depression. Am J Psychiatry 157:2002–2010, 2000

Sallee FR, Sethuraman G, Sine L, et al: Yohimbine challenge in children with anxiety disorders. Am J Psychiatry 157:1236–1242, 2000

Schwartz CE, Snidman N, Kagan J: Adolescent social anxiety as an outcome of inhibited temperament in childhood. J Am Acad Child Adolesc Psychiatry 38:1008–1015, 1999

Sheline YI, Barch DM, Donnelly JM, et al: Increased amygdala response to masked emotional faces in depressed subjects resolves with antidepressant treatment: an fMRI study. Biol Psychiatry 50:651–658, 2001

Silberg JL, Rutter M, Eaves L: Genetic and environmental influences on the temporal association between earlier anxiety and later depression in girls. Biol Psychiatry 49:1040–1049, 2001

Stein MB, Fuetsch M, Muller N, et al: Social anxiety disorder and the risk of depression: a prospective community study of adolescents and young adults. Arch Gen Psychiatry 58:251–256, 2001

Thomas KM, Drevets WC, Dahl RE, et al: Amygdala response to fearful faces in anxious and depressed children. Arch Gen Psychiatry 58:1057–1063, 2001

Weissman MM, Leckman JF, Merikangas KR, et al: Depression and anxiety disorders in parents and children: results from the Yale family study. Arch Gen Psychiatry 41:845–852, 1984

Weissman MM, Warner V, Wickramaratne P, et al: Offspring of depressed parents: 10 years later. Arch Gen Psychiatry 54:932–940, 1997

Wickramaratne PJ, Weissman MM: Onset of psychopathology in offspring by developmental phase and parental depression. J Am Acad Child Adolesc Psychiatry 37:933–942, 1998

Williams JM, Mathews A, MacLeod C: The emotional Stroop task and psychopathology. Psychol Bull 120:3–24, 1996

6

Psychiatric Effects of Disasters and Terrorism

Empirical Basis From Study of the Oklahoma City Bombing

Carol S. North, M.D., M.P.E.

Even though organized research has studied the mental health aftermath of disasters for decades, recent major terrorist incidents—especially the Oklahoma City bombing and the September 11 attacks—have greatly increased professional and public awareness of the need for more knowledge of the impact of such events on the affected population's mental health. To learn more about disasters and mental health, we start by examining the signature diagnosis of disasters, posttraumatic stress disorder (PTSD). First the diagnostic criteria for PTSD are reviewed with an overview of this disorder in the general population to provide a background for special consideration of PTSD following a disaster. Then findings from studies of the effect of the Oklahoma City bombing on the occurrence of PTSD and other disorders are presented to illustrate the value of empirical data in developing clinical directions for assisting populations affected by such events.

DIAGNOSIS OF PTSD

PTSD first appeared as a diagnosis under its current name in DSM-III (American Psychiatric Association 1980). The distinction of being listed in the established diagnostic nomenclature, however, does not ensure full diagnostic

This research was supported by National Institute of Mental Health grant MH40025.

validity by accepted criteria (Robins and Guze 1970)—which has not been achieved for PTSD. According to the current criteria (American Psychiatric Association 2000), diagnosis of PTSD first requires sufficient exposure to the right kind of traumatic event, called the "stressor A criterion" because it is listed under the letter *A* in the outline of criteria. The stressor event must be one that constitutes a threat to life or limb and elicits a response of fear, helplessness, or horror. The exposure can occur through direct involvement in such an event, by being an eyewitness to others experiencing such an event, or indirectly through the sudden and unexpected involvement of a loved one in such an event. This means that after the September 11 attacks, people in the World Trade Center towers who fled for their lives after the planes struck may be candidates for PTSD, those who watched from a safe distance and witnessed the horror unfolding firsthand may also be candidates, and those who lost loved ones in the attacks might also qualify for the diagnosis. The rest of us across the country who saw the event in the repeated images of the planes flying into the towers on TV cannot be candidates for PTSD. Exposure only through TV cannot result in PTSD by definition, although other remarkable forms of distress or disturbance may follow that experience.

Once exposure to a qualifying stressor has been determined, three groups of symptom criteria must also be met to justify the diagnosis of PTSD. These symptom groups are labeled B, C, and D because they follow the stressor A criterion sequentially. The diagnostic criteria require one, three, and two positive symptoms in groups B, C, and D, respectively. Group B symptoms are recurrent reexperience symptoms such as nightmares and flashbacks to the event and unwelcome images intruding into conscious awareness. Group C symptoms are responses reflecting inability to cope with the experience, which sometimes result in considerable effort expended to avoid reminders, and feelings of emotional numbness and distance from others. Group D symptoms are hyperarousal symptoms: feeling keyed up and on edge, being jumpy and easily startled, maintaining ongoing inappropriate vigilance for danger, experiencing trouble sleeping, and having difficulty concentrating.

It should be noted that established diagnostic criteria state that the symptoms must be new after the event to qualify for a diagnosis of PTSD. General populations have endemic rates of many such symptoms, including insomnia and poor concentration, representing preexisting difficulties that do not qualify for contribution to the diagnosis of PTSD and must be subtracted from the prevalence data. Most popular PTSD symptom measures fail to make this distinction, thus inflating the estimates of PTSD. Another requirement for the diagnosis is persistence of the symptoms for more than 1 month. Thus, PTSD by definition cannot be diagnosed within the first month after the event. Many popular PTSD measures fail to specify the 1-month duration in estimations of diagnosis, further inflating the rates. Additionally, to meet full criteria for PTSD, the symptoms must interfere with functioning or cause clinically significant distress. Once the PTSD diagnosis is determined, delayed-onset PTSD is defined as starting at least 6 months after the event, and chronic PTSD is defined as lasting for at least 3 months.

PTSD IN THE POPULATION

Population studies have shown that half of all people will encounter a traumatic event meeting the stressor A criterion during their lives. Of those who experience such an event, as many as one-third may develop PTSD. Women exhibit twice the prevalence of PTSD as men, which is not unexpected given that PTSD is classified as an anxiety disorder, and women have about twice the rates of anxiety and mood disorders as men. PTSD tends to be chronic, lasting on average 3 years, and one-third of cases may go on for a decade or longer. Women appear to experience approximately four times the chronicity of men (Breslau et al. 1998; Kessler et al. 1995).

PTSD is more prevalent than panic disorder and generalized anxiety disorder, but less prevalent than major depression and substance use disorders (Kessler et al. 1994, 1995). Subsets of populations may have differential risk for experiencing traumatic events. For example, combat is largely a male experience, whereas victims of reported rapes are generally female (Kessler et al. 1995). Different types of events may evoke different rates of PTSD. For example, kidnapping and torture evoke very high rates of PTSD, and violent assaults in the community are associated with somewhat lower rates of PTSD. Flooding has been found to be associated with considerably lower rates of PTSD compared with other disaster types (Breslau 1998). In community settings, PTSD tends to be comorbid: Other disorders occur approximately twice as often in the context of PTSD than alone (Kessler et al. 1995).

Studies of disaster allow investigation of the mental health effects of extreme trauma in its most pure form. In community settings, risk for exposure to traumatic events is not random and is confounded with the likelihood of developing psychopathology afterward. Therefore, it is often difficult if not impossible to know what is a direct effect of the event and what is attributable to preexisting characteristics of the individual. Many research studies sample from treatment settings, adding more layers of bias: Treatment populations tend to suffer from psychiatric disorders. In contrast, disasters tend to be more "equal opportunity" events, striking a cross section of the population unselected for characteristics other than their unfortunate physical presence in the path of the disaster agent.

DISASTER TRAUMA THEORY

Psychiatric sequelae of highly traumatic events present as part of a large network of multiple, interrelated relevant factors. Several types and variations of outcomes must be considered (Figure 6–1). Although PTSD is of major interest following disasters, other psychiatric disorders, such as major depression and alcohol abuse, may present important comorbidities or even primary outcomes. Psychopathology may be examined in the acute post-disaster period or over the long term. Although research tends to focus on negative outcomes, positive results such as personal growth and resilience may also result. Failure to inquire into positive outcomes may cause them to be overlooked altogether and paint an especially pessimistic portrait.

Characteristics of the disaster agent may contribute to mental health problems that follow. Disaster typology assumes natural disasters to promote the mildest mental health consequences, technological accidents involving human error to generate greater psychopathology, and acts of terrorism with their willful human origins to be associated with the highest rates of mental health problems (Baum et al. 1983; Beigel and Berren 1985; Frederick 1980). A large database of mental health outcomes following different types of disasters is needed to differentiate empirically differences in associated mental health outcomes for these three types of disasters. Mental health consequences of various disaster types will be most difficult to untangle from aspects that may be inextricably tied to specific disasters and types of events. For example, the scope and magnitude of the terrorism of the Oklahoma City bombing and the September 11 attacks may represent the source of their mental health effects as much as the fact that they represent terrorist acts. Other aspects of the disaster such as how sudden and unexpected it was, the amount of associated terror (fear for one's life) and horror (witnessing grotesque events), the duration of the event, and repetition and recurrence may also be instrumental in generating mental health effects.

Individual characteristics such as demographics may weigh in generating mental health effects. Two of the most robust predictors of PTSD after disasters have been found to be female gender and preexisting psychopathology

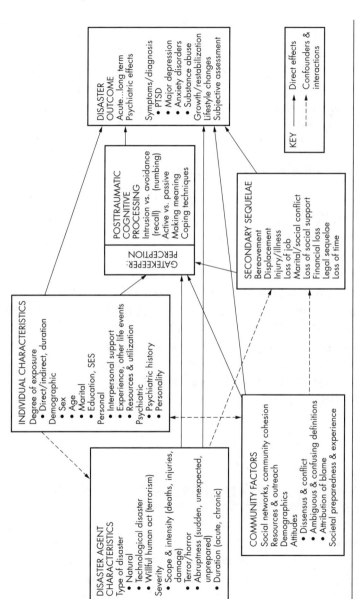

FIGURE 6–1   Disaster trauma theory.

Disaster trauma theory is complex, with many variables from several domains predicting multiple types of outcomes. SES = socioeconomic status, PTSD = posttraumatic stress disorder.

(Weisæth 1985). The community disaster setting may further shape the mental health response of the affected either by the outpouring of support or through conflict over the incident. Subsequent life events may intervene—some resulting from the disaster, such as loss of one's home or job, and others occurring endemically as part of community life, such as divorce, being laid off or fired from one's job, or the inexorable death of loved ones over time. Such events cannot help but affect mental health outcomes. Finally, the gatekeeper or moderator of all these different factors may be how individuals perceive the event, how they process it and make meaning of it, and how successfully they find perspective and move on to heal and resume their lives.

STUDY OF THE OKLAHOMA CITY BOMBING

The Event

The bombing of the Murrah Building in Oklahoma City occurred at 9:02 A.M., April 19, 1995. At the time, it was the most severe act of terrorism ever to occur on American soil. The death toll was 168 (including 19 children and a nurse responder), and injuries numbered approximately 600 (Mallonee et al. 1996; Oklahoma Department of Health 1999). Nearly one-half of the people in the Murrah Building were killed, and most of those who survived were injured. In this close-knit community, 40% of all the townspeople knew someone who was killed in the bombing, and one out of five people in the city attended the funeral of someone who perished in the attack.

Methods

The Washington University disaster research team conducted a study of victims who were in the direct path of the bomb blast (North et al. 1999). The sample of 182 study participants was selected randomly from a registry of survivors of the bomb blast generated by the Oklahoma Health Department, 87% of whom were injured. The data were gathered between 4 and 8 months after the bombing, with approval of the Washington University Human Studies Committee, and written informed consent was obtained from all subjects prior to their participation. A follow-up study was completed at 17 months after the bombing. The participation rate at index was 71% and at follow-up was 75% of the original sample. Instruments used included the Diagnostic Interview Schedule, which generated structured interview research diagnoses both postdisaster and retrospectively, predisaster. The Disaster Supplement obtained data on exposure to the disaster, preexisting and personal factors, ability to function, treatment received, and many variables considered to be important to outcomes. Additionally, Cloninger's Temperament and Character Inventory was used to assess personality.

Findings

The study sample was largely Caucasian, approximately equal in gender representation, middle-aged, and nearly two-thirds married, with 2 years of college on average. Reflecting the resilience of this population, fewer than half of the sample met diagnostic criteria for a postdisaster psychiatric disorder (Figure 6–2). One-third (34%) qualified for a diagnosis of PTSD related to the bombing. The second most prevalent disorder was major depression, diagnosed in approximately one-fourth (23%). A few cases of panic and generalized anxiety disorder were seen as well as a few alcohol and drug use disorder cases. Overall, most postdisaster disorders had been present before the bombing. No new drug or alcohol use cases were observed after the bombing. Many predisaster psychiatric disorders did not recur after the bombing. Examining all the pre- and postdisaster findings together provides a fuller picture and demonstrates the relatively small part played by the new or incident cases after the bombing. It is important to examine the whole picture, including preexisting disorders as well as postdisaster disorders, to obtain a complete understanding of the psychopathology in relation to the event.

The most prevalent symptoms after the bombing were intrusive memories, difficulty sleeping, trouble concentrating, and being jumpy and easily startled. The least prevalent postdisaster symptoms were restricted range of affect and psychogenic amnesia. Overall, 96% of those interviewed reported experiencing at least one PTSD symptom, indicating that the majority of individuals reporting any PTSD symptoms did not have PTSD. Approximately 80% of the victims met DSM criteria for symptom groups B (intrusive reexperience) and D (hyperarousal), and thus experience of these symptoms was normative. Because most symptomatic individuals were not psychiatrically ill, to describe such experiences as symptoms in the absence of illness is inconsistent. It may be more correct to use terminology such as "responses" or "reactions" for these experiences to avoid invoking pathological images in the absence of illness.

Only 36% of the sample met symptom group C criteria. Most (94%) of the individuals in this group also met the full complement of diagnostic

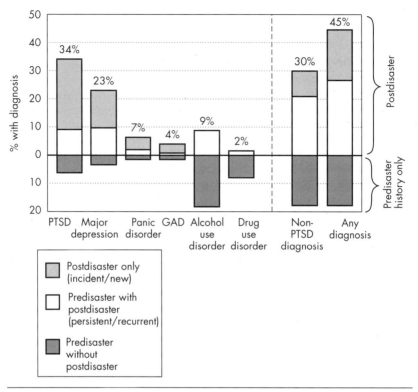

FIGURE 6–2   Predisaster and postdisaster psychiatric diagnoses.

The *light gray* parts of the bars represent the part of disaster psychopathology that was new (incident cases) after the bombing. The sum of the *white* and *light gray* parts of the bars (above the black horizontal dividing line) represents all postdisaster psychopathology. The *dark gray* parts of the bars (below the black horizontal dividing line) represent preexisting psychopathology that did not recur or persist after the bombing. The sum of the *dark gray* and *white* parts of the bars represents all predisaster psychopathology. It is clear that the *light gray* part of the bars, representing new postdisaster psychopathology, was a small part of the overall picture. Notably, no new cases of alcohol or drug use disorders were seen after the bombing. GAD = generalized anxiety disorder, PTSD = posttraumatic stress disorder.

criteria for PTSD. Thus, in this data set, the avoidance and numbing criteria acted as a marker or a gatekeeper for PTSD. Not only were the avoidance and numbing criteria highly concordant with full PTSD, but they were also significantly associated with findings of predisaster psychiatric illness, postdisaster psychiatric comorbidity, seeking mental health treatment, taking medication, drinking alcohol to cope, and functional impairment. In the absence of group C criteria, fulfillment of group B or D criteria was not associated with these indicators of illness.

The postbombing prevalence of PTSD among women was approximately twice the rate in men. History of a predisaster Axis I psychiatric diagnosis approximately doubled the chances of having a postdisaster disorder. Meeting criteria for a personality disorder was associated with more than twice the chance of developing a postdisaster Axis I diagnosis. Other, less robust predictors of PTSD were number of injuries in the bombing, loss of family members or friends in the bombing, and the occurrence of other negative life events after the bombing. The only protective factor was having a college education. When all variables were included in a single multiple stepwise regression model to control for the effects of other variables, only female gender, loss of loved ones in the bombing, other negative life events, and personality disorder showed independent associations with PTSD. Thus, it appears that the association of predisaster Axis I diagnosis with PTSD may have been mediated through personality factors.

The onset of PTSD was rapid. Three-fourths of those with PTSD indicated that the symptoms started the same day as the bombing, 94% within the first week, 98% within the first month, and none after 6 months. By DSM-IV-TR definition, therefore, no cases of delayed PTSD were identified. Asked about the timing of PTSD symptoms in relation to other traumatic events that could have occurred at any time in their lives, study participants provided onset information conforming to a similar time frame, indicating the PTSD had started quickly, and no delayed cases of PTSD were identified. Although 12 new cases of PTSD were identified at follow-up that had not been detected at index, these individuals also described a rapid onset of their symptoms after the disaster. Closer examination of the data revealed that these cases represented subthreshold rather than delayed-onset cases because they lacked only one or two symptoms for the diagnosis and they acquired these symptoms over the next year, crossing the diagnostic threshold. None of the 74 PTSD cases remitted within 3 months, defining all the cases as chronic, and the majority of individuals qualifying for a diagnosis were still suffering with the disorder a year later.

More than one-third of subjects indicated they had problems functioning after the disaster, and more than one-half reported difficulties functioning on the job. Although a diagnosis of PTSD was associated with problems functioning, segregation of the data showed that it was not PTSD alone but comorbidity within PTSD that was associated with self-report of functional problems.

More than one-half of the sample reported having received some form of mental health treatment, exceeding the number of people with diagnosable psychiatric disorders. Nonpsychiatric mental health professionals were the major source of psychological assistance received. Few subjects had consulted psychiatrists, and even fewer had consulted their family physician or their pastor for psychological assistance. It was not so much PTSD but comorbid PTSD that resulted in mental health treatment. Thus, mental health professionals observed PTSD in a nonrepresentative portion of complex cases.

On re-interview a year after the index study, at 17 months postbombing, very similar rates of psychiatric disorders were identified as at index. However, not all information from one interview matched that provided at the other, providing a combined rate of PTSD of 41%. Data from the follow-up assessment indicate that the majority of index cases of major depression were in remission 1 year later, but only a fraction of the index PTSD cases had remitted. No predictors of nonrecovery from PTSD could be identified. Demographic variables, predisaster and postdisaster psychiatric comorbidity, treatment, coping styles, and number of PTSD symptoms in groups B, C, and D were not predictive of recovery from PTSD. However, reduction in the number of symptoms of PTSD over time in group C (and to a smaller extent in group D) was associated with recovery from PTSD. Among those who did not recover, the number of group C symptoms increased.

Clinical Implications of the Oklahoma City Bombing Data

These data have several clinical implications:

- The postdisaster population needs to be divided into those who are psychiatrically ill and those who are subdiagnostically distressed, a dichotomy that can allow effective triage of people to the type of intervention most appropriate for their needs. Because PTSD begins early, assessment can start quickly after the disaster. Those most likely to develop PTSD may be most readily identified by focusing on those with prominent avoidance and numbing symptoms. Disappearance of these symptoms may also be a marker of recovery.
- PTSD is a complex disorder occurring more often as a comorbid condition than alone. This appears to be especially true in treatment settings. The lesson for treatment is that one should not stop looking for psychopathology once a diagnosis of PTSD has been made, because there is likely another diagnosis present that could be more important to course, treatment, and outcome than the PTSD itself.

- In the rush to identify psychiatric cases after a disaster, it is important not to overlook the resilience of the population, as reflected by the fact that the majority of subjects did not develop a psychiatric disorder even after a disaster of the magnitude of the Oklahoma City bombing. At the same time, one should not discount the distress experienced by those who do not have a disorder. These are people with prominent intrusion and hyperarousal symptoms but no avoidance/numbing. They can be reassured that their distressing symptoms do not necessarily indicate signs of impending psychiatric illness but rather are "normal responses to an abnormal event," and that this distress can be expected to diminish with time. These individuals may respond well to interventions to facilitate sharing of their experience and cognitive processing of it. In contrast, those with PTSD, who have by definition prominent avoidance and numbing symptoms, may be retraumatized by therapies forcing them to reexperience the event that they are not emotionally equipped to withstand.
- Because PTSD started quickly and endured in most who met diagnostic criteria, disaster mental health interventions can begin to identify people early but must continue throughout the period of need, which can be expected to be lengthy.
- PTSD that is identified only after some period of time has elapsed should not be automatically assumed to represent delayed-onset PTSD. Rather, these cases should be considered to have been already present but subthreshold at index. Although PTSD does not appear to have occurred in delayed-onset form, delay in seeking treatment may be observed.

Implications for Post–September 11 Planning and Beyond

Findings from the Oklahoma City bombing study may help provide a roadmap to predict the effects of and identify needed interventions after the September 11 attacks. The September 11 situation may have important differences from the Oklahoma City bombing that point to distinct disaster mental health interventions. Differences include the far greater scope and magnitude of the September 11 catastrophe in terms of loss of life and destruction of property, as well as the associated degree of sheer horror. Even though the loss of life was magnitudes greater on September 11, the number of injuries in relation to fatalities was small, and bereavement was widespread. The September 11 attacks represent an assault on the nerve center of the United States and the symbols of its identity. Broadcast media repeatedly played footage of the planes crashing into the buildings and even aired images of people jumping from the towers to their deaths, exposing the general public to the horror. Subsequent upsetting events, including economic difficulties in Manhattan, anthrax attacks, a plane crash in Queens, and threats of future terrorist attacks, served to stir up emotions and keep symptoms active.

It is important to appreciate the distinct populations affected by the September 11 attacks, each of which can be expected to exhibit different mental health profiles and to require different intervention plans. The highest rates of PTSD can be anticipated among the most directly exposed victims who fled for their lives. Those who lost loved ones in the attacks will be at risk for bereavement as well as PTSD. The rescue workers, representing a directly exposed as well as a highly bereaved population, may be at special risk for mental health complications. Additional populations deserving attention include indirectly and secondarily affected groups such as those living nearby and those whose businesses were damaged or lost. The distinct groups can be expected to exhibit different response profiles and may need different mental health intervention planning.

CONCLUSIONS

Data from the Oklahoma City bombing study suggest that disaster victim populations can be subdivided into psychiatrically ill and subdiagnostically distressed categories and triaged accordingly to the appropriate type of mental health interventions. Those with PTSD might be identifiable by their prominent avoidance and numbing profiles, and they may benefit from formal psychiatric treatment. Those with subdiagnostic distress may benefit from sharing, reassurance, and education. Because of delay in seeking treatment, casefinding may be necessary to identify those needing services. Data indicating a great deal of PTSD chronicity suggest the importance of provision of mental health services throughout the period of need.

REFERENCES

American Psychiatric Association: Diagnostic and Statistical Manual of Mental Disorders, 3rd Edition. Washington, DC, American Psychiatric Association, 1980

American Psychiatric Association: Diagnostic and Statistical Manual of Mental Disorders, 4th Edition, Text Revision. Washington, DC, American Psychiatric Association, 2000

Baum A, Fleming R, Davidson LM: Natural disaster and technological catastrophe. Environ Behav 15:333–354, 1983

Beigel A, Berren M: Human-induced disasters. Psychiatr Ann 15:143–150, 1985

Breslau N: Epidemiology of trauma and posttraumatic stress disorder, in Psychological Trauma. Edited by Yehuda R. Washington, DC, American Psychiatric Press, 1998, pp 1–29

Breslau N, Kessler RC, Chilcoat HD, et al: Trauma and posttraumatic stress disorder in the community. Arch Gen Psychiatry 55:626–632, 1998

Frederick CJ: Effects of natural vs. human-induced violence upon victims. Evaluation and Change (special issue):71–75, 1980

Kessler RC, McGonagle KA, Zhao S, et al: Lifetime and 12-month prevalence of DSM-III-R psychiatric disorders in the United States. Arch Gen Psychiatry 51:8–19, 1994

Kessler RC, Sonnega A, Bromet E, et al: Posttraumatic stress disorder in the National Co-morbidity Survey. Arch Gen Psychiatry 52:1048–1060, 1995

Mallonee S, Shariat S, Stennies G, et al: Physical injuries and fatalities resulting from the Oklahoma City bombing. JAMA 276:382–387, 1996

North CS, Nixon SJ, Shariat S, et al: Psychiatric disorders among survivors of the Oklahoma City bombing. JAMA 282:755–762, 1999

Oklahoma Department of Health: 1995 Oklahoma City bombing injuries data base. Oklahoma City, OK, 1999

Robins E, Guze SB: Establishment of diagnostic validity in psychiatric illness: its application to schizophrenia. Am J Psychiatry 126:983–987, 1970

Weisæth L: Post-traumatic stress disorder after an industrial disaster, in Psychiatry: The State of the Art. Edited by Pichot P, Berner P, Wolf R, et al. New York, Plenum, 1985, pp 299–307

7

Neuroanatomy of Panic Disorder

Implications of Functional Imaging in Fear Conditioning

David Gutman, M.D.
Jack M. Gorman, M.D.
Joy Hirsch, Ph.D.

Panic disorder is a common and disabling illness characterized by recurrent unexpected panic attacks along with one or more of the following symptoms: persistent concern about having additional attacks, worry about the implications of the attack or its consequences, or a significant change in behavior related to the attacks (American Psychiatric Association 2000). Several models have been proposed to explain the neuroanatomy and pathophysiology of panic disorder. These have ranged from explanations based on dysfunction of regions in the brainstem to aberrant interaction between regions of the cortex and limbic system (Gorman et al. 1989, 2000; Klein 1993). Functional brain imaging studies in humans may now help to clarify which elements of these models are accurate and thereby lead to more effective treatments.

Functional imaging studies can be grouped by technology or method. Imaging technologies include single photon emission computed tomography (SPECT), positron emission tomography (PET), and functional magnetic resonance imaging (fMRI). Methods include paradigms that observe state (e.g., resting blood flow studies), trait (e.g., provocation studies in which a panic attack occurs in the scanner), or related traits (e.g., displaying traumatic pictures to subjects with posttraumatic stress disorder [PTSD]). Studies of panic disorder have used pharmacological methods such as administration of doxapram, lactate, and CCK-4 (Dager et al.

1999; Javanmard et al. 1999; J.M. Kent, unpublished data, 2002; Layton et al. 2001) to elicit panic attacks in panic disorder patients and healthy control subjects. Although informative, the use of panicogens in human brain imaging is limited by the difficulty of temporally synchronizing a scan with the onset of panic symptoms, the potential for motion artifact induced by a panic attack, and the difficulty of repeating the study once the subject has panicked. Therefore, methods that can differentiate the brain functioning of panic patients versus healthy subjects without inducing a panic attack are important. This review focuses on the use of classical conditioning in imaging studies as a potential method to explore the neuroanatomy of panic disorder.

The well-studied paradigm of classical conditioning can serve as a model for panic disorder (Bouton et al. 2001; Goldstein and Chambless 1978; Razran 1961). Although there is some controversy about conditioning as an explanation for panic disorder—for example, its ability to explain nocturnal panic attacks—it can still serve as a testable model for understanding panic disorder (McNally 1990). In classical conditioning, a conditioned stimulus (CS) is paired with an unconditioned stimulus (US) and subsequently begins to elicit behavior usually associated with the US. The familiar example is derived from Pavlov's work with animals (Pavlov 1927). After repeated pairings of a bell (CS) with food (US), the bell alone begins to elicit a conditioned response (CR), such as salivation. Spatial and temporal contexts are important in regulating the expression of these acquired relationships. For example, a response to a cue that may make sense in one environment may not be appropriate in another. Although these learned associations fade with repeated exposure to the CS without the US (extinction), they can be recovered with contextual retrieval cues (Rescorla and Heth 1975). In panic disorder, interoceptive cues (e.g., racing heart) and exteroceptive cues (e.g., crowded elevator, bridge) that occur during the initial panic attacks (USs) can become CSs that trigger anticipatory anxiety (CR) or panic attacks. Furthermore, a CS (e.g., racing heart) that elicits panic or anticipatory anxiety (CR) in the environment in which the association was initially acquired can begin to generalize to other environments. For example, a patient may experience a racing heart prior to a panic attack on the subway and then develop anticipatory anxiety every time he or she has a racing heart on the subway (the original, "appropriate" context). This can then generalize so that having a racing heart on the elevator (a novel, "inappropriate" context) also elicits anticipatory anxiety, even though this relationship (racing heart leading to anticipatory anxiety) was not acquired in this context. Such a relationship has been observed in patients with implantable cardioverter/

defibrillators who have an increased rate of anxiety disorder after implantation, which is correlated with the frequency of repeated defibrillations they receive (Godemann et al. 2001). An effective treatment for panic disorder, cognitive-behavioral therapy (CBT), also supports conditioned fear as a model of panic disorder (Barlow et al. 2001). The therapist uses repeated exposures to a CS, such as dizziness, to extinguish the conditioned response (panic attack) (Furst and Cooper 1970).

Gorman et al. (2000) described a neuroanatomical model of panic disorder based on preclinical and basic research in conditioned fear. Animal studies of fear conditioning have elaborated a network of brain regions that make up a "fear system" (LeDoux 1996). The amygdala has been demonstrated to be a crucial part of the fear system in animal models of fear and anxiety. Sensory stimuli initially project to the thalamus and are then relayed via two pathways to the lateral nucleus of the amygdala. One pathway is from the thalamus to the frontal cortex to the amygdala, and the other directly from the thalamus to the amygdala (de Olmos 1990; LeDoux et al. 1990) (Figure 7–1). LeDoux has termed these pathways the "high road" and the "low road," respectively (LeDoux 1996). The amygdala receives sensory information from all over the body and projects to areas of the brain that produce the fear response (Davis 1992; LeDoux et al. 1988, 1990). Efferents of the central nucleus of the amygdala project to multiple areas: to the periaqueductal gray, responsible for producing defensive behaviors such as freezing and pain modulation (De Oca et al. 1998); the parabrachial nucleus, causing an increase in respiratory rate (Takeuchi et al. 1982); the lateral nucleus of the hypothalamus, activating the sympathetic nervous system and causing autonomic arousal and sympathetic discharge (Price and Amaral 1981); the paraventricular nucleus, activating the hypothalamic-pituitary-adrenal axis, thereby increasing the release of adrenocorticoids (Dunn and Whitener 1986); and the locus ceruleus, causing an increase in norepinephrine release, resulting in an increased fear response, and elevation in blood pressure and heart rate (Cedarbaum and Aghajanian 1978). In addition, the hippocampus mediates contextual information during conditioning (Kim and Fanselow 1992).

Several paradigms have been used in different imaging modalities to explore the role of these structures in the experience of fear and anxiety in humans. Much research has focused on the amygdala, and human facial expressions have been frequently used as stimuli for imaging studies of the amygdala. An early PET study by George et al. (1993) that used a visual stimulus of human facial expressions demonstrated activity in the right anterior cingulate and the bilateral inferior frontal gyri. Morris et al. (1996) demonstrated amygdala sensitivity to type and degree of emotion displayed

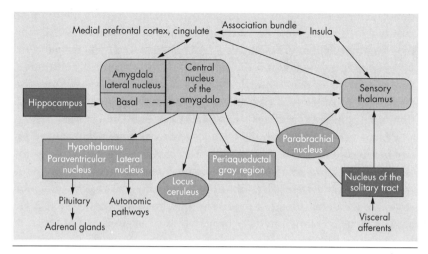

FIGURE 7–1 Neuroanatomical pathways of viscerosensory information in the brain.

Viscerosensory information is conveyed to the amygdala by two major pathways: downstream, from the nucleus of the solitary tract via the parabrachial nucleus or the sensory thalamus; and upstream, from the primary viscerosensory cortices and via corticothalamic relays allowing for higher-level neurocognitive processing and modulation of sensory information. Contextual information is stored in memory in the hippocampus and conveyed directly to the amygdala. Major efferent pathways of the amygdala relevant to anxiety include the following: the locus ceruleus (increases norepinephrine release, which contributes to physiological and behavioral arousal), the periaqueductal gray region (controls defensive behaviors and postural freezing), the hypothalamic paraventricular nucleus (activates the hypothalamic-pituitary-adrenal axis, releasing adrenocorticoids), the hypothalamic lateral nucleus (activates the sympathetic nervous system), and the parabrachial nucleus (influences respiratory rate and timing).

For a color version of this figure, please see the color insert at the back of this book.

Source. Adapted from Gorman JM, Kent JM, Sullivan GM, et al.: "Neuroanatomical Hypothesis of Panic Disorder, Revised." *American Journal of Psychiatry* 157:493–505, 2000. Used with permission.

by a facial expression, with the left amygdala being progressively activated with increasingly fearful faces compared with happy faces. When subjects performed a gender discrimination task while viewing either fearful or happy faces, they showed increased activity with fearful faces in the left amygdala, left pulvinar, left anterior insula, and bilateral anterior cingulate gyri (Morris et al. 1998a). Phillips et al. (1997) also demonstrated amygdala activation with presentation of fearful faces, noting that this activation did not occur with presentation of neutral or disgust expressions. Children also have been shown to have amygdala activation during a task with fearful faces (Baird et al. 1999). Vocal expressions of fear, but not disgust, also activate the amygdala (Phillips et al. 1998). One study suggests that the amygdala may not necessarily be activated by the fearful expressions themselves, but by the intensity of the expression (Breiter et al. 1996).

Activation of the amygdala can occur without an individual's conscious knowledge of the stimulus, as has been demonstrated in a visual masking paradigm with fearful faces (Whalen et al. 1998a). Visual masking occurs when a visual stimulus is shown briefly, followed by another visual stimulus of longer duration. Although individuals may demonstrate a CR to the first image, they will be aware only of the second image (Esteves and Ohman 1993). Subjects demonstrate a lateralized amygdala response to a CS, correlated with the level of masking of the stimulus (Morris et al. 1998b). Several studies have found evidence of lateralization of amygdala activity. When subjects viewed an angry face previously conditioned with a burst of white noise, they had increased activity in the left amygdala; but when the face was masked, activity increased in the right amygdala. The response of the amygdala is also time dependent and seems to decrease over continued presentations of the CS during acquisition (Breiter et al. 1996; Buchel et al. 1998; Whalen et al. 1998a). LaBar et al. (1998) showed a similar temporally related decrease in activity in the amygdala during extinction. Increased activity in the amygdala is also correlated with biological markers, such as skin conductance (Buchel et al. 1998; LaBar et al. 1998). The left amygdala responds to instructed fear (e.g., a subject is told a stimulus signals the onset of a shock), but the right amygdala has been noted to be more active during fear conditioning (LaBar et al. 1998; Morris et al. 1998b; Phelps et al. 2001; Pine et al. 2001). Furthermore, the right amygdala response to fearful faces decreases more rapidly than that of the left amygdala (Phillips et al. 2001; Wright et al. 2001). Although there is abundant evidence of possible lateralization of amygdala activity during conditioning, this has not been established in all studies (Buchel et al. 1998).

Different sensory modalities in addition to visual stimuli can be used to probe the fear and anxiety system. Aversive olfactory stimuli produce increases in regional cerebral blood flow (rCBF) in the left amygdala and left orbitofrontal cortex; these increases are correlated with each other and with the degree of aversive intensity (Zald and Pardo 1997). Morris et al. (1999) played neutral, fearful, happy, and sad vocalizations to healthy volunteers and demonstrated decreased response in the right amygdala to the fear stimulus with a fear-specific inhibitory interaction with the left anterior insula. The pons also had a fear-specific interaction with the amygdala. This again reveals the importance of using various sensory stimuli in the evaluation of networks of brain regions involved in processing fear and anxiety.

Several groups have made use of higher cognitive processes to engage the fear system, for example, using a Stroop task that involves reading neutral versus threatening words. The results differ somewhat, with one group noting increased activity in the anterior cingulate and another finding activation of the amygdala bilaterally, along with the left lingual gyrus, posterior parahippocampal gyrus, and left premotor area (Isenberg et al. 1999; Whalen et al. 1998b).

In addition to studies with cognitive tasks, information about the fear system in humans can be gleaned from the observation of subjects with brain injuries. People with bilateral amygdala damage have difficulty perceiving fear and anger in vocal intonations and pictures of facial affect (Adolphs et al. 1994; Scott et al. 1997). Some studies have shown that a bilaterally functioning amygdala is necessary for the perception of fearful faces (Adolphs et al. 1995), but others have found that the perception of aversive words is reduced in subjects with left but not right amygdalectomies (Anderson and Phelps 2001). Temporal lobectomy also impairs CR acquisition (LaBar et al. 1995).

The amygdala plays an important role in the production of fear and anxiety and has been the focus of much imaging research in these two important emotions. Yet it is only one area in a group of regions that control the fear response. The prefrontal cortex (PFC) and anterior cingulate also play a role in the fear network and have been implicated in imaging studies of human subjects.

Tasks that require higher-level processing of emotion, such as naming a feeling, lead to increased cortical activity with reciprocally decreased activity in the amygdala. Hariri et al. (2000) noted that a task requiring matching fearful or angry facial expressions increased activity in the amygdala bilaterally. When subjects were asked to label these expressions, activity in the amygdala was diminished but correlated with increased activity in the right PFC.

Like the amygdala, PFC activity can be modulated by repeated exposure to an emotional stimulus or during fear conditioning. However, the stimuli that lead to habituation differ between the two regions. For example, the left PFC habituates more rapidly to happy faces than to fearful faces (Wright et al. 2001). With repeated exposure to a reinforced CS (CS+) associated with an electric shock, activity in the anterior cingulate increases as measured by active tissue volume and the timing of the peak signal shifts toward CS onset. The active tissue volume decreases with repeated exposures to a nonreinforced CS (CS−) unassociated with electric shock (Knight et al. 1999). Likewise, Fredrikson et al. (1995) found that exposure to a visual snake stimulus that had been previously paired with an electric shock led to increased rCBF in the left anterior and posterior cingulate gyrus, the left primary somatosensory cortex, and the left premotor cortex as well as bilaterally in the parietal area, ventromedial thalamus, posterior hypothalamus, and central gray of the midbrain. Using fMRI, Buchel et al. (1998) observed activation of bilateral anterior cingulate gyri, bilateral anterior insulae, and medial parietal cortex during conditioning. Studies in patients with PTSD further support the role of the anterior cingulate and PFC in the control of anxiety symptoms. Patients with PTSD have decreased activity in the thalamus, anterior cingulate, and medial frontal gyrus compared with traumatized subjects without PTSD (Lanius et al. 2001).

As mentioned previously, the type of stimulus and sensory modality used in a study can have an impact on the brain regions observed to be active during a study. In particular, the sensory system used to present a CS and US may have an effect on areas that are activated and may be included as part of a fear network. When a visual CS is used with an auditory US, increased activity is noted in the auditory cortex when the CS+ is seen (Morris et al. 2001). An auditory CS paired with a corneal air puff US leads to increased activity in the somatosensory cortex and contralateral cerebellum when the CS+ is heard (Ramnani et al. 2000).

fMRI INVESTIGATION OF FEAR CONDITIONING

In a pilot fMRI study using a fear conditioning paradigm, we explored long-range cortical networks associated with fear and anxiety. To examine networked brain regions associated with cognitive tasks without signals associated from sensory input (Hirsch et al. 2001), we employed a method that requires the conjunction of activity associated with identical or nearly identical tasks presented in various sensory modalities within a subject and the conservation of that activity across multiple subjects. Thus, prior knowledge of specific regions of interest is not necessary, and the technique allows for a search for systems involved in higher-level emotional and cognitive functions.

fMRI was used to localize areas relevant to classical conditioning. Five healthy (without panic disorder) volunteer subjects underwent classical conditioning in the fMRI scanner. The US was an aversive auditory stimulus (Lang et al. 1999a). A CS+ of a red square was used as well as a CS– of a green square. The study consisted of two baseline habituation runs of two CSs, a CS+ (red square) and a CS– (green square), presented in a random order (preconditioning run) (Figure 7–2). This was followed by two conditioning runs in which the CS+ was paired with an aversive tone and the CS– was not (conditioning run). A third set of two runs presented the CS+ and CS– without a paired sound (postconditioning run). Evidence of classical conditioning was taken as the difference between functional images acquired prior to the conditioning experience (runs 1 and 2) and the same paradigm run after the conditioning experience (runs 5 and 6). Four additional subjects underwent the same procedure, but without classical conditioning (the CS+ was not paired with a US), to serve as a control group. These data served to confirm that there were no changes in the images due to repeated testing.

An additional subject underwent classical conditioning using the afore-mentioned procedure. This was followed by another classical conditioning paradigm that used aversive pictures (Lang et al. 1999b) as a US and a high-pitched tone and a low-pitched tone for the CS+ and CS–, respectively. The use of different sensory modalities for the US and CS provides the ability to analyze the data for areas that are active during stages of classical conditioning regardless of the sensory modality used to perceive the stimuli. This analysis is performed using logical equations that examine images for areas that are either activated in common (an AND function) during two separate trials or active during one trial but not another (a NOT function).

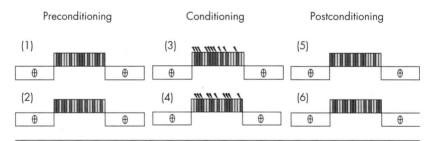

FIGURE 7–2   Sequence of imaging runs.

Forty-six images of the whole brain were acquired during each run (21 contiguous slices/image), which lasted 3 minutes and 4 seconds. A standard block design was used, in which 13 images (52 seconds) were acquired during an initial baseline epoch, followed by a task epoch of 20 images (80 seconds) and a recovery baseline epoch of 13 images (52 seconds). A total of six runs were acquired. Each baseline consisted of a crosshair. Each task epoch consisted of a randomized presentation of 10 *red* (CS+ [reinforced stimulus]) and 10 *green* (CS– [nonreinforced stimulus]) squares. Each square was presented for 3 seconds with an interstimulus interval of 0.5 seconds, during which a crosshair was presented. During the task epochs of runs 3 and 4, an aversive auditory stimulus was paired with the CS+ for 2.5 seconds.

For a color version of this figure, please see the color insert at the back of this book.

A 1.5 T General Electric magnetic resonance scanner was used to obtain T2*-weighted images with a gradient echo pulse sequence that was sensitive to magnetic resonance signal changes induced by alteration in the proportion of deoxyhemoglobin in the local vasculature accompanying neuronal activation (TR = 4,000 seconds, TE = 60 seconds, flip angle = 60 degrees). The in-plane resolution was 1.5 mm by 1.5 mm, and slice thickness was 4.5 mm. Twenty-one contiguous axial slices of the brain, which covered the entire cortex, were taken parallel to the anterior-posterior commissure line. Forty-six images were acquired for each run: a baseline (resting) period of 10 images (40 seconds), a stimulation period of 20 images (80 seconds), and a baseline (recovery) period of 10 images (40 seconds).

Activation of each voxel was determined by a multistage statistical analysis that compared mean amplitude of signals acquired during stimulation and baseline periods. This technique also required statistically significant signal changes on two identical runs resulting in an empirically determined false-positive rate of $P < 0.0001$ for each condition (Kim et al. 1997).

After voxels were identified as active for each condition (preconditioning, conditioning, postconditioning), a logical analysis was used to identify areas activated by the CS after conditioning, but not activated by the CS before conditioning. A "logical exclusion" AND NOT operation was employed to segregate activity associated with response to the CS after conditioning from that before conditioning, presumably yielding activity associated with classical conditioning. The cross-modality study also employed a logical AND operation to include activity associated with conditioning, but not activity pertaining to the specific sensory modality in which it was induced. A measure of brain activity was obtained by summing all active voxels in the imaged brain volume.

Assignments of anatomical labels were based on correspondence between the anatomy on the images and the Human Brain Atlas (Talairach and Tournoux 1988). Conventional high-resolution (T1-weighted) images were also acquired along the same plane locations as the T2*-weighted images and served as anatomical references. The stages of assignment included: identification of the brain slice passing through the anterior-posterior commissure line, assignment of an atlas plate to each acquired brain slice, and assignment of the corresponding anatomical labels. This process was achieved in the same manner for all subjects and yielded a summary tabulation containing anatomical regions for each of the clusters of activated voxels. An area was considered "conserved" if it was present for all subjects in the experiment.

The images in Figures 7–3, 7–4, and 7–5 show 17 contiguous slices of brain for one subject. Figures 7–3 and 7–4 demonstrate regions active when the CS is experienced after conditioning and not active when the CS

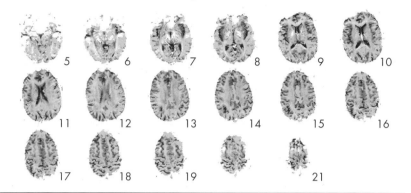

FIGURE 7–3 Classical conditioning with an auditory US and a visual CS. Each colored region indicates a significant increase in the fMRI T2* signal from baseline ($P \leq 0.0001$, $P \leq 0.0003$, and $P \leq 0.0005$; depicted as *yellow, orange,* and *red,* respectively, on brain images).

For a color version of this figure, please see the color insert at the back of this book.

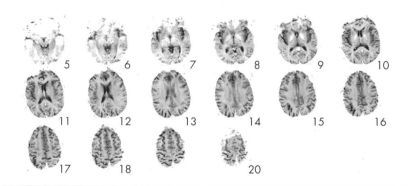

FIGURE 7–4 Classical conditioning with a visual US and an auditory CS. Each colored region indicates a significant increase in the fMRI T2* signal from baseline ($P \leq 0.0001$, $P \leq 0.0003$, and $P \leq 0.0005$; depicted as *yellow, orange,* and *red,* respectively, on brain images).

For a color version of this figure, please see the color insert at the back of this book.

is presented prior to conditioning. Areas active across sensory modalities when the subject was presented with a CS after classical conditioning are seen in Figure 7–5. The images in Figure 7–5 (the result of a logical AND operation of the activity in Figures 7–3 and 7–4) illustrate activity associated

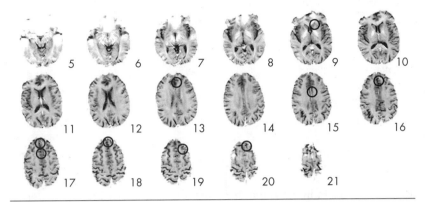

FIGURE 7–5 Long-range cortical networks activated by classical conditioning with an aversive unconditioned stimulus (a cross–sensory modality conjunction).

Active areas are highlighted with a circle. Each colored region indicates a significant increase in the fMRI T2* signal from baseline ($P \leq 0.0001$, $P \leq 0.0003$, and $P \leq 0.0005$; depicted as *yellow, orange,* and *red,* respectively, on brain images).
For a color version of this figure, please see the color insert at the back of this book.

with classical conditioning but not related to sensory processing. Regions active in Figure 7–4 that were conserved across all five subjects when viewing a visual CS after classical conditioning with an aversive auditory US are listed in Table 7–1.

Subjects demonstrated significantly increased brain activity when viewing the CS+ after conditioning compared with viewing the CS+ during habituation (preconditioning run). The total number of active voxels in the experimental group (CS+ paired with US) when the postconditioning trial was compared with baseline increased by a mean of 3,914.6 (standard error of the mean [SEM] 1,349.39). The control group had a mean average decrease of 4,772.5 (SEM 3,283.83) in total number of active voxels. This was statistically significant (two-tailed t test: $P = 0.03$, $t = 2.660723$, $df = 7$) (Figure 7–6). This implies that the conditioning procedure had an effect. In the future, simultaneous monitoring of physiological variables, such as heart rate and skin conductance, could provide further corroboration of a conditioning effect.

Classical conditioning results in increased brain activity on viewing a conditioned stimulus. Furthermore, we observe specific neuroanatomical regions that are associated with classical conditioning in healthy subjects using a noninvasive, nonpainful aversive stimulus. Our results are consistent with animal models (LeDoux 1996) and prior classical conditioning

TABLE 7–1 Regions conserved across subjects in classical conditioning

Left	Right
Cingulate gyrus	Cingulate gyrus
Middle occipital gyrus	Middle occipital gyrus
Superior temporal gyrus	Superior temporal gyrus
Middle temporal gyrus	Middle temporal gyrus
Inferior parietal gyrus	Inferior parietal gyrus
Inferior frontal gyrus	Caudate
Superior frontal gyrus	
Supramarginal gyrus	

imaging studies in humans that have demonstrated activity in the anterior cingulate, frontal cortex, and parietal cortex (Buchel et al. 1998; Fredrikson et al. 1995; Knight et al. 1999). Furthermore, we observed lateralization of function in particular regions, such as activity in the right caudate and left inferior frontal, superior frontal, and supramarginal gyri. It is notable that the amygdala was not observed to be active in this study. It is possible that the block design used in the study made this observation difficult, because there is evidence that the amygdala becomes active briefly and then rapidly accommodates (Labar et al. 1998). Also, the analysis concentrates on activity after acquisition of conditioning, not during acquisition, in which the amygdala may play a more important role. These preliminary findings suggest the need for replication as well as the comparison of psychiatrically healthy control subjects with patients with panic disorder.

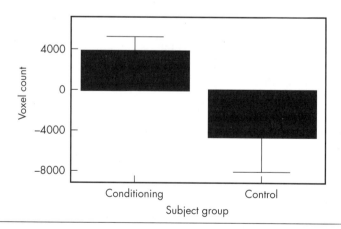

FIGURE 7–6 Change in total active voxels after conditioning.

Error bars show mean ± 1.0 standard error.

CONCLUSIONS

The improved spatial and temporal resolution of fMRI allows for testing of proposed neural networks based on animal studies. fMRI has the further advantage of a high degree of safety and the ability to perform test-retest studies. Our understanding of the anatomy of fear in animals can be used to begin to map a human network of normal and pathological fear and anxiety. In panic disorder, we can now test theoretical models that may lead to improved psychological and pharmacological treatments. Classical conditioning offers particular advantages, including a well-detailed animal model and strong theoretical support, as a system to understand panic disorder.

REFERENCES

Adolphs R, Tranel D, Damasio H, et al: Impaired recognition of emotion in facial expressions following bilateral damage to the human amygdala. Nature 372:669–672, 1994

Adolphs R, Tranel D, Damasio H, et al: Fear and the human amygdala. J Neurosci 15:5879–5891, 1995

American Psychiatric Association: Diagnostic and Statistical Manual of Mental Disorders, 4th Edition, Text Revision. Washington, DC, American Psychiatric Association, 2000

Anderson AK, Phelps EA: Lesions of the human amygdala impair enhanced perception of emotionally salient events. Nature 411:305–309, 2001

Baird AA, Gruber SA, Feir DA, et al: Functional magnetic resonance imaging of facial affect recognition in children and adolescents. J Am Acad Child Adolesc Psychiatry 38:195–199, 1999

Barlow DH, Gorman JM, Shear MK, et al: Cognitive-behavioral therapy, imipramine, or their combination for panic disorder: a randomized controlled trial. JAMA 283:2529–2536, 2001

Bouton ME, Mineka S, Barlow DH: A modern learning theory perspective on the etiology of panic disorder. Psychol Rev 108:4–32, 2001

Breiter HC, Etcoff NL, Whalen P, et al: Response and habituation of the human amygdala during visual processing of facial expression. Neuron 17:875–887, 1996

Buchel C, Morris J, Dolan RJ, et al: Brain systems mediating aversive conditioning: an event-related fMRI study. Neuron 20:947–957, 1998

Cedarbaum JM, Aghajanian GK: Afferent projections to the rat locus coeruleus as determined by a retrograde tracing technique. J Comp Neurol 178:1–16, 1978

Dager SR, Friedman SD, Heide A, et al: Two-dimensional proton echo-planar spectroscopic imaging of brain metabolic changes during lactate-induced panic. Arch Gen Psychiatry 56:70–77, 1999

Davis M: The role of the amygdala in fear and anxiety. Annu Rev Neurosci 15:353–375, 1992

De Oca BM, DeCola JP, Maren S, et al: Distinct regions of the periaqueductal gray are involved in the acquisition and expression of defensive responses. J Neurosci 18:3426–3432, 1998

de Olmos J: Amygdaloid nuclear gray complex, in The Human Nervous System. Edited by Paxinos G. San Diego, CA, Academic Press, 1990, pp 583–710

Dunn JD, Whitener J: Plasma corticosterone responses to electrical stimulation of the amygdaloid complex: cytoarchitectural specificity. Neuroendocrinology 42:211–217, 1986

Esteves F, Ohman A: Masking the face: recognition of emotional facial expressions as a function of the parameters of backward masking. Scand J Psychol 34:1–18, 1993

Fredrikson M, Wik G, Fischer A, et al: Affective and attentive neural networks in humans: a PET study of Pavlovian conditioning. Neuroreport 7:97–101, 1995

Furst JB, Cooper A: Combined use of imaginal and interoceptive stimuli in desensitizing fear of heart attacks. J Behav Ther Exp Psychiatry 1:87–89, 1970

George MS, Ketter TA, Gill DS, et al: Brain regions involved in recognizing facial emotion or identity: an oxygen-15 PET study. J Neuropsychiatry Clin Neurosci 5:384–394, 1993

Godemann F, Ahrens B, Behrens S, et al: Classic conditioning and dysfunctional cognitions in patients with panic disorder and agoraphobia treated with an implantable cardioverter/defibrillator. Psychosom Med 63:231–238, 2001

Goldstein AJ, Chambless DL: A reanalysis of agoraphobia. Behav Ther 9:47–59, 1978

Gorman JM, Liebowitz MR, Fyer AJ, et al: A neuroanatomical hypothesis for panic disorder. Am J Psychiatry 146:148–161, 1989

Gorman JM, Kent JM, Sullivan GM, et al: Neuroanatomical hypothesis of panic disorder, revised. Am J Psychiatry 157:493–505, 2000

Hariri AR, Bookheimer SY, Mazziotta JC: Modulating emotional responses: effects of a neocortical network on the limbic system. Neuroreport 11:43–48, 2000

Hirsch J, Moreno DR, Kim KH: Interconnected large-scale systems for three fundamental cognitive tasks revealed by functional MRI. J Cogn Neurosci 13:389–405, 2001

Isenberg N, Silbersweig D, Engelien A, et al: Linguistic threat activates the human amygdala. Proc Natl Acad Sci U S A 96:10456–10459, 1999

Javanmard M, Shlik J, Kennedy SH, et al: Neuroanatomic correlates of CCK-4-induced panic attacks in healthy humans: a comparison of two time points. Biol Psychiatry 45:872–882, 1999

Kim JJ, Fanselow MS: Modality-specific retrograde amnesia of fear. Science 256:675–677, 1992

Kim KH, Relkin NR, Lee KM, et al: Distinct cortical areas associated with native and second languages. Nature 388:171–174, 1997

Klein DF: False suffocation alarms, spontaneous panics, and related conditions: an integrative hypothesis. Arch Gen Psychiatry 50:306–317, 1993

Knight DC, Smith CN, Stein EA, et al: Functional MRI of human Pavlovian fear conditioning: patterns of activation as a function of learning. Neuroreport 10:3665–3670, 1999

LaBar KS, LeDoux JE, Spencer DD, et al: Impaired fear conditioning following unilateral temporal lobectomy in humans. J Neurosci 15:6846–6855, 1995

LaBar KS, Gatenby JC, Gore JC, et al: Human amygdala activation during conditioned fear acquisition and extinction: a mixed-trial fMRI study. Neuron 20:937–945, 1998

Lang P, Bradley M, Cuthbert BN: International Affective Digitized Sounds (IADS): Stimuli, Instruction Manual and Affective Ratings. Technical Report A-4. Center for Research in Psychophysiology, University of Florida, Gainesville, 1999a

Lang PJ, Bradley MM, Cuthbert BN: International Affective Picture System (IAPS): Instruction manual and affective ratings. Technical Report A-4. Center for Research in Psychophysiology, University of Florida, Gainesville, 1999b

Lanius RA, Williamson PC, Densmore M, et al: Neural correlates of traumatic memories in posttraumatic stress disorder: a functional MRI investigation. Am J Psychiatry 158:1920–1922, 2001

Layton ME, Friedman SD, Dager SR, et al: Brain metabolic changes during lactate-induced panic: effects of gabapentin treatment. Depress Anxiety 14:251–254, 2001

LeDoux J: The Emotional Brain: The Mysterious Underpinnings of Emotional Life. New York, Simon and Schuster, 1996

LeDoux JE, Iwata J, Cicchetti P, et al: Different projections of the central amygdaloid nucleus mediate autonomic and behavioral correlates of conditioned fear. J Neurosci 8:2517–2529, 1988

LeDoux JE, Cicchetti P, Xagoraris A, et al: The lateral amygdaloid nucleus: sensory interface of the amygdala in fear conditioning. J Neurosci 10:1062–1069, 1990

McNally RJ: Psychological approaches to panic disorder: a review. Psychol Bull 108:403–419, 1990

Morris JS, Frith CD, Perrrett DI, et al: A differential neural response in the human amygdala to fearful and happy facial expressions. Nature 383:812–815, 1996

Morris JS, Friston KJ, Buchel C, et al: A neuromodulatory role for the human amygdala in processing emotional facial expressions. Brain 121:47–57, 1998a

Morris JS, Ohman A, Dolan RJ: Conscious and unconscious emotional learning in the human amygdala. Nature 393:467–470, 1998b

Morris JS, Scott SK, Dolan RJ: Saying it with feeling: neural responses to emotional vocalizations. Neuropsychologia 37:1155–1163, 1999

Morris JS, Buchel C, Dolan RJ: Parallel neural responses in amygdala subregions and sensory cortex during implicit fear conditioning. Neuroimage 13:1044–1052, 2001

Pavlov IP: Conditioned Reflexes. New York, Dover, 1927

Phelps EA, O'Connor KJ, Gatenby JC, et al: Activation of the left amygdala to a cognitive representation of fear. Nat Neurosci 4:437–441, 2001

Phillips ML, Young AW, Senior C, et al: A specific neural substrate for perceiving facial expressions of disgust. Nature 389:495–498, 1997

Phillips ML, Young AW, Scott SK, et al: Neural responses to facial and vocal expressions of fear and disgust. Proc R Soc Lond B Biol Sci 265:1809–1817, 1998

Phillips ML, Medford N, Young AW, et al: Time courses of left and right amygdalar responses to fearful facial expressions. Hum Brain Mapp 12:193–202, 2001

Pine DS, A. Fyer A, Grun J, et al: Methods for developmental studies of fear conditioning circuitry. Biol Psychiatry 50:225–228, 2001

Price JL, Amaral DG: An autoradiographic study of the projections of the central nucleus of the monkey amygdala. J Neurosci 1:1242–1259, 1981

Ramnani N, Toni I, Josephs O, et al: Learning- and expectation-related changes in the human brain during motor learning. J Neurophysiol 84:3026–3035, 2000

Razran G: The observable unconscious and the inferable conscious in current Soviet psychophysiology: interoceptive conditioning, semantic conditioning, and the orienting reflex. Psychol Rev 68:87–89, 1961

Rescorla RA, Heth CD: Reinstatement of fear to an extinguished conditioned stimulus. J Exp Psychol Anim Behav Process 1:88–96, 1975

Scott SK, Young AW, Calder AJ, et al: Impaired auditory recognition of fear and anger following bilateral amygdala lesions. Nature 385:254–257, 1997

Takeuchi Y, McLean JH, Hopkins DA: Reciprocal connections between the amygdala and parabrachial nuclei: ultrastructural demonstration by degeneration and axonal transport of horseradish peroxidase in the cat. Brain Res 239:583–588, 1982

Talairach J, Tournoux P: Co-planar Stereotaxic Atlas of the Human Brain. New York, Thieme Medical, 1988

Whalen PJ, Rauch SL, Etcoff NL, et al: Masked presentations of emotional facial expressions modulate amygdala activity without explicit knowledge. J Neurosci 18:411–418, 1998a

Whalen PJ, Bush G, McNally RJ, et al: The emotional counting Stroop paradigm: a functional magnetic resonance imaging probe of the anterior cingulate affective division. Biol Psychiatry 44:1219–1228, 1998b

Wright CI, Fischer H, Whalen PJ, et al: Differential prefrontal cortex and amygdala habituation to repeatedly presented emotional stimuli. Neuroreport 12:379–383, 2001

Zald DH, Pardo JV: Emotion, olfaction, and the human amygdala: amygdala activation during aversive olfactory stimulation. Proc Natl Acad Sci U S A 94:4119–4124, 1997

8

Neuroimaging Studies in Nonhuman Primates Reared Under Early Stressful Conditions

Implications for Mood and Anxiety Disorders

Sanjay J. Mathew, M.D.
Dikoma C. Shungu, Ph.D.
Xiangling Mao, M.S.
Leonard A. Rosenblum, Ph.D.
Jeremy D. Coplan, M.D.
Jack M. Gorman, M.D.

A major challenge in psychiatric research is the development of animal models that are useful in developing pathophysiological conceptualizations of illness. Nonhuman primate studies offer useful guides toward building a comprehensive neurobiology of the range of normal and impaired fear and anxiety responses, although they are necessarily limited as homologous disease models of human disorders (Gorman et al. 2002). For the past 30 years, our primate behavioral laboratory has studied the bonnet macaque (*Macaca radiata*), a highly gregarious species that exhibits stable adult and maternal-infant relationships, demonstrates both cooperative and competitive interactions, and manifests playful interactions throughout infancy and adolescence (Coplan et al. 1995). On the other hand, when individual or group pressures are applied, these social

The authors wish to thank Shirne Baptiste, Douglas Rosenblum, Manuel de al Nuez, Eric Smith, Mark Perera, Holly Lisanby, and Lawrence Kegeles for their valuable contributions to this work.

interactions can break down, with increases in hostility, hierarchical relations, and individual stress (Mathew et al. 2001). Following imposition of environmental stressors, systematic behavioral change has been observed in these primates (Andrews and Rosenblum 1991a, 1991b; Rosenblum and Paully 1984), whose mediating neurobiology is experimentally accessible (Coplan et al. 1996). This particular primate model (termed variable foraging demand [VFD]) has potential relevance to human psychiatric disorders marked by fearful avoidance of social interaction, separation anxiety, and depressive affect, and is potentially useful in its suggestion that early insecure maternal attachment may shift behavior and neurobiology toward a traitlike socially anxious and timid profile.

This chapter reviews the major behavioral and biological abnormalities reported in the VFD primate, and then discusses findings from more recent neuroimaging investigations utilizing proton magnetic resonance spectroscopic imaging (^{1}H MRSI) and volumetric magnetic resonance imaging (MRI). The brain regions initially investigated in these studies—the medial temporal lobe and anterior cingulate—reflect these regions' presumed importance in the mediation of emotional and cognitive processes in a variety of animal species (Allman et al. 2001; McEwen 2000). Future areas of investigation involving additional brain regions of interest, such as the corpus striatum, and utilizing newer neuroimaging modalities, such as diffusion tensor imaging (DTI), are then discussed. The ultimate goal of this series of nonhuman primate neuroimaging experiments is to develop viable neuroanatomical models of social behavior as a function of early adverse rearing stress conditions, with potential applicability to human mood and anxiety disorders.

THE VARIABLE FORAGING DEMAND MODEL

Rosenblum and Paully (1984) found that exposing nursing mothers to unpredictable foraging demand conditions induced unstable patterns of attachment to their infants, resulting in a wide range of persistent behavioral and neurobiological abnormalities in the offspring. In this model, genetically random, group-living mother-infant dyads are placed in environments where the mother is confronted with alternating 2-week periods in which ample food is readily obtainable with little or no effort (low foraging demand [LFD]) and in which food, although still ample, requires considerably more time and effort to obtain (high foraging demand [HFD]). Control subjects face only LFD conditions over a comparable period, and both groups are on ad libitum feeding before and after the experimental conditions. Six to eight 2-week alterations in foraging demand in the VFD subjects provide a level of salient environmental uncertainty that alters normal maternal response patterns, with profound consequences for the offspring. All subjects are permanently separated from their mothers and maintained in peer groups at 1 year of age.

BEHAVIORAL AND BIOLOGICAL ABNORMALITIES IN VFD PRIMATES

Grown primates raised under VFD conditions, in comparison with predictably reared control subjects, showed stable increases in levels of social timidity, including behaviors such as social subordination, avoidance of agonistic encounters, and decreased species-typical huddling (Andrews and Rosenblum 1991b). Other disturbances evident in VFD subjects at various stages of development include greater expression of depressive episodes upon maternal separation, diminished autonomous functioning, and decreased exploratory behavior when challenged by novel stimuli. This cluster of behaviors is closely akin to the description of young children manifesting as "behaviorally inhibited to the unfamiliar" (Kagan et al. 1987, p. 1459), who are predisposed to developing a range of anxiety disorders (Hirshfeld et al. 1992). Thus, the VFD model suggests that early environmental rearing stress conditions may shift behavior toward a trait-like social inhibition profile.

Investigations of the brain neurochemistry in VFD-reared subjects have revealed specific abnormalities in biological systems important in stress responsivity and affect regulation. Overlapping with the cohorts of VFD-reared subjects from the behavioral studies described previously, VFD-reared subjects showed sustained elevations in cisternal cerebrospinal fluid (CSF) corticotropin-releasing factor (CRF) concentrations into young adulthood (Coplan et al. 2001), replicating earlier findings from the same subjects in juveniles (Coplan et al. 1996). Moreover, significant within-group stability of CRF over a 30-month period was noted within the longitudinally assessed VFD-reared group (Coplan et al. 2001). Despite high levels of juvenile CSF CRF, these VFD subjects showed lower CSF cortisol levels (Coplan et al. 1996), a pattern of abnormalities observed in some studies of posttraumatic stress disorder (PTSD) (Yehuda et al. 1995). Elevations of CSF CRF in juvenile VFD subjects were positively correlated with contemporaneous levels of CSF somatostatin, as well as the metabolites of serotonin (5-hydroxyindoleacetic acid [5-HIAA]) and dopamine (homovanillic acid [HVA]) (Coplan et al. 1998). Finally, VFD subjects displayed exaggerated behavioral responses to the noradrenergic probe yohimbine and blunted behavioral responses to the 5-hydroxytryptamine (5-HT) probe *m*-chlorophenylpiperazine (Rosenblum et al. 1994). The overall suggestion from these neurochemical and neurohormonal data is that early rearing disturbances in nonhuman primates produce enduring changes in biogenic amines and components of the hypothalamic-pituitary-adrenal (HPA) axis resembling many of the abnormalities seen in humans who suffer from pathological anxiety and mood disorders.

RATIONALE FOR NEUROIMAGING STUDIES IN VFD PRIMATES

Although the aforementioned studies suggest broad neurobiological impairments into adulthood as a consequence of early adverse rearing stress conditions, very little was deduced from these initial CSF and challenge studies about the specific brain regions pathologically implicated in the VFD primate. Guided by various rodent (Helmeke et al. 2001a, 2001b), primate (Czeh et al. 2001; Lyons et al. 2001), and human clinical studies (De Bellis et al. 2000) of early stressful experiences, initial neuroanatomical investigations of VFD focused on the anterior cingulate cortex and the medial temporal lobe, which contains key structures such as the hippocampus. Neuroimaging investigations in VFD primates offer several advantages over clinical patient populations in developing a functional anatomy of early adverse rearing stress: 1) the ready potential for repeated longitudinal neuroimaging and social-behavioral assessments that can be controlled over the primate's lifetime; 2) the absence of confounding influences of medication, disease comorbidity, substance abuse, and family history (controlled for by random assignment to rearing groups) on measures of neuronal structure and integrity; and 3) the potential for guided postmortem studies that would enable correlations of developmental brain imaging findings, behavior, and neuropathology. Indeed, terminal neuropathological investigations of VFD primates, including analyses of neurogenesis, glial proliferation, and hippocampal mossy fiber sprouting, have the potential to offer important histological correlates of in vivo neuroimaging findings with broad applicability to many neurological and psychiatric conditions.

PROTON MAGNETIC RESONANCE SPECTROSCOPIC IMAGING

^{1}H MRSI is a brain imaging technique that provides a noninvasive means of quantifying endogenous brain chemistry and examining regional cellular energetics and function in living subjects. Employing the physical principles used in MRI, ^{1}H MRSI routinely measures several chemical spe-

cies, including *N*-acetyl aspartate (NAA); choline; the combination of glutamate, glutamine, and gamma-aminobutyric acid (GABA), designated Glx; myoinositol; and creatine. Initial VFD primate studies have employed ^{1}H MRSI, in contrast to phosphorus magnetic resonance spectroscopy (MRS) methods, due to ^{1}H MRSI's greater applicability to measurements of neuronal integrity, much greater sensitivity, and better spatial resolution (Henry et al. 2001).

The major ^{1}H MRS metabolites investigated in the VFD primate are as follows:

- NAA is a cell marker whose concentration correlates with neuronal density (Barker 2001). The precise role of NAA is controversial, but it has been speculated to be a source of acetyl groups for lipid synthesis, a regulator of protein synthesis, a storage form of acetyl-CoA or aspartate, an osmolyte, and a breakdown product of *N*-acetyl-aspartyl glutamate (Barker 2001). A reduction in NAA concentration has been interpreted most commonly as a marker for neuronal loss, even in the absence of volumetric MRI reduction, as recently shown in adult PTSD (Schuff et al. 2001). Perhaps the most apt description of NAA is an "in vivo marker of neurometabolic fitness, reflecting a level of neural viability that can recover after insult" (Valenzuela and Sachdev 2001, p. 593).

- The choline resonance reflects a pool of choline composed of acetylcholine and the by-products of phosphatidylcholine hydrolysis, phosphocholine and glycerophosphocholine. Abnormalities in the choline resonance have been linked to abnormalities in myelination, cerebral oxidative metabolism, intraneuronal signaling, or endocrine status (Jung et al. 2002). Because choline is found in much higher concentrations in oligodendrocytes and astrocytes than in neurons (Urenjak et al. 1993), one interpretation of choline elevations is glial proliferation, or gliosis.

- Glutamate is the predominant compound in the MRSI resonance designated Glx (Prost et al. 1997), which also contains the amino acid derivatives glutamine and GABA. Because there is growing preclinical evidence that glutamatergic neurotransmission is heightened in several brain regions during stressful periods, and that enhanced glutamate release could contribute to glucocorticoid-induced neurotoxicity (Moghaddam 2002; Moghaddam et al. 1994), assessments of the MRSI Glx resonance might be informative in illuminating the potential role of persistent glutamate excitotoxicity in brain regions vulnerable to stress-induced damage following adverse early rearing.

Likewise, NAA and choline might be particularly sensitive to perturbations in stress conditions, as was demonstrated in adult male tree
shrews exposed to chronic psychosocial stress (an animal model reported to have high validity for major depression), which resulted in
significantly decreased whole brain concentrations of NAA and choline (Czeh et al. 2001).

* Creatine reflects systemic energy use and storage, and is generally held
to be an internal standard in ratio analyses of neurometabolic change
(Ross and Michaelis 1994).

RATIONALE FOR INVESTIGATIONS OF MEDIAL TEMPORAL LOBE AND ANTERIOR CINGULATE

The medial temporal lobe, with voxels centered on the hippocampus, and
the anterior cingulate, two structures composing Papez's circuit (Papez
1937), an anatomical circuit believed to subserve emotional experience,
were selected as the initial regions of interest. On the basis of neuroimaging data suggestive of regionally specific neuronal vulnerability as a function of early traumatic experiences (De Bellis et al. 2000) and experimental data suggesting direct neurotoxic effects of CRF in the hippocampus
(Brunson et al. 2001), a decreased NAA/creatine ratio was predicted in
the medial temporal lobe and anterior cingulate in a group of adult male
bonnet macaques who had undergone VFD stress rearing conditions approximately 10 years previously in infancy, reflecting impaired neuronal
metabolism and function. In addition, reductions in hippocampal volume
in VFD-reared subjects were hypothesized, presumably reflective of glucocorticoid and excitatory amino acid (glutamate) contributions to neuronal
cell death. These regionally specific hypotheses would suggest long-term
morphological and functional deficits in vulnerable hippocampal neurons
as a function of stressful early rearing conditions, a pattern of neuroanatomical deficits found in adult PTSD (Bremner et al. 1997; Schuff et al.
2001; Stein et al. 1997).

Neuroimaging investigations in PTSD have revealed a convergence of
structural and functional abnormalities involving cortical regions such as
the anterior cingulate, as well as the hippocampus (reviewed in Pitman et
al. 2001). Regarding hippocampal function, at least two clinical reports in
adult PTSD have documented reductions in NAA in hippocampal or medial temporal lobe regions in the absence of morphometric MRI deficits
(Freeman et al. 1998; Schuff et al. 2001). Schuff et al. (2001) speculated that
the decreased hippocampal NAA in the absence of volume deficits might

reflect glial proliferation that attenuates potential volumetric effects of atrophy detectable on MRI. Bremner et al. (1999a) also reported decreased blood flow in the right hippocampus in adult women with a history of childhood sexual abuse. In the VFD primate, previous CSF investigations (Coplan et al. 1996, 2001) suggested that a primary mediating factor contributing to hippocampal dysfunction might be excessive CRF. Notably, administration of corticotropin-releasing hormone (CRH) to the brains of immature rats was associated with a progressive loss of hippocampal CA3 neurons and exuberant growth of mossy fibers, which are the axons of the dentate gyrus granule cells that normally innervate the CA3 neurons (Brunson et al. 2001).

For the anterior cingulate, we utilized a MRSI sequence allowing for determination of the Glx resonance, hypothesizing that VFD-reared subjects would concomitantly display both elevations in Glx/creatine and lowered NAA/creatine concentrations compared with normal control subjects. A convergence of preclinical data points to the importance of alterations in GABA and glutamatergic neurotransmission in the anterior cingulate in early rearing stress conditions. For example, maternally deprived and socially isolated rodents were found to have a significant decrease in nicotinamide adenine dinucleotide phosphate (NADPH)-diphorase-reactive neurons in the anterior cingulate (Poeggel et al. 1999, 2000). These neurons have been found to be GABAergic, suggestive of reduced GABA inhibitory function in this region. This same research laboratory has extensively studied the trumpet-tailed rat *(Octodon degus)* and found that disturbances of the early emotional environment (parental deprivation and social isolation) significantly elevated spine densities on the basal dendrites in dorsal anterior cingulate cortex, suggestive of elevated excitatory synaptic input in this brain region (Helmeke et al. 2001a, 2001b). Primary malfunctioning of glutamate and/or GABA neurotransmission in the anterior cingulate, which is contained in the medial prefrontal cortex (mPFC), might have neuroendocrine consequences. Decreased GABA inhibitory projections from the mPFC to the amygdala (and/or increased glutamatergic input to amygdala) might render the CRF-rich central nucleus of the amygdala hyperactive, which would result in the persistent CRF elevations noted in VFD primates (Coplan et al. 2001).

Because the majority of the Glx resonance is composed of glutamate, heightened Glx in VFD-reared primates was hypothesized, reflecting the increasing evidence that activation of the HPA axis (as observed in VFD primates) is mediated in part by heightened glutamate neurotransmission in the prefrontal cortex (Moghaddam 2002). Heightened Glx might also be consistent with the notion that a diffuse excitatory influence in VFD subjects may account for the tandem increases in the various neurochemicals correlating with CSF CRF (Coplan et al. 1998). Alternatively, heightened Glx resonance in the anterior cingulate might also reflect alterations in GABA levels at a field strength of 1.5 T (Auer et al. 2000). Clinically, convergent data support the notion of impairments of anterior cingulate function in trauma-related conditions. A MRSI study in children with abuse-related PTSD was consistent with decreased NAA/creatine in the anterior cingulate (De Bellis et al. 2000), and several neuroimaging studies suggest a diminished regional CBF (rCBF) in the anterior cingulate in the presence of emotionally relevant stimuli in PTSD (Bremner et al. 1999b; Shin et al. 2001).

PROTON MAGNETIC RESONANCE SPECTROSCOPIC IMAGING FINDINGS IN VFD-REARED PRIMATES

All studies were conducted on a 1.5 T General Electric Signa magnetic resonance system using the multislice method of Duyn et al. (1993). Subjects were scanned under anesthesia induced by an intramuscular injection of althesin, a neurosteroid. Spectra were quantified using a nonlinear least-squares fitting algorithm, by an operator blind to subject rearing group. Of the 22 subjects undergoing examinations, viable scans were obtained for 19 subjects (10 VFD, 9 control).

Figure 8–1 displays a representative MRSI spectrum of a VFD subject obtained from the medial temporal lobe. The major finding from this region is that the choline/creatine ratios in the medial temporal lobe (averaged across both hemispheres) were significantly elevated in VFD subjects compared with control subjects. Contrary to the initial hypotheses, there were no significant rearing group differences in medial temporal lobe NAA/creatine ratios. There was a significant positive correlation between the NAA/creatine and choline/creatine ratios in this region.

In the anterior cingulate, short-echo time analyses allowed derivation of the Glx resonance, in addition to the other metabolites described. In this region, the male VFD subjects, approximately 10 years after the initial stress paradigm, displayed significantly decreased NAA/creatine and increased Glx/creatine ratios in the anterior cingulate, compared with age- and gender-matched normal control subjects, with no overlap between groups (Figure 8–2).

Among all subjects, there was a significant negative correlation between the NAA/creatine and Glx/creatine ratios in the anterior cingulate. The choline/creatine ratio in the anterior cingulate did not differ between

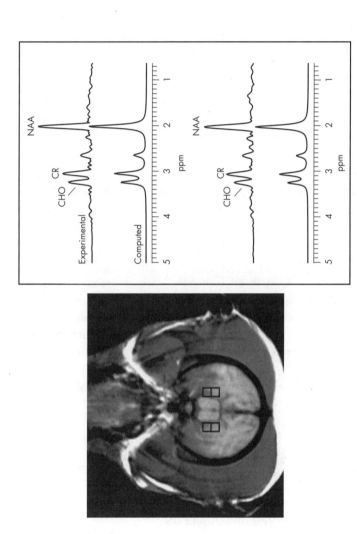

FIGURE 8–1　　Representative proton magnetic resonance (^{1}H MR) spectra from two voxels covering the medial temporal lobe. Experimentally measured spectrum and component resonance curves were selected to obtain nonlinear least-squares fit to experimental curves. Resonance spectral peaks identified are *N*-acetyl aspartate (NAA), choline (CHO), and creatine (CR). ppm = parts per million.

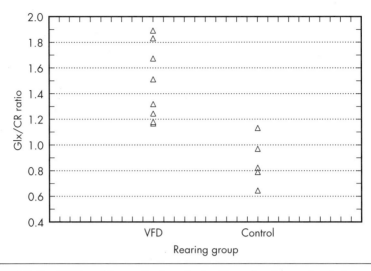

FIGURE 8–2 VFD subjects displayed significantly elevated Glx/creatine ratios compared with age-matched control subjects in the anterior cingulate, approximately 10 years after the initiation of the early rearing stressor. Glx = glutamate/glutamine/GABA, Cr = creatine, VFD = variable foraging demand.

rearing groups; however, with the removal of one outlier control subject, the VFD group displayed significantly elevated choline/creatine ratios compared with the control group. There was a significant negative correlation between the NAA/creatine and choline/creatine ratios in this region, in contrast to the positive correlation observed in the medial temporal lobe.

In summary, highly significant MRSI differences between VFD and control primates were observed in two brain regions deemed important in regulating emotional experiences, approximately 10 years after the initial adverse rearing stressor. These preliminary neuroimaging findings add to the growing evidence of traitlike neurobiological and behavioral abnormalities in VFD-reared primates.

MRI VOLUMETRY OF THE VFD HIPPOCAMPUS

The main rationale for volumetric investigations in conjunction with MRSI studies is to generate hypotheses about the relationship between baseline morphometry and neuronal metabolic function derived from MRSI. If, for example, NAA reductions were observed in the absence of volume loss (as observed in the hippocampus in PTSD subjects [Schuff et al. 2001]), this profile would be suggestive of neuronal metabolic impairments without neuronal loss. Another interpretation of this finding might be the presence of reactive glial proliferation, which would attenuate atrophy as detected on volumetric MRI, but not affect NAA concentration, because NAA is thought to be neuron specific (Birken and Oldendorf 1989).

Preliminary analyses of the VFD volumetric data failed to reveal significant hippocampal volumetric differences in this region between the VFD and control subjects, results that are consistent with reports showing negative hippocampal volumetric MRI differences in primates undergoing early stressful conditions (Lyons et al. 2001; Sanchez et al. 1998). Further volumetric studies with larger samples of differentially reared primates are necessary before more definitive conclusions can be drawn.

FUTURE DIRECTIONS

Investigations of Corpus Striatum

There are two primary future directions regarding neuroimaging studies in VFD primates: 1) the addition of striatal subregions as a region of interest, and 2) the use of multimodal imaging, particularly the novel use of DTI in the primate cohort. Because the complex social-behavioral and affective processes described in the VFD are clearly not localizable to just one brain region or circuit, it is imperative to examine other regions that might play a pivotal role in mediating reward-related processing of social and cognitive stimuli. We are thus particularly interested in examining the corpus striatum, a key component of the basal ganglia that has been implicated in a host of anxiety and mood conditions in humans. The striatum receives projections from neurons of the entire cerebral cortex and thalamus, as well as dopaminergic projections from the substantia nigra compacta, and serotonergic fibers from the dorsal raphe nuclei of the midbrain (Gonzalo et al. 2001). Additionally, several types of interneurons within the striatum have been described, with varied neurotransmitter and neuropeptide expression (Kawaguchi et al. 1995).

Recent high-spatial-resolution positron emission tomography (PET) studies have permitted improved delineation of striatal subregions in human (Drevets et al. 2001; Kegeles et al. 2002) and nonhuman primates (Drevets et al. 1999). The anteroventral striatum (AVS) is composed of nucleus accumbens, ventromedial caudate, and anteroventral putamen, and the dorsal striatum (DS) is composed of dorsal caudate and putamen. As discussed by Drevets et al. (2001), the AVS is innervated by the amygdala and the prefrontal cortical regions involved in reward-related and emotional processing, whereas the DS receives afferent connections primarily from cortical areas involved in sensorimotor function. Distinguishing across striatal subregions has enabled recent understanding about the relationships between regional dopaminergic tone and euphoria (Drevets et al. 2001) and cognitive functioning (Mozley et al. 2001), processes germane to social behavioral regulation. High-resolution MRI acquisitions that enable striatal subregion identification, employed in PET co-registration protocols (Mawlawi et al. 2001), can be utilized in the bonnet macaque.

The overlap between the AVS and the accumbens, a region implicated in brain reward mechanisms and the reinforcing aspects of drugs of abuse, suggests a hypothesis related to the observed baseline differences in social affiliative behaviors across members of the same species. Insel and Winslow (1999) have suggested that the neural substrates of social attachment are those pathways that couple social recognition (as manifested by olfactory, auditory, and visual stimuli) with the neural pathways for reinforcement, principally the dopaminergic projections from the ventral tegmental area to the nucleus accumbens and prefrontal cortex. Pathological conditions associated with impaired social dexterity and contingently appropriate social responses, as has been suggested in social anxiety disorder (Stein 1998), have been hypothesized to be related to dopaminergic dysfunction within reinforcement/reward pathways that subserve prosocial, affiliative behavior. At least two single photon emission computed tomography (SPECT) studies in social anxiety disorder have found deficits of dopaminergic innervation into the striatum (Schneier et al. 2000; Tiihonen et al. 1997), whereas an early MRSI study reported abnormalities in choline and NAA in striatal subregions, including caudate (Davidson et al. 1993). A recent functional MRI (fMRI) study in normal subjects further suggests that ventral striatal regions are involved in the evaluation of stimuli relevant to social interaction, such as eye gaze (Kampe et al. 2001). Thus, high-resolution neuroimaging examinations of striatal subregions offers the potential of characterizing the neurobiological underpinnings of social reward systems (and indirectly, dopaminergic function) in VFD-reared primates.

Diffusion Tensor Imaging

Preliminary data showing significant elevations in the choline/creatine resonance in two brain regions in VFD primates has prompted an exploration of strategies to explain this finding's significance in socially mediated processes.

A potential novel approach to this question is offered by DTI, a MRI technique that allows investigation of neural structural integrity, including white matter structures such as myelin (Steel et al. 2001). The choline resonance in MRSI includes precursors and breakdown products of myelin, and has been speculated to reflect greater myelin turnover (Jung et al. 1999). In further support of this hypothesis are the developmental changes observed in constituents of the choline resonance (such as phosphorylcholine and phosphorylethanolamine) that are linked to developmental myelination (Bluml et al. 1999). If VFD primates have increased choline resonance due to abnormal myelin turnover, DTI can test this notion directly, because it provides a noninvasive tool to quantitatively examine white matter organization. Measures of diffusion anisotropy (the DTI index of neuronal structural integrity) can be correlated with related measures from other modalities, such as the NAA concentration in MRSI (Steel et al. 2001). Investigations of potential white matter structural abnormalities in VFD subjects, resulting in "miswiring" of frontal-striatal-limbic connections, provide another level of functional analysis beyond morphometry and neurochemistry. These multimodal imaging studies can be used to guide subsequent postmortem investigations of brain structural pathology in striatum and the other regions, including anterior cingulate and hippocampus.

CONCLUSIONS

Nonhuman primate models of stressful early rearing have provided important clues regarding how an organism's early emotional environment may be a predisposing factor toward subsequent psychopathology. Neuroimaging studies in differentially reared nonhuman primates affords the opportunity to correlate brain structure and function with contemporaneous behavioral measures, CSF and plasma neurochemistry, and other relevant biological measures. Perhaps most important, these studies offer the potential of correlating in vivo neuroimaging data with directive postmortem analyses to enable a fuller understanding of the neuroanatomical basis of complex measures such as NAA and choline.

REFERENCES

Allman JM, Hakeem A, Erwin JM, et al: The anterior cingulate cortex: the evolution of an interface between emotion and cognition. Ann N Y Acad Sci 935:107–117, 2001

Andrews MW, Rosenblum LA: Dominance and social competence in differentially reared bonnet macaques, in Primatology Today: XIIIth Congress of the International Primatological Society. Edited by Ehara A. Amsterdam, Elsevier, 1991a, pp 347–350

Andrews MW, Rosenblum LA: Attachment in monkey infants raised in variable- and low-demand environments. Child Dev 62:686–693, 1991b

Auer DP, Putz B, Kraft E, et al: Reduced glutamate in the anterior cingulate cortex in depression: an in vivo proton magnetic resonance spectroscopy study. Biol Psychiatry 47:305–313, 2000

Barker PB: *N*-acetyl aspartate—a neuronal marker? Ann Neurol 49:423–424, 2001

Birken DL, Oldendorf WH: *N*-acetyl-L-aspartic acid: a literature review of a compound prominent in ¹H-NMR spectroscopic studies of brain. Neurosci Biobehav Rev 13:23–31, 1989

Bluml S, Seymour KJ, Ross BD: Developmental changes in choline- and ethanolamine-containing compounds measured with proton-decoupled 31P MRS in in vivo human brain. Magn Reson Med 42:653–654, 1999

Bremner JD, Randall P, Vermetten E, et al: MRI-based measurement of hippocampal volume in posttraumatic stress disorder related to childhood physical and sexual abuse: a preliminary report. Biol Psychiatry 41:23–32, 1997

Bremner JD, Narayan M, Staib L, et al: Neural correlates of memories of childhood sexual abuse in women with and without posttraumatic stress disorder. Am J Psychiatry 156:1787–1795, 1999a

Bremner JD, Staib L, Kaloupek D, et al: Neural correlates of exposure to traumatic pictures and sounds in Vietnam combat veterans with and without posttraumatic stress disorder (PTSD): a positron emission tomography study. Biol Psychiatry 45:806–816, 1999b

Brunson KL, Eghbal-Ahmadi M, Bender R, et al: Long-term, progressive hippocampal cell loss and dysfunction induced by early life administration of corticotropin-releasing hormone reproduce the effects of early life stress. Proc Natl Acad Sci U S A 98:8856–8861, 2001

Coplan JD, Rosenblum LA, Gorman JM: Primate models of anxiety: longitudinal perspectives. Psychiatr Clin North Am 18:727–743, 1995

Coplan JD, Andrews MW, Rosenblum LA, et al: Persistent elevations of cerebrospinal fluid concentrations of corticotropin-releasing factor in adult nonhuman primates exposed to early life stressors: implications for the pathophysiology of mood and anxiety disorders. Proc Natl Acad Sci U S A 93:1619–1623, 1996

Coplan, JD, Trost, RC, Owens MJ, et al: Cerebrospinal fluid concentrations of somatostatin and biogenic amines in grown primates reared by mothers exposed to manipulated foraging conditions. Arch Gen Psychiatry 55:473–477, 1998

Coplan JD, Smith ELP, Altemus M, et al: Variable foraging demand: sustained elevations in cisternal cerebrospinal fluid corticotropin releasing factor concentrations in adult primates. Biol Psychiatry 50:200–204, 2001

Czeh B, Michaelis T, Watanabe T, et al: Stress-induced changes in cerebral metabolites, hippocampal volume, and cell proliferation are prevented by antidepressant treatment with tianeptine. Proc Natl Acad Sci U S A 98:12796–12801, 2001

Davidson JR, Krishnan KR, Charles HC, et al: Magnetic resonance spectroscopy in social phobia: preliminary findings. J Clin Psychiatry 54 (suppl):19–25, 1993

De Bellis MD, Keshavan MS, Spencer S, et al: *N*-acetylaspartate concentration in the anterior cingulate of maltreated children and adolescents with PTSD. Am J Psychiatry 157:1175–1177, 2000

Drevets WC, Price JC, Kupfer DJ, et al: PET measures of amphetamine-induced dopamine release in ventral versus dorsal striatum. Neuropsychopharmacology 21:694–709, 1999

Drevets WC, Gautier C, Price JC, et al: Amphetamine-induced dopamine release in human ventral striatum correlates with euphoria. Biol Psychiatry 49:81–96, 2001

Duyn JH, Gillen J, Sobering G, et al: Multisection proton MR spectroscopic imaging of the brain. Radiology 188:277–282, 1993

Freeman TW, Cardwell D, Karson CN, et al: In vivo proton magnetic resonance spectroscopy of the medial temporal lobes of subjects with combat-related posttraumatic stress disorder. Magn Reson Med 40:66–71, 1998

Gonzalo N, Moreno A, Erdozain MA, et al: A sequential protocol combining dual neuroanatomical tract-tracing with the visualization of local circuit neurons within the striatum. J Neurosci Methods 111:59–66, 2001

Gorman JM, Mathew S, Coplan J: Neurobiology of early life stress: nonhuman primate models. Semin Clin Neuropsychiatry 7:96–103, 2002

Helmeke C, Ovtscharoff W, Poeggel G, et al: Juvenile emotional experience alters synaptic inputs on pyramidal neurons in the anterior cingulate cortex. Cereb Cortex 11:717–727, 2001a

Helmeke C, Poeggel G, Braun K: Differential emotional experience induces elevated spine densities on basal dendrites of pyramidal neurons in the anterior cingulate cortex of Octodon degus. Neuroscience 104:927–931, 2001b

Henry ME, Frederick BD, Moore CM, et al: Magnetic resonance spectroscopy in psychiatric illness, in Psychiatric Neuroimaging Research: Contemporary Strategies. Edited by Dougherty DD, Rauch SL. Washington, DC, American Psychiatric Press, 2001, pp 291–333

Hirshfeld DR, Rosenbaum JF, Biederman J, et al: Stable behavioral inhibition and its association with anxiety disorder. J Am Acad Child Adolesc Psychiatry 31:103–111, 1992

Insel TR, Winslow JT: The neurobiology of social attachment, in Neurobiology of Mental Illness. Edited by Charney DS, Nestler EJ, Bunney BS. New York, Oxford University Press, 1999, pp 880–890

Jung RE, Brooks WM, Yeo RA, et al: Biochemical markers of intelligence: a proton MR spectroscopy study of normal human brain. Proc R Soc Lond B Biol Sci 266:1375–1379, 1999

Jung RE, Yeo RA, Love TM, et al: Biochemical markers of mood: a proton magnetic resonance spectroscopy study of normal human brain. Biol Psychiatry 51:224–229, 2002

Kagan J, Reznick JS, Snidman N: The physiology and psychology of behavioral inhibition in children. Child Dev 58:1459–1473, 1987

Kampe KK, Frith CD, Dolan RJ, et al: Reward value of attractiveness and gaze. Nature 413:589, 2001

Kawaguchi Y, Wilson CJ, Augood SJ, et al: Striatal interneurones: chemical, physiological and morphological characterization. Trends Neurosci 18:527–535, 1995

Kegeles LS, Martinez D, Kochan LD, et al: NMDA antagonist effects on striatal dopamine release: positron emission tomography studies in humans. Synapse 43:19–29, 2002

Lyons DM, Yang C, Sawyer-Glover AM, et al: Early life stress and inherited variation in monkey hippocampal volumes. Arch Gen Psychiatry 58:1145–1151, 2001

Mathew SJ, Coplan JD, Gorman JM: Neurobiological mechanisms of social anxiety disorder. Am J Psychiatry 158:1558–1567, 2001

Mawlawi O, Martinez D, Slifstein M, et al: Imaging human mesolimbic dopamine transmission with positron emission tomography, I: accuracy and precision of D2 receptor parameter measurements in ventral striatum. J Cereb Blood Flow Metab 21:1034–1057, 2001

McEwen BS: Effects of adverse experiences for brain structure and function. Biol Psychiatry 48:721–731, 2000

Moghaddam B: Stress activation of glutamate neurotransmission in the prefrontal cortex: implications for dopamine-associated psychiatric disorders. Biol Psychiatry 51:775–787, 2002

Moghaddam B, Bolinao ML, Stein-Behrens B, et al: Glucocorticoids mediate the stress-induced extracellular accumulation of glutamate. Brain Res 655:251–254, 1994

Mozley LH, Gur RC, Mozley PD, et al: Striatal dopamine transporters and cognitive functioning in healthy men and women. Am J Psychiatry 158:1492–1499, 2001

Papez J: A proposed mechanism of emotion. Arch Neurol Psychiatry 38:725–743, 1937

Pitman RK, Shin LM, Rauch SL: Investigating the pathogenesis of posttraumatic stress disorder with neuroimaging. J Clin Psychiatry 62 (suppl 17):47–54, 2001

Poeggel G, Lange E, Hase C, et al: Maternal separation and early social deprivation in *Octodon degus:* quantitative changes of nicotinamide adenine dinucleotide phosphate-diaphorase-reactive neurons in the prefrontal cortex and nucleus accumbens. Neuroscience 94:497–505, 1999

Poeggel G, Haase C, Gulyaeva N, et al: Quantitative changes in reduced nicotinamide adenine dinucleotide phosphate-diaphorase-reactive neurons in the brain of *Octodon degus* after periodic maternal separation and early social isolation. Neuroscience 99:381–387, 2000

Prost R, Mark L, Mewissen M, et al: Detection of glutamate/glutamine resonances by ^{1}H magnetic resonance spectroscopy at 0.5 tesla. Magn Reson Med 37:615–618, 1997

Rosenblum LA, Paully GS: The effects of varying environmental demands on maternal and infant behavior. Child Dev 55:305–314, 1984

Rosenblum LA, Coplan JD, Friedman S, et al: Adverse early experiences affect noradrenergic and serotonergic functioning in adult primates. Biol Psychiatry 35:221–227, 1994.

Ross BD, Michaelis T: Clinical applications of magnetic resonance spectroscopy. Magn Reson Q 10:191–247, 1994

Sanchez MM, Hearn EF, Do D, et al: Differential rearing affects corpus callosum size and cognitive function in rhesus monkeys. Brain Res 812:38–49, 1998

Schneier FR, Liebowitz MR, Abi-Dargham A, et al: Low dopamine D2 receptor binding potential in social phobia. Am J Psychiatry 157:457–459, 2000

Schuff N, Neylan TC, Lenoci MA, et al: Decreased hippocampal *N*-acetylaspartate in the absence of atrophy in posttraumatic stress disorder. Biol Psychiatry 50:952–959, 2001

Shin LM, Whalen PJ, Pitman R, et al: An fMRI study of anterior cingulate function in posttraumatic stress disorder. Biol Psychiatry 50:932–942, 2001

Steel RM, Bastin ME, McConnell S, et al: Diffusion tensor imaging (DTI) and proton magnetic resonance spectroscopy (1H MRS) in schizophrenic subjects and normal controls. Psychiatry Research: Neuroimaging 106:161–170, 2001

Stein MB: Neurobiological perspectives on social phobia: from affiliation to zoology. Biol Psychiatry 44:1277–1285, 1998

Stein MB, Koverola C, Hanna C, et al: Hippocampal volume in women victimized by childhood sexual abuse. Psychol Med 27:951–959, 1997

Tiihonen J, Kuikka J, Bergstrom K, et al: Dopamine reuptake site densities in patients with social phobia. Am J Psychiatry 154:239–242, 1997

Urenjak J, Williams SR, Gadian DG, et al: Proton nuclear magnetic resonance spectroscopy unambiguously identifies different neural cell types. J Neurosci 13:981–989, 1993

Valenzuela MJ, Sachdev P: Magnetic resonance spectroscopy in AD. Neurology 56:592–598, 2001

Yehuda R, Boisoneau D, Lowy MT, Giller EL Jr: Dose-response changes in plasma cortisol and lymphocyte glucocorticoid receptors following dexamethasone administration in combat veterans with and without posttraumatic stress disorder. Arch Gen Psychiatry 52:583–593, 1995

9

Neurotoxic Effects of Childhood Trauma

Magnetic Resonance Imaging Studies of Pediatric Maltreatment-Related Posttraumatic Stress Disorder Versus Nontraumatized Children With Generalized Anxiety Disorder

Michael D. De Bellis, M.D., M.P.H.

Maltreatment during childhood, defined as neglect, physical abuse, sexual abuse, or emotional maltreatment, constitutes a chronic and extreme childhood stress. Furthermore, for the child victim, various forms of maltreatment tend to coexist (Kaufman et al. 1994; Levy et al. 1995; McGee et al. 1995; Widom 1989). Child maltreatment is a common contributor to child and adult mental illness (Felitti et al. 1998).

Posttraumatic stress disorder (PTSD) is commonly seen in maltreated children, especially during the period immediately following maltreatment disclosure (Famularo et al. 1996; McLeer et al. 1998). PTSD is a debilitating chronic mental illness with enormous social and economic costs (Kessler 2000). As described in DSM-IV-TR, the essential feature (criterion A) of PTSD is exposure to an extreme traumatic stressor in which the person experienced, witnessed, or was confronted with events that involved actual or threatened death or serious injury, or a threat to the physical integrity of self or others; and responded with intense fear, helplessness, horror, or, in children, disorganized or agitated behaviors (American Psychiatric Association

This work was supported by National Institute of Mental Health grant 5 K08 MH01324-02 (M.D.D., Principal Investigator) and a 1998 National Alliance for Research on Schizophrenia and Depression Young Investigator Award (M.D.D., Principal Investigator).

2000). The diagnosis of PTSD is made when criterion A is experienced and when three clusters of categorical symptoms—intrusive reexperiencing of the trauma(s) (criterion B), persistent avoidance of stimuli associated with the trauma(s) (criterion C), and persistent symptoms of increased physiological arousal (criterion D)—are present for more than 1 month after the traumatic event(s).

Children are more likely to be diagnosed with PTSD after experiencing trauma than their adult counterparts (Fletcher 1996). The diagnostic picture of PTSD in children and adolescents is similar to that in adults (De Bellis 1997), with the exception of children younger than 4 years, in whom identification of symptoms is based on observable behaviors instead of relying only on a child's verbal report (Scheeringa et al. 1995). Maltreated children and adolescents manifest high rates of PTSD symptoms, depression, suicidal thoughts and behaviors, aggressive and antisocial behaviors, and cognitive deficits (for a review, see De Bellis 2001). Furthermore, sub–disorder-level PTSD symptoms are commonly seen in victims of childhood maltreatment (Armsworth and Holaday 1993; Famularo et al. 1994; Hillary and Schare 1993; Mannarino et al. 1994; Wolfe and Charney 1991; Wolfe et al. 1994). Even children with sub–disorder-level PTSD symptoms show substantial functional impairment and distress (Carrion et al. 2001b).

PTSD is an anxiety disorder. The causes of the high rates of anxiety and mood disorders in maltreated children are both familial/genetic and environmental. Increased rates of mood and anxiety disorders are found in parents involved in their children's maltreatment (De Bellis et al. 2001a; Famularo et al. 1992; Kaplan et al. 1983). However, some scientists believe that child abuse is causally and independently related to increased risk for disorders in adulthood. For example, a study of twins discordant for child abuse exposure demonstrated that even after controlling for family background and parental psychopathology, the twin exposed to abuse was subject to an increased risk for adult psychopathology (Kendler et al. 2000). Consequently, maltreatment is seen as a most extreme form of dysfunctional family and interpersonal functioning on a continuous spectrum of adverse life circumstances and dysfunctional relationships. Maltreated children grow under the psychological influence of chronic stress. This stress is associated with neurobiological differences between maltreated and non-maltreated individuals. These neurobiological differences likely contribute to psychopathology.

On the other hand, anxiety disorders are a common form of childhood psychopathology. Pediatric generalized anxiety disorder (GAD) affects approximately 6% of American children (Shaffer et al. 1996). The essential symptoms of GAD are intrusive uncontrollable worry about everyday life circumstances and social competence, and associated autonomic hyperarousal. Kagan's concept of behavioral inhibition to the unfamiliar is thought to be an extreme inherent temperamental trait (Kagan et al. 1988). Behaviorally inhibited children have increased sympathetic tone, increased excretion of urinary catecholamines after completion of cognitive tasks, and higher levels of baseline and laboratory salivary cortisol measures compared with control subjects (Kagan et al. 1988). In prospective investigations, behaviorally inhibited children were shown to be predisposed to generalized social anxiety (Schwartz et al. 1999) and to depression (Caspi et al. 1996).

Consequently, pediatric PTSD and GAD share the following characteristics: genetic/familial predispositions, a later vulnerability to anxiety and mood disorders, an inability to control upsetting thoughts, and physiological hyperarousal. In this chapter, we review current research findings on the neurobiology of childhood maltreatment and maltreatment-related PTSD (for a more extensive review see De Bellis 2001). We compare these findings to those of nontraumatized children who suffer from GAD. The data to be presented support evidence for adverse brain development in maltreatment-related pediatric PTSD, whereas children with GAD may have an inherent dysmorphometry of neurobiological structures implicated in anxiety disorders. This dysmorphometry may represent a vulnerability to childhood GAD.

THE NEUROBIOLOGY OF ANXIETY

Several neurobiological systems are implicated in anxiety disorders. These include subcortical structures (amygdala and related nuclei and circuitry) and cortical structures (medial prefrontal cortex, superior temporal gyrus [STG], and right hemisphere).

The amygdala consists of several cell groups and many efferent projections involved in fear and anxiety. The functional anatomy of anxiety disorders is complex. Most studies to date are preclinical. Direct projections from the central nucleus of the amygdala to a variety of regions (lateral hypothalamus and paraventricular nucleus, parabrachial nucleus, the ventral tegmental area, the locus ceruleus, central gray, nucleus reticularis pontis caudalis, and trigeminal and facial nerve) are associated with many fearful and anxious behaviors (for a review, see Davis 1997; see also Chapter 1, "Synaptic Self: Conditioned Fear, Developmental Adversity, and the Anxious Individual"). In primate studies, the amygdala is involved in social inhibition (see Chapter 14, "The Amygdala and Social Behavior: What's Fear Got to Do With It?"). Results from human neuroimaging studies suggest that bilateral amygdala activation is involved in the color naming of threat words (Isenberg et al. 1999), during viewing of masked fearful faces (Whalen et al. 1998), and during both conditioned fear acquisition and extinction in healthy subjects (LaBar et al. 1998). In the latter study, this activation was right-hemisphere dominant.

The amygdala and its projections to the STG, thalamus, and prefrontal cortex are thought to constitute the neural basis of our abilities to interpret others' behavior in terms of mental states (e.g., thoughts, intentions, desires, beliefs). This process has also been called theory of mind or social intelligence (Brothers 1990). The STG and amygdala are involved in processing social information (see Chapter 14, "The Amygdala and Social Behavior: What's Fear Got to Do With It?"; Baron-Cohen et al. 1999). Apprehensive expectations in patients with GAD usually involve social and or personal concerns (e.g., worries about work or school performance, worries about appearance or what others think of them). In primate studies, the STG is involved in identifying facial expressions (Desimone 1991; Hasselmo et al. 1989). In a human functional magnetic resonance imaging (MRI) study, the amygdala, STG, and prefrontal cortex were activated during the performance of a social intelligence task in healthy volunteers (Baron-Cohen et al. 1999). Based on studies of experimental conditioning, the STG is thought to be involved in higher cognitive processing of the fear experience and modulation of amygdala activity (Quirk et al. 1997).

The prefrontal cortex is activated during novel or dangerous situations (Posner and Petersen 1990). LeDoux has shown that the medial prefrontal cortex inhibits activation of the amygdala and related nuclei and circuitry (see Chapter 1, "Synaptic Self: Conditioned Fear, Developmental Adversity, and the Anxious Individual"; LeDoux 1998). The anterior cingulate cortex, a region of the medial prefrontal cortex, is involved in the extinction of conditioned fear responses and has been implicated in the pathophysiology of PTSD (for a review, see Hamner et al. 1999). Recent neuroimaging studies provide evidence for medial prefrontal and anterior cingulate dysfunction in adult PTSD and other anxiety disorders (for a review, see De Bellis 2001 and Rauch et al. 1997). The role of the medial prefrontal cortex and PTSD is discussed in more detail later in this chapter. See Figure 9–1.

Finally, there is a substantial literature indicating the involvement of the right cerebral hemisphere in social processing and anxiety. The right hemisphere is involved in identifying facial expressions (Etcoff 1986). Several studies have demonstrated right-sided prefrontal activation in temperamentally

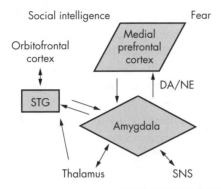

FIGURE 9–1 Schematic of two neurobiological systems implicated in anxiety disorders.

DA=dopamine, NE = norepinephrine, SNS = sympathetic nervous system, STG = superior temporal gyrus.

fearful monkeys (Kalin et al. 1998) and in behaviorally inhibited children (for a review, see Kagan et al. 1988). Behaviorally inhibited children are predisposed to develop childhood anxiety disorders (Kagan and Snidman 1999). Several electroencephalography investigations have shown greater electrical activity in the right hemisphere of anxious and anxious/depressed adults, especially greater posterior right-hemispheric activity in persons with high-trait anxiety (Davidson et al. 1999; Heller et al. 2000; Keller et al. 2000; Stapleton et al. 1997).

The neurodevelopment of childhood anxiety disorders is not well understood. To date, there are few published neuroimaging studies of pediatric anxiety disorders. In light of these research studies, studies of children with anxiety disorders who have no histories of traumatic life events offer an opportunity to apply translational thinking to clinical studies. The core symptoms of GAD are exaggerated worry about social circumstances and associated autonomic hyperactivity. Interestingly, nontraumatized children with GAD were found to have dysmorphometry of the amygdala and the STG. In one study, children and adolescents with GAD were found to have significantly larger right and total amygdala volumes than healthy comparison subjects (De Bellis et al. 2000a). Intracranial, cerebral, and cerebral gray and white matter volumes; right and left temporal lobe, hippocampal, caudate, and putamen volumes; and total corpus callosum area and its comparison regional measures did not differ between groups. In another study, nontraumatized children and adolescents with GAD were found to have significantly larger total gray matter and white matter STG volumes than healthy comparison subjects whereas prefrontal cortex and thalamus volumes did not differ between groups (De Bellis et al. 2002c). There was a more pronounced right > left asymmetry in total and white matter STG volumes in GAD subjects compared with control subjects. Furthermore, the STG white matter percentage asymmetry index correlated significantly with child reports of anxiety symptoms. Although these were pilot studies and more research on this topic is warranted, right-sided dysmorphometry of the amygdala and the STG may index some genetic trait such as increased sensitivity to social or threat cues, which could create a vulnerability for pediatric GAD. However, each pediatric anxiety disorder subtype may have its own unique neurobiology. We now review and contrast the neurobiology of pediatric maltreatment-related PTSD.

THE NEUROBIOLOGY OF PEDIATRIC MALTREATMENT TRAUMA

There is little research on the neurobiological effects of maltreatment or of PTSD in developing children and adolescents. Studies of the neurobiological effects of stress in laboratory animal models and of the psychobiology of adult PTSD are critically important because these studies provide comparative models. Cannon (1929) was the first to demonstrate the "fight or flight or freeze" reaction in response to life-threatening stress. He showed that either physical or emotional stress triggered the same response from an organism. This response involves activation of the peripheral sympathetic nervous system (SNS). Hans Selye then studied the effects of chronic stress on the hypothalamic-pituitary-adrenal (HPA) axis and the immune system and postulated the idea of "homeostatic balance." Selye said that successful coping to a stressor is followed by a restoration of homeostatic balance, and unsuccessful adaptation may result in significant deviations from this normative balance (Selye 1973). McEwen went further and called the latter balance "allostasis," an equilibrium that places severe strain on an organism that may be impossible to sustain indefinitely (see Chapter 2, "Does Stress Damage the Brain?"; McEwen 1995). Contemporary theories of the neurobiology of stress and PTSD have been extensively reviewed (Friedman et al. 1995). PTSD symptoms are thought to be mediated by dysregulation of biological stress systems (e.g., the neural circuits and neurotransmitter and neuroendocrine stress systems) that mediate the fear or anxiety response. The main physiological mechanisms for coping with stress and fear are extensive and are described throughout this book. These systems are interconnected at many levels to coordinate the individual's responses and adaptations to acute and chronic environmental stressors. In this chapter, we briefly review only the locus ceruleus–norepinephrine/SNS or catecholamine system and the limbic-hypothalamic-pituitary-adrenal (LHPA) axis. These major neurobiological stress response systems significantly influence arousal, stress reactions, emotional regulation, and physical, cognitive, and brain development.

A brief review of these major biological stress response systems is important because 1) these are the major systems implicated in anxiety and mood disorders (for a review, see Charney et al. 1999); 2) there are pharmacological treatments to target these systems (De Bellis et al. 1999a); and 3) alcohol and various illicit substances also "self-medicate" or target these systems by damping hyperarousal or dysregulated biological stress system(s), contributing to the high rates of teenage substance abuse in maltreated individuals (for a review, see De Bellis 2002). An understanding of the psychobiology of maltreatment may also lead to early psychotherapeutic and psychopharmacological treatment, and early treatment can lead to secondary prevention of the chronic mental disorders and the comorbidity commonly seen in maltreated children.

Traumatic stress is perceived by our senses as overwhelming fear. Interpersonal traumatic reminders (e.g., adults physically or verbally fighting, a loud voice, a particular facial expression, or the face of a perpetrator) can lead to PTSD reexperiencing and intrusive symptoms through the learning mechanisms of classical conditioning. The initial fear response is associated with the original fear-producing stimuli or stressor (unconditioned stimuli). However, the traumatic anxiety is associated with the conditioned stimuli, also known as the "traumatic reminders or triggers." These fear-associated sensory inputs are relayed through the thalamus and to primary sensory cortical brain regions (i.e., occipital [vision] and temporal [auditory]). These brain regions project to the amygdala, which in turn projects to the locus ceruleus and the hypothalamus.

Accordingly, traumatic stress increases the activity of the locus ceruleus, the major catecholamine- or norepinephrine-containing nucleus in the brain. Activation of locus ceruleus neurons increases norepinephrine in specific brain regions (locus ceruleus, hypothalamus, hippocampus, amygdala, and cerebral cortex). Traumatic stress also results in the simultaneous activation of another very basic and ancient cell body, the paragigantocellularis (for a review, see Aston-Jones et al. 1994). The paragigantocellularis has major inputs to the locus ceruleus but also controls and activates the SNS, causing the biological changes of the "fight or flight or freeze" reaction. The locus ceruleus, via its connections through the amygdala, activates the LHPA axis. Therefore, intense fear or anxiety activates the amygdala, which in turn activates the hypothalamus, and hypothalamic corticotropin-releasing hormone (CRH) (or factor [CRF]) is released. CRH activates the LHPA axis by stimulating the pituitary to secrete adrenocorticotropic hormone (ACTH), but CRH also activates cortical brain regions. These events promote cortisol release from the adrenal gland, reciprocally stimulate the SNS, and centrally cause behavioral activation and intense arousal (for a review, see Chrousos and Gold 1992). These processes lead to direct and indirect effects of the "fight or flight or freeze" reaction, including increases in heart rate, blood pressure, metabolic rate, alertness, and circulating catecholamines (epinephrine, norepinephrine, and dopamine). Other effects include dilated pupils; sweating; inhibition of renal sodium excretion; redistribution of the blood to the heart, brain, and skeletal muscle and away from skin, gut, and kidneys; enhanced blood coagulation as a result of increased platelet aggregability; increased glycogenolysis; and increased metabolic rate and alertness. Activation of the catecholamine system and CRH in animals results in behaviors consistent with PTSD cluster D symptoms of anxiety, such as hyperarousal and hypervigilance. In summary, traumatic stress causes increases in catecholamines and CRH in the body and the brain.

BIOLOGICAL STRESS RESPONSE SYSTEMS AND HUMAN DEVELOPMENT

Traumatized children and adults manifest dysregulation of biological stress response systems (for a review, see De Bellis 2001). Hence, it is not surprising that traumatized children and adults with or without PTSD evidence this dysregulation, at baseline, when confronted with "traumatic triggers" and novel life stressors. Adult combat veterans with PTSD have elevated levels of central CRH (Baker et al. 1999; Bremner et al. 1997). Additionally, adults with PTSD have elevated 24-hour urinary excretion of catecholamines (Southwick et al. 1995). Depressed women with histories of child abuse evidence autonomic hyperarousal at baseline and hypersensitivity of the LHPA axis in response to a social stressor (Heim et al. 2000). These data provide evidence of dysregulation in baseline functioning of the CRH and the catecholamine system in adult PTSD (for a review, see Southwick et al. 1998).

Although limited, the psychobiological data in maltreated children and adolescents suggest that those with mood and anxiety symptoms (i.e., PTSD symptoms) show evidence of elevated LHPA axis and catecholamine activity. Results from pediatric studies suggest that maltreated children have hypersecretion of CRH. These include findings of hypersecretion of morning cortisol in sexually abused girls (Putnam et al. 1991),

dysregulation of the diurnal 24-hour cortisol rhythm in depressed maltreated children (Hart et al. 1996; Kaufman 1991), and lower baseline
ACTH and blunted ACTH response to ovine CRH in dysthymic sexually
abused girls (De Bellis et al. 1994a). A recent study identified significantly
greater concentrations of urinary free cortisol over 24 hours in medication-naïve children with maltreatment-related PTSD than in non-maltreated healthy comparison subjects (De Bellis et al. 1999a). In another recent study, higher levels of salivary cortisol throughout the day were found
in children with maltreatment-related PTSD or subthreshold PTSD compared with archival control subjects (Carrion et al. 2002).

Results from pediatric studies suggest that maltreated children show
evidence of enhanced catecholamine activity. These include findings of
greater 24-hour urinary norepinephrine concentrations in neglected depressed males (Queiroz et al. 1991) and greater 24-hour urinary catecholamine and catecholamine metabolite concentrations in dysthymic
sexually abused girls (De Bellis et al. 1994b). Children and adolescents
with maltreatment-related PTSD show evidence of increased catecholamine activity. Findings of decreased platelet adrenergic receptors and
increased heart rate following orthostatic challenge in physically and sexually abused children with PTSD compared with non-maltreated subjects
were reported (Perry 1994). A recent study identified significantly greater
concentrations of urinary dopamine and norepinephrine concentrations
over 24 hours in medication-naïve children with maltreatment-related
PTSD than in nontraumatized children with GAD and healthy control
children (De Bellis et al. 1999a). In the latter study, all children adhered
to a low-monoamine diet for 3 days prior to and on the day of the 24-hour
catecholamine collection. Therefore, catecholamine activity in pediatric
PTSD may differ from that in pediatric GAD.

FEAR, BIOLOGICAL STRESS SYSTEMS, AND THE DEVELOPING BRAIN

Birth to adulthood is marked by progressive changes in brain maturation.
Although these processes are influenced primarily by genetics, positive
and negative environmental experiences also play an important role. In
the developing brain, elevated levels of catecholamines and cortisol may
lead to adverse brain development through the mechanisms of accelerated
loss (or metabolism) of neurons (Edwards et al. 1990; Sapolsky et al. 1990;
Simantov et al. 1996; Smythies 1997), delays in myelination (Dunlop et al.
1997), abnormalities in developmentally appropriate pruning (Lauder
1988; Todd 1992), or the inhibition of neurogenesis (Gould et al. 1997,

1998; Tanapat et al. 1998). Furthermore, stress decreases brain-derived neurotrophic factor expression (Smith et al. 1995). Accordingly, the chronic stress of child maltreatment experiences may have adverse influences on a child's brain development. Understanding these complexities may be the key to understanding pediatric maltreatment-related PTSD as well as the brain developmental, cognitive functioning, and psychopathological consequences of childhood maltreatment.

Until recently, investigators have generally studied childhood brain function with psychoeducational instruments (i.e., intelligence and achievement tests). The results of these studies suggest that maltreated children demonstrate a variety of intellectual and academic impairments, including lower IQ (Augoustinos 1987; Carrey et al. 1995; Money et al. 1983; Perez and Widom 1994; Pianta et al. 1989; Trickett et al. 1994). However, studies applying neuropsychological methods suggest that children and adolescents with PTSD show deficits in executive functioning and attention (Beers and De Bellis 2002) and everyday memory (Moradi et al. 1999).

More recently, MRI has provided a safe and novel approach to measure brain maturation in healthy and psychologically traumatized living children. To date, fewer than 10 studies involving maltreated children have been reported. The results of these studies suggest that child abuse-related PTSD is associated with adverse brain development. These include findings of smaller intracranial and cerebral volumes, smaller total midsagittal area and middle and posterior regions of the corpus callosum, and larger lateral ventricular volumes than in nonabused control subjects (De Bellis et al. 1999b). In this research study, 43 maltreated children and adolescents with PTSD and 61 matched control subjects underwent comprehensive clinical assessments and an anatomical MRI brain scan (De Bellis et al. 1999b). Maltreated subjects with PTSD had 7.0% smaller intracranial volumes and 8.0% smaller cerebral volumes than control subjects. The total midsagittal area of the corpus callosum, the major interconnection between the two hemispheres that is broadly conceptualized as facilitating intercortical communication, and the middle and posterior regions of the corpus callosum were smaller in abused subjects. In contrast, right, left, and total lateral ventricles were proportionally larger than controls, after adjustment for intracranial volume. Intracranial volume robustly correlated positively with age at onset of PTSD trauma (i.e., smaller cerebral volumes were associated with earlier onset of trauma) and negatively with duration of abuse. The positive correlation of intracranial volumes with age at onset of PTSD trauma suggests that traumatic stress is associated with disproportionately negative consequences if it occurs during early childhood. The negative correlation of intracranial volumes with abuse duration suggests that childhood maltreatment has global adverse influences on brain development that may be cumulative. Symptoms of intrusive thoughts, avoidance, hyperarousal, and dissociation correlated positively with ventricular volume, and negatively with intracranial volume and total corpus callosum and regional measures.

There was some indication that maltreated males with PTSD show more evidence of adverse brain development than maltreated females with PTSD. A significant sex by diagnosis effect revealed greater total corpus callosum area reduction and trends for smaller cerebral volume and corpus callosum region 6 (isthmus) in maltreated males with PTSD compared with maltreated females with PTSD (De Bellis et al. 1999b). These findings suggest that males are more vulnerable to the effects of severe stress in global brain structures than females. However, both males and females showed evidence of adverse brain development. Thus, the overwhelming stress of child maltreatment experiences may have adverse influences on a child's brain maturation. In another study from a separate research group, smaller brain and cerebral volumes and attenuation of frontal lobe asymmetry in children with maltreatment-related PTSD or subthreshold PTSD were found compared with archival control subjects (Carrion et al. 2001a). However, these two MRI studies did not control for low socioeconomic status, which may also influence brain maturation through ecological variables. In another study from our group, which controlled for socioeconomic status, 28 psychotropic-naïve children and adolescents with abuse-related PTSD and 66 sociodemographically similar healthy control subjects underwent comprehensive clinical assessments and anatomical MRI brain scans (De Bellis et al. 2002b). Subjects with PTSD had smaller intracranial, cerebral and prefrontal cortex, prefrontal cortical white matter, and right temporal lobe volumes and areas of the corpus callosum and its subregions (2, 4, 5, 6, and 7) and larger frontal lobe CSF volumes than control subjects. The total midsagittal area of corpus callosum and middle and posterior regions remained smaller, whereas right, left, and total lateral ventricular and frontal lobe CSF volumes were proportionally larger than in control subjects, after adjustment for cerebral volume. Brain volumes were positively correlated with age at onset of PTSD trauma and negatively correlated with duration of abuse. Significant sex by group effect demonstrated greater lateral ventricular volume increases in maltreated males with PTSD than in maltreated females with PTSD. Unlike findings in adult PTSD, in all three cross-sectional studies and one longitudinal pediatric PTSD study (De Bellis et al. 2001b), no hippocampal differences were seen. Instead global differences were seen. Findings of decreased intracranial volumes and cerebral volumes in maltreated children with PTSD may be indicative of neuronal loss associated with severe stress. This process may be associated with the global developmental deficits and pervasive emotional and behavioral problems commonly seen in maltreated children and adolescents with anxiety and mood disorders. Consequently, these data provide further evidence that maltreatment-related PTSD and subthreshold PTSD are associated with adverse brain development. These data also suggest that male children may be more vulnerable to these effects (De Bellis et al. 1999b, 2002b).

However, PTSD is an anxiety disorder. Unlike the findings discussed earlier in children and adolescents with non–trauma-related GAD (De Bellis et al. 2000a, 2002c), maltreated children and adolescents with PTSD showed global adverse brain development and no anatomical changes in limbic (hippocampal or amygdala) structures (Carrion et al. 2001a; De Bellis et al. 1999b, 2001b, 2002b). These results provide indirect evidence that PTSD in maltreated children may be regarded as a complex, environmentally induced developmental disorder. In these cross-sectional studies, however, causal relationships between maltreatment, psychiatric symptoms, and brain changes cannot be ascertained. An important mission for the field of developmental traumatology research is to unravel these complex interactions. One method of examining these differences is to study the subcortical structures (amygdala and related nuclei and circuitry) as well as cortical structures (medial prefrontal cortex, STG, and right hemisphere) implicated in pediatric anxiety disorders.

THE PREFRONTAL CORTEX, SUPERIOR TEMPORAL GYRUS, AND PEDIATRIC POSTTRAUMATIC STRESS DISORDER

Exposure to mild to moderate uncontrollable stress particularly impairs prefrontal cortical function according to studies of humans and animals (for a review, see Arnsten and Goldman-Rakic 1998). Severe stress and the associated increased activation of catecholamines (especially norepinephrine and dopamine) can "turn off" frontal inhibition of the limbic system, leading to anxiety symptoms (for a review, see Arnsten 1998). Impairment of prefrontal cortical functioning has profound effects on thinking and decision making, and may be responsible not only for PTSD symptoms but also for the lower IQ and cognitive impairments seen in adults with PTSD (Macklin et al. 1998) and the prefrontal cognitive deficits seen in pediatric maltreatment-related PTSD (Beers and De Bellis 2002; Perez and Widom 1994).

Recent neuroimaging studies provide evidence for medial prefrontal and anterior cingulate dysfunction in adult PTSD. Positron emission tomography

(PET) investigations comparing women who had been sexually abused as children and who had PTSD with women with similar history who did not have PTSD found a lower level of anterior cingulate blood flow during traumatic reminder imagery (Shin et al. 1999) and during recalled memories of sexual abuse (Bremner et al. 1999a). A lower level of anterior cingulate blood flow has also been seen in Vietnam combat veterans with PTSD compared with those without PTSD during traumatic reminder exposure to combat imagery (Bremner et al. 1999b). In these studies, subjects with PTSD activated the amygdala but not the medial frontal cortex, whereas subjects without PTSD activated the medial frontal cortex but did not show the same degree of amygdala activation.

PET investigations are currently not feasible in developing children. However, new technologies, such as magnetic resonance spectroscopy (MRS), a safe and novel approach, have been used to study the in vivo neurochemistry of the medial frontal cortex in the brains of living children. The N-acetyl signal in the proton (^{1}H) spectrum consists mainly of N-acetyl aspartate (NAA) and is considered a marker of neuronal integrity. Decreased NAA concentrations are associated with increased metabolism and loss of neurons (for a review, see Prichard 1996). A preliminary investigation suggested that maltreated children and adolescents with PTSD have lower NAA/creatine ratios compared with sociodemographically matched control subjects (De Bellis et al. 2000b). These findings suggest neuronal loss in the anterior cingulate region of the medial prefrontal cortex and were not specific to the gender of the child and adolescent subjects. Neuronal loss in the anterior cingulate of pediatric PTSD patients is consistent with the adult neuroimaging studies, which provide evidence for medial prefrontal and anterior cingulate dysfunction in adult PTSD. Interestingly, studies of adult primates whose mothers underwent a variable foraging demand paradigm during their early development also showed decreased NAA in the prefrontal cortex as well as dysregulation of the LHPA axis and increased central CRH (see Chapter 3, "Neuropsychobiology of the Variable Foraging Demand Paradigm in Nonhuman Primates," and Chapter 8, "Neuroimaging Studies in Nonhuman Primates Reared Under Early Stressful Conditions: Implications for Mood and Anxiety Disorders").

The STG is a relatively large and complex cortical region. Maltreated but medically healthy children and adolescents with a diagnosis of PTSD had significantly larger unadjusted STG gray matter volumes and smaller STG white matter volumes than comparison subjects (De Bellis et al. 2002a). After adjustment for differences in cerebral volume, right, left, and total STG volumes were found to be larger in PTSD subjects compared with control subjects. Regression analysis showed that PTSD subjects had significantly greater gray matter volumes in most, and particularly right-sided, STG measurements. Furthermore, findings of significant side by diagnosis interactions for STG and STG gray but not white matter volumes suggest that there is a more pronounced right > left asymmetry in total and posterior STG volumes, but a lack of the left > right asymmetry seen in total, anterior, and posterior STG gray matter volumes in PTSD compared with control subjects. These data suggest developmental alterations in the STG in pediatric PTSD. The finding of a relatively large brain structure in maltreated children and adolescents with PTSD, who had previously reported smaller intracranial, cerebral, and corpus callosum structures, is interesting and is similar to the findings in pediatric GAD (De Bellis et al. 2002c). However, the nature of the larger STG differed between pediatric subjects with PTSD (STG gray matter asymmetry) and GAD (STG white matter asymmetry). The STG is involved in processing social information, and maltreatment is a social trauma. "Traumatic triggers" in maltreated children are interpersonal in nature (e.g., raised or lowered tone of voice, facial expressions). Thus, social cues may trigger PTSD symptoms of hypervigilance. The STG is involved in the temporolimbic and neocortical association circuits, which have reciprocal connections. Therefore, one may speculate that auditory traumatic reminders outside a maltreated child's conscious awareness may lead to enhanced anxiety and hypervigilance, and behavioral dyscontrol. Taken together, these preliminary STG findings suggest complex developmental alterations in pediatric GAD and PTSD. See Figure 9–2.

CONCLUSIONS

MRI studies to date provide indirect evidence that PTSD in maltreated children may be regarded as a complex, environmentally induced developmental disorder. In contrast, GAD in nontraumatized children may represent an inherent propensity for larger right amygdala volume and "connectivity" to larger STG volume, creating some predispositional trait such as increased sensitivity to social cues with anxious arousal. Thus, maltreated children with PTSD may be "conditioned" to be more fearful of social cues. Future anatomical and functional MRI brain studies of childhood GAD and PTSD and of children at risk for anxiety disorders, which target medial prefrontal cortex, STG, amygdala, and other brain regions involved in processing social cues, and of the relationship of these findings to symptoms and cognitive function are warranted. Because we now know that there is neurogenesis in the primate brain (Gould et al. 1999), effective

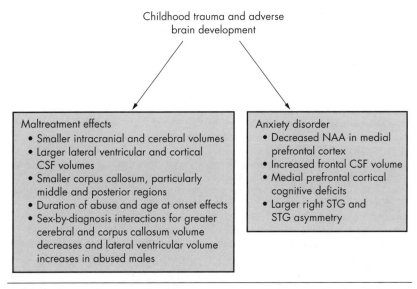

FIGURE 9–2   Outline of the complexities of MRI findings in developmental traumatology.

Pediatric maltreatment-related PTSD is associated with findings of adverse (global) brain development as well as findings associated with dysmorphometry in the neurobiological regions implicated in anxiety disorders. CSF = cerebrospinal fluid, NAA = *N*-acetyl aspartate, STG = superior temporal gyrus.

treatments for maltreatment-related anxiety and depressives disorders are an important area for future investigations regarding therapeutic reversibility. Although early trauma may be toxic to the human brain, early interventions could attenuate these changes. When rescued from extremely neglectful and abusive environments, some profoundly delayed maltreated children have been found to be capable of accelerated rates of catch-up growth, including remission of severe psychopathology and normalization of cognitive function (Koluchova 1972, 1976; Money et al. 1983). Brain maturation studies in traumatized and nontraumatized children with anxiety disorders are noninvasive and timely.

REFERENCES

American Psychiatric Association: Diagnostic and Statistical Manual of Mental Disorders, 4th Edition, Text Revision. Washington, DC, American Psychiatric Association, 2000

Armsworth MW, Holaday M: The effects of psychological trauma on children and adolescents. J Couns Dev 72:49–56, 1993

Arnsten AFT: The biology of being frazzled. Science 280:1711–1712, 1998

Arnsten AFT, Goldman-Rakic PS: Noise stress impairs cortical function: evidence for a hyperdopaminergic mechanism. Arch Gen Psychiatry 55:362–368, 1998

Aston-Jones G, Valentino RJ, Van Bockstaele EJ, et al: Locus coeruleus, stress, and PTSD: neurobiological and clinical parallels, in Catecholamine Function in Posttraumatic Stress Disorder: Emerging Concepts. Washington, DC, American Psychiatric Press, 1994, pp 17–62

Augoustinos M: Developmental effects of child abuse: a number of recent findings. Child Abuse Negl 11:15–27, 1987

Baker DG, West SA, Nicholson WE, et al: Serial CSF corticotropin-releasing hormone levels and adrenocortical activity in combat veterans with posttraumatic stress disorder. Am J Psychiatry 156:585–588, 1999

Baron-Cohen S, Ring HA, Wheelwright S, et al: Social intelligence in the normal and autistic brain: an fMRI study. Eur J Neurosci 11:1891–1898, 1999

Beers SR, De Bellis MD: Neuropsychological function in children with maltreatment-related posttraumatic stress disorder. Am J Psychiatry 159:483–486, 2002

Bremner JD, Licinio J, Darnell A, et al: Elevated CSF corticotropin-releasing factor concentrations in posttraumatic stress disorder. Am J Psychiatry 154:624–629, 1997

Bremner JD, Narayan M, Staib L, et al: Neural correlates of memories of childhood sexual abuse in women with and without posttraumatic stress disorder. Am J Psychiatry 156:1787–1795, 1999a

Bremner JD, Staib L, Kaloupek D, et al: Neural correlates of exposure to traumatic pictures and sound in Vietnam combat veterans with and without posttraumatic stress disorder: a positron emission tomography study. Biol Psychiatry 45:806–816, 1999b

Brothers L: The social brain: a project for integrating primate behavior and neurophysiology in a new domain. Concepts in Neuroscience 1:27–51, 1990

Cannon WB: The wisdom of the body. Physiol Rev 9:399–431, 1929

Carrey NJ, Butter HJ, Persinger MA, et al: Physiological and cognitive correlates of child abuse. J Am Acad Child Adolesc Psychiatry 34:1067–1075, 1995

Carrion VG, Weems CF, Eliez S, et al: Attenuation of frontal asymmetry in pediatric posttraumatic stress disorder. Biol Psychiatry 50:943–951, 2001a

Carrion VG, Weems CF, Ray RD, et al: Toward an empirical definition of pediatric PTSD: the phenomenology of PTSD symptoms in youth. J Am Acad Child Adolesc Psychiatry 41:166–173, 2001b

Carrion VG, Weems CF, Ray RD, et al: Diurnal salivary cortisol in pediatric posttraumatic stress disorder. Biol Psychiatry 51:575–582, 2002

Caspi A, Moffitt TE, Newman DL, et al: Behavioral observations at age 3 years predict adult psychiatric disorders. Arch Gen Psychiatry 53:1033–1039, 1996

Charney DS, Nestler EJ, Bunney BS: Neurobiology of Mental Illness. New York, Oxford University Press, 1999

Chrousos GP, Gold PW: The concepts of stress and stress system disorders: overview of physical and behavioral homeostasis. JAMA 267:1244–1252, 1992

Davidson RJ, Abercrombie H, Nitschke JB, et al: Regional brain function, emotion and disorders of emotion. Curr Opin Neurobiol 9:228–234, 1999

Davis M: Neurobiology of fear responses: the role of the amygdala. J Neuropsychiatry Clin Neurosci 9:382–402, 1997

De Bellis MD: Posttraumatic stress disorder and acute stress disorder, in Handbook of Prevention and Treatment With Children and Adolescents. Edited by Ammerman RT, Hersen M. New York, Wiley, 1997, pp 455–494

De Bellis MD: Developmental traumatology: the psychobiological development of maltreated children and its implications for research, treatment, and policy. Dev Psychopathol 13:537–561, 2001

De Bellis MD: Developmental traumatology: a contributory mechanism for alcohol and substance use disorders. Psychoneuroendocrinology 27:155–170, 2002

De Bellis MD, Chrousos GP, Dorn LD, et al: Hypothalamic-pituitary-adrenal axis dysregulation in sexually abused girls. J Clin Endocrinol Metab 78:249–255, 1994a

De Bellis MD, Lefter L, Trickett PK, et al: Urinary catecholamine excretion in sexually abused girls. J Am Acad Child Adolesc Psychiatry 33:320–327, 1994b

De Bellis MD, Baum A, Birmaher B, et al: Developmental traumatology, part I: biological stress systems. Biol Psychiatry 45:1259–1270, 1999a

De Bellis MD, Keshavan M, Clark DB, et al: Developmental traumatology, part II: brain development. Biol Psychiatry 45:1271–1284, 1999b

De Bellis MD, Casey BJ, Dahl R, et al: A pilot study of amygdala volumes in pediatric generalized anxiety disorder. Biol Psychiatry 48:51–57, 2000a

De Bellis MD, Keshavan MS, Spencer S, et al: N-acetylaspartate concentration in the anterior cingulate in maltreated children and adolescents with PTSD. Am J Psychiatry 157:1175–1177, 2000b

De Bellis MD, Broussard E, Wexler S, et al: Psychiatric co-morbidity in caregivers and children involved in maltreatment: a pilot research study with policy implications. Child Abuse Negl 25:923–944, 2001a

De Bellis MD, Hall J, Boring AM, et al: A pilot longitudinal study of hippocampal volumes in pediatric maltreatment-related posttraumatic stress disorder. Biol Psychiatry 50:305–309, 2001b

De Bellis MD, Keshavan M, Frustaci K, et al: Superior temporal gyrus volumes in maltreated children and adolescents with PTSD. Biol Psychiatry 51:544–552, 2002a

De Bellis M.D, Keshavan M, Shifflett H, et al: Brain structures in pediatric maltreatment-related posttraumatic stress disorder: a sociodemographically matched study. Biol Psychiatry 52:1066–1078, 2002b

De Bellis MD, Keshavan M, Shifflett H, et al: Superior temporal gyrus volumes in pediatric generalized anxiety disorder. Biol Psychiatry 51:553–562, 2002c

Desimone R: Face-selective cells in the temporal cortex of monkeys. J Cogn Neurosci 3:1–8, 1991

Dunlop SA, Archer MA, Quinlivan JA, et al: Repeated prenatal corticosteroids delay myelination in the ovine central nervous system. J Matern Fetal Med 6:309–313, 1997

Edwards E, Harkins K, Wright G, et al: Effects of bilateral adrenalectomy on the induction of learned helplessness. Neuropsychopharmacology 3:109–114, 1990

Etcoff NL: The neuropsychology of emotional expression, in Advances in Clinical Neuro-psychology, Vol 3. Edited by Goldstein G, Tarter RE. New York, Plenum, 1986, pp 127–179

Famularo R, Kinscherff R, Fenton T: Psychiatric diagnoses of abusive mothers. J Nerv Ment Dis 180:658–661, 1992

Famularo R, Fenton T, Kinscherff R: Maternal and child posttraumatic stress disorder in cases of maltreatment. Child Abuse Negl 18:27–36, 1994

Famularo R, Fenton T, Augustyn M, et al: Persistence of pediatric post traumatic stress disorder after 2 years. Child Abuse Negl 20:1245–1248, 1996

Felitti VJ, Anda RF, Nordenberg D, et al: Relationship of childhood abuse and household dysfunction to many of the leading causes of death in adults. Am J Prev Med 14:245–258, 1998

Fletcher KE (ed): Childhood posttraumatic stress disorder, in Child Psychopathology. New York, Guilford, 1996, pp 242–276

Friedman MJ, Charney DS, Deutch AY: Neurobiological and Clinical Consequences of Stress. Philadelphia, PA, Lippincott-Raven, 1995

Gould E, Tanapat P, Cameron HA: Adrenal steroids suppress granule cell death in the developing dentate gyrus through an NMDA receptor–dependent mechanism. Brain Res Dev Brain Res 103:91–93, 1997

Gould E, Tanapat P, McEwen BS, et al: Proliferation of granule cell precursors in the dentate gyrus of adult monkeys is diminished by stress. Proc Natl Acad Sci U S A 95:3168–3171, 1998

Gould E, Reeves AJ, Graziano MSA, et al: Neurogenesis in the neocortex of adult primates. Science 286:548–552, 1999

Hamner MB, Lorberbaum JP, George MS: Potential role of the anterior cingulate cortex in PTSD: review and hypothesis. Depress Anxiety 9:1–14, 1999

Hart J, Gunnar M, Cicchetti D: Altered neuroendocrine activity in maltreated children related to symptoms of depression. Dev Psychopathol 8:201–214, 1996

Hasselmo ME, Rolls ET, Baylis GC: The role of expression and identity in the face-selective responses of neurons in the temporal visual cortex of the monkey. Behav Brain Res 32:203–218, 1989

Heim C, Newport DJ, Heit S, et al: Pituitary-adrenal and autonomic responses to stress in women after sexual and physical abuse in childhood. JAMA 284:592–597, 2000

Heller W, Nitschke JB, Etienne MA, et al: Patterns of regional brain activity differentiate types of anxiety. J Abnorm Psychol 106:376–385, 2000

Hillary BE, Schare ML: Sexually and physically abused adolescents: an empirical search for PTSD. J Clin Psychol 49:161–165, 1993

Isenberg N, Silbersweig D, Engelien A., et al: Linguistic threat activates the human amygdala. Proc Natl Acad Sci U S A 96:10456–10459, 1999

Kagan J, Snidman N: Early childhood predictors of adult anxiety disorders. Biol Psychiatry 46:1536–1541, 1999

Kagan J, Reznick JS, Gibbons J: Biological basis of childhood shyness. Science 240:167–171, 1988

Kalin NH, Larson C, Shelton SE, et al: Asymmetric frontal brain activity, cortisol, and behavior associated with fearful temperament in rhesus monkeys. Behav Neurosci 112:286–292, 1998

Kaplan S, Pelkovitz D, Saltzinger S, et al: Psychopathology of parents of abused and neglected children and adolescents. J Am Acad Child Adolesc Psychiatry 22:238–244, 1983

Kaufman J. Depressive disorders in maltreated children. J Am Acad Child Adolesc Psychiatry 30:257–265, 1991

Kaufman J, Jones B, Stieglitz E, et al: The use of multiple informants to assess children's maltreatment experiences. J Fam Violence 9:227–248, 1994

Keller J, Nitschke JB, Bhargava T, et al: Neuropsychological differentiation of depression and anxiety. J Abnorm Psychol 109:3–10, 2000

Kendler KS, Bulik CM, Silberg J, et al: Childhood sexual abuse and adult psychiatric and substance use disorders in women: an epidemiological and cotwin control study. Arch Gen Psychiatry 57:953–959, 2000

Kessler, RC: Posttraumatic stress disorder: the burden to the individual and to society. J Clin Psychiatry 61 (suppl 5):4–12, 2000

Koluchova J: Severe deprivation in twins: a case study. J Child Psychol Psychiatry 13:107–114, 1972

Koluchova J: The further development of twins after severe and prolonged deprivation: a second report. J Child Psychol Psychiatry 17:181–188, 1976

LaBar KS, Gatenby JC, Gore JC, et al: Human amygdala activation during conditioned fear acquisition and extinction: a mixed-trial fMRI study. Neuron 20:937–945, 1998

Lauder JM: Neurotransmitters as morphogens. Prog Brain Res 73:365–388, 1988

LeDoux J: Fear and the brain: where have we been, and where are we going? Biol Psychiatry 44:1229–1238, 1998

Levy HB, Markovic J, Chaudry U, et al: Reabuse rates in a sample of children followed for 5 years after discharge from a child abuse inpatient assessment program. Child Abuse Negl 11:1363–1377, 1995

Macklin ML, Metzger LJ, Litz BT, et al: Lower precombat intelligence is a risk factor for posttraumatic stress disorder. J Consult Clin Psychol 66:232–236, 1998

Mannarino AP, Cohen JA, Berman SR: The relationship between preabuse factors and psychological symptomatology in sexually abused girls. Child Abuse Negl 18:63–71, 1994

McEwen BS: Adrenal steroid actions on brain: dissecting the fine line between protection and damage, in Neurobiological and Clinical Consequences of Stress: From Normal Adaptation to PTSD. Edited by Charney DS, Friedman MJ, Deutch AY. New York, Raven, 1995, pp 135–151

McGee R, Wolfe D, Yuen S, et al: The measurement of maltreatment. Child Abuse Negl 19:233–249, 1995

McLeer SV, Dixon JF, Henry D, et al: Psychopathology in non–clinically referred sexually abused children. J Am Acad Child Adolesc Psychiatry 37:1326–1333, 1998

Money J, Annecillo C, Kelly JF: Abuse-dwarfism syndrome: after rescue, statural and intellectual catchup growth correlate. J Clin Child Psychol 12:279–283, 1983

Moradi AR, Doost HTN, Taghavi MR, et al: Everyday memory deficits in children and adolescents with PTSD: performance on the Rivermead Behavioral Memory test. J Child Psychol Psychiatry 40:357–361, 1999

Perez C, Widom CS: Childhood victimization and long-term intellectual and academic outcomes. Child Abuse Negl 18:617–633, 1994

Perry BD: Neurobiological sequelae of childhood trauma: PTSD in children, in Catecholamine Function in Posttraumatic Stress Disorder: Emerging Concepts. Edited by Murburg MM. Washington, DC, American Psychiatric Press, 1994, pp 233–255

Pianta R, Egeland B, Erickson MF: Results of the mother-child interaction research project, in Child Maltreatment: Theory and Research on the Causes and Consequences of Child Abuse and Neglect. Edited by Cicchetti D, Carlson V. Cambridge, MA, Cambridge University Press, 1989, pp 203–253

Posner MI, Petersen SE: The attention system of the human brain. Annu Rev Neurosci 13:25–42, 1990

Prichard JW: MRS of the brain: prospects for clinical application, in MR Spectroscopy: Clinical Applications and Techniques. Edited by Young IR, Charles HC. London, Livery House, 1996, pp 1–25

Putnam FW, Trickett PK, Helmers K, et al: Cortisol abnormalities in sexually abused girls, in Program, 144th Annual Meeting of the American Psychiatric Association, New Orleans, LA, May 11–16, 1991. Washington, DC, American Psychiatric Press, 1991

Queiroz EA, Lombardi AB, Santos Furtado CRH, et al: Biochemical correlate of depression in children. Arq Neuropsiquiatr 49:418–425, 1991

Quirk GJ, Armony JL, LeDoux JE: Fear conditioning enhances different temporal components of tone-evoked spike trains in auditory cortex and lateral amygdala. Neuron 19:613–624, 1997

Rauch SL, Savage CR, Alpert NM, et al: The functional neuroanatomy of anxiety: a study of three disorders using positron emission tomography and symptom provocation. Biol Psychiatry 42:446–452, 1997

Sapolsky RM, Uno H, Rebert CS, et al: Hippocampal damage associated with prolonged glucocorticoid exposure in primates. J Neurosci 10:2897–2902, 1990

Scheeringa MS, Zeanah CH, Drell MJ, et al: Two approaches to the diagnosis of posttraumatic stress disorder in infancy and early childhood. J Am Acad Child Adolesc Psychiatry 34:191–200, 1995

Schwartz CE, Snidman N, Kagan J: Adolescent social anxiety as an outcome of inhibited temperament in childhood. J Am Acad Child Adolesc Psychiatry 38:1008–1015, 1999

Selye H: Homeostasis and heterostasis. Perspect Biol Med 16:441–445, 1973

Shaffer D, Fisher P, Dulcan MK, et al: The NIMH diagnostic interview schedule for children version 2.3 (DISC-2.3): description, acceptability, prevalence rates, and performance in the MECA study. J Am Acad Child Adolesc Psychiatry 35:865–877, 1996

Shin LM, McNally RJ, Kosslyn SM, et al: Regional cerebral blood flow during script-imagery in childhood sexual abuse-related PTSD: a PET investigation. Am J Psychiatry 156:575–584, 1999

Simantov R., Blinder E, Ratovitski T, et al: Dopamine induced apoptosis in human neuronal cells: inhibition by nucleic acids antisense to the dopamine transporter. Neuroscience 74:39–50, 1996

Smith MA, Makino S, Kvetnansky R, et al: Effects of stress on neurotrophic factor expression in the rat brain. Ann N Y Acad Sci 771:234–239, 1995

Smythies JR: Oxidative reactions and schizophrenia: a review-discussion. Schizophr Res 24:357–364, 1997

Southwick SM, Yehuda R, Morgan CA: Clinical studies of neurotransmitter alterations in post-traumatic stress disorder, in Neurobiological and Clinical Consequences of Stress: From Normal Adaptation to Post-traumatic Stress Disorder. Edited by Friedman MJ, Charney DS, Deutch AY. Philadelphia, PA, Lippincott-Raven, 1995, pp 335–349

Southwick SS, Yehuda R, Wang S: Neuroendocrine alterations in posttraumatic stress disorder. Psychiatr Ann 28:436–442, 1998

Stapleton JM, Morgan MJ, Liu X, et al: Cerebral glucose utilization is reduced in second test session. J Cereb Blood Flow Metab 17:704–712, 1997

Tanapat P, Galea LA, Gould E: Stress inhibits the proliferation of granule cell precursors in the developing dentate gyrus. Int J Dev Neurosci 16:235–239, 1998

Todd RD: Neural development is regulated by classical neuro-transmitters: dopamine D2 receptor stimulation enhances neurite outgrowth. Biol Psychiatry 31:794–807, 1992

Trickett PK, McBride-Chang C, Putnam FW: The classroom performance and behavior of sexually abused girls. Dev Psychopathol 6:183–194, 1994

Whalen PJ, Rauch SL, Etcoff NL, et al: Masked presentations of emotional facial expressions modulate amygdala activity without explicit knowledge. J Neurosci 18:411–418, 1998

Widom CS: The cycle of violence. Science 244:160–166, 1989

Wolfe DA, Sas L, Wekerle C: Factors associated with the development of posttraumatic stress disorder among victims of sexual abuse. Child Abuse Negl 18:37–50, 1994

Wolfe J, Charney DS: Use of neuropsychological assessment in posttraumatic stress disorder. Psychol Assess 3:573–580, 1991

10

Scientific Basis of Psychological Treatments for Anxiety Disorders

Past, Present, and Future

David H. Barlow, Ph.D.
Laura B. Allen, M.A.

Beginning in the 1960s, psychological approaches to treating anxiety and related disorders were derived from basic psychological science, specifically, theories and data pertaining to learning, emotional development and regulation, and, somewhat later, cognitive science. Recently, these basic science approaches have become increasingly integrated with findings from neuroscience. These exciting developments from translational research have led to comprehensive theoretical models of the development of anxiety and related emotional disorders that have profound implications for psychological treatment (Barlow 2002; Bouton et al. 2001; Öhman and Mineka 2001).

Before projecting the development of future psychological procedures for treating emotional disorders, we should examine where we have been (the past) and where we are now (the present) based on translational research as represented in Table 10–1. The past, beginning approximately in the early 1960s, is best represented by Wolpe's systematic desensitization

Portions of this chapter were presented at the Annual Meeting of the American Psychopathological Association, March 7–9, 2002, in New York City, and the Annual Meeting of the Anxiety Disorders Association of America, March 22, 2002, in Austin, Texas.

as well as the development of situational exposure for phobic behavior (Agras et al. 1968; Marks 1971; Wolpe 1958). This stage was followed by what we refer to as the present, beginning in the 1980s, when a variety of individual cognitive-behavioral protocols were developed to address the increasingly sophisticated knowledge of the different pathological processes defining individual anxiety and related disorders. We see these stages as a prelude to the future, of which we are beginning to get a glimpse, in which psychological procedures will directly target the emotional dysregulation at the heart of emotional disorders by utilizing a set of powerful core procedures. We describe each of these stages in turn, concluding with our speculations and projections of the future of psychological procedures for emotional disorders emanating from basic behavioral science, cognitive theory, and neuroscience.

THE PAST

The work of Joseph Wolpe (1958) represents perhaps the most visible beginning of behavior therapy. He based his procedure, systematic desensitization, on the notion that phobic behavior specifically, and neurosis in general, most likely represent conditioned emotional responses. Therapy, then, consists of eliminating these conditioned emotional responses. Wolpe utilized a variety of procedures from basic science laboratories thought relevant at that time, including extinction and counterconditioning. But he added a theoretical twist by suggesting the process of reciprocal inhibition as a theoretical underpinning for the success of systematic desensitization. This theoretical model, proposing that a peripheral inhibition of the physiological activity underlying arousal could be effected by utilizing incompatible responses such as relaxation, was considered untenable even then. The more satisfactory learning mechanism offered at that time to account for the success of systematic desensitization was counterconditioning. In this process, an alternative response to anxiety or fear is systematically associated with the anxiety-producing stimulus to replace the maladaptive emotional response. In the typical paradigm, Wolpe would treat someone with a specific phobia, for example, by arranging for the person to imagine mild representations of the phobic object or situation while deeply relaxed, and progress in a hierarchical fashion to the most frightening representation of the phobic object or situation. Wolpe chose relaxation for its convenience. Similarly, he chose imaginal representations rather than realistic exposure because of the added flexibility it afforded to the treatment process.

TABLE 10–1   Stages of treatment development

- **The past (circa 1960s–1970s)**
  Wolpe's systematic desensitization and situational exposure

- **The present (late 1980s–today)**
  Individual cognitive–behavioral treatment protocols

- **The future**
  Talking to the amygdala

In fact, Wolpe was doing several things during systematic desensitization that, in retrospect, are important. He was systematically exposing the patient to a variety of cues associated with the phobic object or situation, albeit in imagination. In addition, he was preventing escape (at least in imagination) by prolonging the imaginal exposure until the individual experienced some decrease in anxiety, although subsequent research suggests that imaginal representations of phobia stimuli were only about 50% as efficient and effective as real-life (in vivo) exposure (Barlow et al. 1969). Interestingly, Wolpe also utilized a variety of additional procedures that have largely gone unnoticed. For example, he commonly administered mixtures of 40%–65% CO_2 and air to patients, not to increase anxiety or to produce panic attacks as in the current laboratory paradigm, but rather to take advantage of the deep state of relief and relaxation that occurred after CO_2 was effectively blown off (Wolpe 1958, 1973). Of course, at the same time, by administering CO_2, Wolpe was conducting what we now call interoceptive exposure. In any case, these procedures proved effective for specific phobia, but relatively ineffective for more broad-ranging, ubiquitous phobias such as agoraphobia (Barlow 1988).

In the mid-1960s, scientists began experimenting with some different therapeutic strategies (e.g., Agras et al. 1968). Specifically, they encouraged individuals with what we would now call panic disorder with agoraphobia to expose themselves to real-life frightening situations. Experimenters would motivate them to do so by systematically facilitating and praising (reinforcing) longer and more intense exposure. At the same time, Isaac Marks in London was testing similar procedures (Marks 1971). This approach was innovative because the tenor of the times assumed that experiencing anything more than minimal anxiety might result in some harm to the patient. In addition to psychodynamic explanations as to why this might happen, Wolpe himself cited Pavlovian studies on transmarginal inhibition in which animals would "shut down" under too much stimulation (Wolpe 1958). Of course, this proved not to be the case. Since that time, investigators around the world have clearly demonstrated that situational exposure is an effective treatment for agoraphobia and that the process is substantially more effective than any number of credible alternative procedures (Barlow 2002). Nevertheless, the exact mechanisms by which these treatments produced their effects remained something of a mystery, although it seemed that significant changes were occurring at a very basic level. These early studies continued to apply theoretical concepts of learning derived from animal research to the treatment of different disorders. Some remarkable findings would, at times, emerge from the data.

Preliminary Exposure-Based Studies

The study by Agras et al. (1968) examined the effects of selective positive social reinforcement on agoraphobic behavior. Reinforcement was chosen because of its success in studies of animal behavior and human verbal behavior (Agras et al. 1968). It was speculated that, because agoraphobia was considered an avoidant response to fearful stimuli, utilizing these basic components of learning (reinforcement) would facilitate behavior change in these individuals. To test this hypothesis, researchers instructed patients with relatively severe agoraphobia to walk successively farther from the treatment center. Therapists utilized alternating patterns of reinforcement and nonreinforcement to examine the effects of positive social reinforcement on two separate behavioral indicators: time spent away from the center and distance walked. In this case, reinforcement consisted of verbal praise from the therapist including statements such as "Good… you're doing well…excellent," whereas therapists only offered a generally supportive attitude for nonreinforced trials (Agras et al. 1968, p. 424). This method made it possible to distinguish the effects of selective social reinforcement from those of general support. Reinforcement for time spent away from the center was implemented on two separate phases, after a baseline phase. One subject received two additional phases of reinforcement, in which distance walked from the center was the criterion for reinforcement. As expected, each individual made significant behavioral improvements during the reinforcement periods (as compared with no reinforcement), and the patient receiving differential reinforcement was able to adapt her behavior to the particular reinforcement contingency (although she was not necessarily consciously aware of it). In other words, when time spent away from the clinic was reinforced, the individual increased time spent away, but when the criterion changed to distance walked, she increased how far she walked away from the center. The authors concluded that therapeutic support and positive verbal reinforcement were both successful in modifying phobic behavior. Further, they noted that the success of a variety of different therapeutic techniques might be related to these very basic components of many treatments.

However, the most interesting finding at the time was that some of the individuals began to improve during the baseline phase of the study, *prior* to the addition of any reinforcement from the therapist. Investigators began to realize that the baseline phase itself served as an exposure exercise for the patients. That is, during this time, the patients repeatedly encountered the feared physical sensations (inevitably experiencing some anxiety and panic) as they were instructed to walk away from the clinic. Thus, it seemed as though mere exposure to the feared stimuli resulted in at least some of the behavior change, although the positive reinforcement was successful perhaps in facilitating the exposure.

In 1971, Watson and Marks reported another inadvertent discovery. The original purpose of their study was to examine the effects of imaginal exposure to relevant and irrelevant cues on the treatment of specific phobia and agoraphobia. Specifically, they hypothesized that exposure to specific phobic stimuli was necessary for fear reduction, and confronting general fearful stimuli would not lead to a decrease in fear responding. The authors recruited a group of 16 individuals (6 with specific phobia and 10 with agoraphobia) and treated them through two separate treatment phases of imaginal exposure, consisting of eight 50-minute treatment sessions within each phase. One imaginal exposure phase consisted of sessions in which a therapist read a vivid description of the individual's particular phobic situation to produce a high level of anxiety for the full 50 minutes (flooding procedure). The other imaginal exposure phase was procedurally similar, but the story contained irrelevant fear cues in which the therapist described the person being eaten by a tiger—a situation that would invoke fear in most individuals. A counterbalanced crossover design allowed for testing of any order effects. In addition, the authors obtained physiological (heart rate and skin conductance), subjective (anxiety and fear), and objective (assessor report) measures prior to, during, and after the exposure treatment. Contrary to the authors' predictions, the flooding and irrelevant fear treatments were equally effective. The authors offered a number of explanations for this puzzling outcome.

One possibility is that flooding resulted in habituation (or a decrease in physiological responding) to anxiety. If this were the case, then the degree of positive outcome, or improvement of the treatment, should be related to the degree of emotional arousal (anxiety) experienced during the procedure. However, when the data were examined more closely, this proved not to be the case. Specifically, positive gains were associated with subjective anxiety experienced during the sessions *only* for the irrelevant fear condition, and not for the flooding procedure. On the other hand, good outcome to the flooding condition was related to physiological activity *prior* to the start of treatment. These data argue against assuming a general habituation explanation, because only the outcome from the irrelevant fear exposure seems to support such an interpretation. Thus, it appeared as though the anxiety reduction experienced in each condition might be operating through different mechanisms.

In support of this notion, the study also found that when irrelevant fear was introduced as the second phase of treatment, the level of anxiety reported during those sessions was less than when flooding (relevant fear) constituted the second phase. Essentially, it seemed as though presenting the flooding condition first had some sort of "protective" effect on the patients, such that they experienced less anxiety thereafter. Exposure to the irrelevant fear first had no such protective effect. These differential results also seemed to suggest that the two conditions operated on separate fear contexts. For example, the authors proposed that "irrelevant fear experiences might have nonspecific abreactive or general fear-habituative effects or both.... Relevant fear (flooding) might habituate patients to fear in general, but could also act more specifically by blocking avoidance of the phobic stimulus" (Watson and Marks 1971, p. 289). Although the investigators did not recognize the full implications of their findings, their results pointed the way to an important discovery. Basically, their findings suggest that irrelevant fear exposure may result in reduction in anxiety generally. Flooding may also accomplish this, in addition to reducing fear to the specific stimulus. This would explain why experiencing the flooding procedure in the first treatment phase resulted in less overall anxiety during the second phase. By the time the individuals experienced the irrelevant fear in the second phase, they had habituated somewhat to the anxiety response *and* to the specific phobic stimulus, so the irrelevant cue was much less frightening. However, those who experienced the irrelevant fear during the first phase had only the benefit of general anxiety reduction. When the flooding procedure was later introduced, the fear association with the specific phobic stimulus remained. Therefore, these individuals still demonstrated some anxiety at this point in the treatment process.

Together, these examples began to illustrate the complexity of the process of fear reduction. Yet Watson and Marks may have provided the first experimental analysis of what is now a key feature of treatment: interoceptive exposure. More recent research has shown that the essence of successful treatment of panic disorder involves induction of and exposure to the somatic sensations associated with panic. Although early studies such as Wolpe's (1958) CO_2 inhalation procedures and the Watson and Marks

(1971) study discussed above were originally following different hypotheses and formulations of treatment for patients with panic disorder, it is possible that the results from these case studies and experiments were due mostly to the induction of somatic sensations during the treatment.

Even though these and other early studies demonstrated the effectiveness of exposure-based procedures for reducing anxiety and fear, most early clinical trials lacked "clinical significance." By this we are referring to the effectiveness of a particular treatment for an individual patient. The best estimates of outcome by the early 1980s suggested that 60%–75% of people receiving exposure-based treatments for panic disorder and agoraphobia (PDA) showed some clinical benefit. However, in a review of 24 studies of exposure-based treatments for PDA, it is clear that as many as 35% of those entering treatment received little or no benefit (Jansson and Öst 1982). Furthermore, of those receiving some benefit, only 10%–20% could be said to have achieved somewhat normal functioning. The remainder continued to suffer from anxiety, panic, and residual avoidance (Barlow 1994).

Theories of Anxiety Reduction

By the mid-1980s, a number of theoretical explanations for the success of exposure-based treatments, some emanating from the aforementioned theories of learning, had been proposed. Leading theoretical candidates for the mechanisms of action underlying the psychological treatments included habituation, extinction, cognitive schema change, increases in self-efficacy, and emotional processing.

Habituation

Habituation refers to the idea that psychophysiological responses will decrease in intensity with repeated exposure to the fearful situation. Additionally, lower levels of physiological arousal prior to exposure facilitate habituation; extremely high levels can even "sensitize" the individual to the feared stimulus. There are a number of concerns with the theory of habituation resulting from research on anxiety and fear. Most of the animal literature on habituation notes that the effects are relatively short-lived, and fear often returns after a period of time. Known as "return of fear," this phenomenon has been studied in relation to treatments for anxiety disorders (Craske and Rachman 1987; Grey et al. 1981; Lang and Craske 2000; Lang et al. 1999). Rachman's research has consistently demonstrated that the only difference between those who experience return of fear and those who do not is increased heart rate *before* treatment among those who habituate (a physiological measure of anticipatory anxiety). Habituation theory fails to account for these findings; in fact, it suggests that an elevated physiological response prior to treatment would result in less habituation. Additionally, habituation theory posits that all indices of fear will return, when actually only subjective accounts of fear return; physiological response to the feared stimuli remains low after treatment. This finding suggests both a physiological and a cognitive (as well as, perhaps, behavioral) component to fear reduction (Lang 1985).

Similarly, when psychophysiological levels are extremely high at baseline (as is often the case in PDA), habituation theory states that sensitization will likely occur, whereby the individual actually becomes *more* afraid of the stimulus with repeated exposure. Contrary to this view, individuals with PDA also improve with exposure. Furthermore, Watson and Marks (1971) demonstrated that level of physiological arousal prior to flooding correlated with good treatment outcome. Thus, it seems that habituation is not an adequate explanation for successful treatment.

Extinction

Another process, known as extinction, was thought to also play a role in anxiety reduction as a result of exposure. Unlike habituation, extinction theories postulated that anxiety responses are *learned,* and that reducing them is a direct result of decreasing the strength of these learned responses. Therefore, exposure to the feared stimuli results in the learning of a new, non-fearful response, whereas avoidance of a situation negatively reinforces the learned feared response, because anxiety is reduced. Whereas habituation examines anxiety reduction from a physiological standpoint, extinction came to be associated with cognitive processes, because learning is believed to play an active role in reducing anxiety.

Models of extinction proved more popular than habituation theories, because even animal studies have demonstrated some active learning process involved in fear reduction (e.g., Rescorla 1979). Although it is unclear exactly what is learned during this process, more recent accounts of anxiety treatments have stressed the importance of examining information processing during exposure. Some researchers have theorized that extinguishing the avoidance behavior in individuals with anxiety disorders results in their learning that threatening consequences are unlikely to occur. In other words, the situation is no longer frightening because the expected outcome does not occur. Repeated learning of this new association results in an overall decrease in fearful responding.

However, extinction models are not without their limitations. For example, certain studies have demonstrated that even when individuals are allowed to escape a feared situation before maximum anxiety is reached, anxiety reduction can still occur (e.g., Agras et al. 1968; Barlow 1988; Emmelkamp 1982). Extinction theory postulates that the act of escape would reinforce the idea that the situation is indeed harmful. Additionally, this theory fails to account for the recurring problem of inexplicable return of fear after seemingly successful extinction.

Self-Efficacy

In reaction to the perceived inadequacies of basic learning theories circa 1980 to fully account for the effectiveness of exposure treatment, more explicitly cognitively based theories soon developed. Bandura's (1977) theory of self-efficacy is one example. He proposed that increasing one's self-efficacy, or sense of mastery over one's environment, is the basis for the success of any treatment for anxiety. Conquering fearful situations during exposure is likely to increase self-efficacy maximally, but Bandura noted that self-efficacy can be increased in a number of other ways, including verbal support from others during attempts to cope, and observing others master the situation.

Critics of this theory have claimed that the theory is circular, in that self-efficacy increases as a *result* of behavior change, instead of causing a change in behavior. In fact, some early studies demonstrated that the most important predictor of outcome is anxiety reduction, not increased self-efficacy (Barlow 1988). Bandura augmented his original description of self-efficacy by stating that this concept may indeed be related to perceived vulnerability and control, although the connection between these concepts is not well understood. Recent developments have underscored the importance of strengthening the closely related concepts of self-efficacy and a sense of controllability (Barlow 2000).

Altering Cognitive Schemas

Aaron T. Beck developed cognitive therapy out of his observations of the role of deep-seated negative thinking as a principal characteristic of emotional disorders (Beck 1967; Young et al. 2001). In this very influential theory, Beck assumed that the heart of anxiety and other negative emotions lay in what he termed "hypervalent cognitive schemata." Information about one's self, the world, and the future (the cognitive triad) is continually processed in a distorted way as dangerous. The state of anxiety, then, is associated with automatic thoughts and images reflecting this view of the world. This theory was innovative because it did not depend on conscious rational appraisal, but was closer to a "verbal mediational" model of learning. This twist circumvented the difficulties that other cognitive approaches had with irrational anxiety. Thus, anxiety reduction consists of correcting inappropriate attributions and appraisals, and substituting more rational and realistic thoughts. In the 1980s, this theory generated enormous interest because it was tied directly to an innovative method for modifying inappropriate cognitions, cognitive therapy. Early difficulties with this theory revolved around the fact that if the individual could not recognize these cognitions, they must still be there but "unconscious." However, evidence for this state of affairs was based entirely on self-report, rendering the theory untestable. Later developments in cognitive science have obviated this difficulty to some extent.

Emotional Processing Theories

Around this time, emotional processing theories were developed to explain anxiety reduction (Lang 1977a, 1977b, 1979, 1985). These models also emphasized cognitive and emotional components of anxiety. Although emotional processing accounts agree that exposure is essential to anxiety reduction, they note that the effective processing of emotion during exposure is the key ingredient or "mechanism of action" determining outcome.

According to this model, anxiety and fear are action tendencies stored in memory and comprise a number of different factors: stimulus, response, and emotional meaning. Each of these aspects must be accessed and processed for significant fear reduction to result. Increased physiological response to anxiety-provoking stimuli is a sign of successful access, although accessing the physiological component will not necessarily address the entire emotional structure. Thus, retrieving the association between the stimuli and fearful response (anxiety or panic) may indeed result in a decrease in anxious physiological responding (habituation), but it is still possible that the subjective account of fear will remain high. The theory of emotional processing explains these findings by stating that the emotional-cognitive response structure, or emotional network, was not fully accessed during exposure. Therefore, subjective fear does not have the opportunity to decrease, and other components of the response will likely return.

Foa and Kozak (1986) also suggested that for an exposure-based treatment to be successful, the individual must be provided with information incompatible with the existing fear and memory structure (the emotional meaning component). Emotional change can be facilitated as a result of the integration of these new concepts into the fear structure (Foa and Kozak 1986). In the context of extinction and emotional processing, it is understandable why methods such as distraction and cognitive avoidance can lead to poor outcome for exposure-based treatments: individuals who avoid thinking about the situation will also fail to access the emotional fear structure. In fact, cognitive avoidance seems to be an important predictor of poor outcome (White and Barlow 2002).

Like the other theories discussed, emotional processing theory has some limitations. A primary difficulty is the common finding of a significant discrepancy between self-reported fear and actual physiological responding. After successful treatment, patients often report significantly decreased fear, but objective measures of physiological levels of fear indicate that very little change has occurred. One might conclude that the emotional structure was not completely processed; however, early studies did not necessarily support this interpretation, since benefits seemed to be enduring even in the context of heightened physiological responding (Barlow 1988).

THE PRESENT

Treatments for Anxiety Disorders

The varied theories of anxiety reduction led directly to a variety of interventions that came to be known as cognitive-behavioral therapy (CBT). In addition to exposure-based procedures developed in the late 1960s and 1970s, cognitive therapy became a staple of anxiety reduction procedures, although it was modified to fit the specific anxiety disorder that was the target of treatment. In addition to situational exposure, interoceptive exposure was developed specifically for patients with panic disorder. In this procedure, somatic sensations resembling the anxiety-provoking panic attack were re-created in the clinical setting until the anxiety response to these internal cues was "extinguished" (Barlow 1986a, 1986b; Barlow and Cerny 1988).

Individual CBT Protocols

In the 1980s, controlled studies had begun to demonstrate significant empirical support for the effectiveness of CBT (Barlow 1988). As a consequence, in the late 1980s, treatments for anxiety disorders were increasingly characterized by specific individual protocols for the different anxiety disorders. Specific strategies for cognitive restructuring, coping skills, and exposure were specified for each disorder, because clinicians and researchers viewed the different anxiety disorders as distinct, separate conditions stemming from specific experiences unique to each disorder. Thus, it seemed necessary to vary the treatments accordingly.

For example, psychoeducation for an individual with panic disorder would focus specifically on the fear of physical sensations that might cause the person to believe he or she was going to have a panic attack. The clinician would help the patient understand how the sensations lead to a catastrophic thought, and this would eventually lead to avoidance of situations or activities that elicited paniclike sensations. On the other hand, for a client being treated for social anxiety, it would be more relevant to discuss how thoughts of negative evaluation by others lead to anxious feelings and avoidance of social interaction. In addition, anxiety disorders such as generalized anxiety disorder and obsessive-compulsive disorder present differently than the phobic disorders or panic disorder, so individualized treatments were developed and standardized. These treatments were then tested empirically in a variety of formats, uses, and settings. Demonstration of the efficacy of these CBT protocols reached its zenith in the late 1990s with the publication of results of large-scale clinical trials, many of which were conducted across several sites. We will briefly describe two examples: cognitive-behavioral treatment of panic disorder, and cognitive-behavioral group treatment (CBGT) of social phobia.

Panic Disorder

In a large-scale clinical trial, four different research sites examined the effectiveness of CBT, medication (imipramine), and their combination as treatments for panic disorder (Barlow et al. 2000). Specifically, individuals participating in the study were randomly assigned to one of five treatment groups: CBT alone, imipramine alone, pill placebo, CBT plus imipramine, and CBT plus placebo. All patients received 3 months of weekly treatment. After the treatment phase, "responders" (as evidenced by an independent rating of "much improved" or "mild" severity of panic symptoms) continued participating in a maintenance phase, in which they were seen monthly for the next 6 months. After the discontinuation of treatment, these individuals were followed for another 6 months. The data yield some interesting findings.

The investigators hypothesized that the combined treatment of CBT plus imipramine would be most effective in reducing panic disorder severity. Results at posttreatment and postmaintenance are presented in Figure 10–1. An examination of data post–acute treatment shows that the combined treatment was more effective than CBT alone but did not differ from any other condition, including CBT plus placebo. Among responders only, medication seemed to produce a more broad-based effect. After the maintenance phase, the combined CBT-imipramine group was significantly better than the other three treatment conditions (CBT alone, imipramine alone, and CBT plus placebo), at least on one measure. Thus, the investigators' speculations seemed to have been supported, albeit weakly, at least for the 6 months following treatment. Yet when data were analyzed during follow-up, 6 months after the maintenance phase (no treatment at all had been received during this time), the outcome had shifted. At this point, the only treatment conditions showing superiority over placebo were CBT alone and CBT plus placebo. The effects of the two medication conditions had diminished in the 6 months after the maintenance phase. Moreover, when relapse rates were examined for each treatment condition (as measured by an independent evaluator's rating of global improvement), the combined-treatment group had the highest relapse rate at 6-month follow-up (48.28%). Imipramine alone had he next highest relapse rate (40%), with CBT plus placebo showing comparable rates to CBT alone (16.67% and 17.86%, respectively). Thus, there were no data to indicate that medication alone or a combined treatment was superior to CBT 6 months following treatment discontinuation. In fact, CBT seemed to fare better than all the other conditions (excluding CBT plus placebo) in that the results were more durable.

Regarding the assumption that the combined effect of CBT and medication would be superior at follow-up, this was not the case. In fact, it seems as if the addition of the medication actually prevented CBT from achieving its full effect. Although we may speculate that similar results would be obtained in comparable studies focusing on other anxiety disorders, the treatment protocol, therapists, and outcome measures for this investigation were limited exclusively to panic disorder.

Social Phobia

A study examining the effectiveness of CBGT for social phobia found similar results (Heimberg et al. 1998; Liebowitz et al. 1999). In this investigation, the authors compared CBGT (an empirically supported group therapy) for social phobia with phenelzine, pill placebo, and educational-supportive group therapy (a placebo for CBGT). When assessed at mid-treatment, the individuals taking phenelzine evidenced a more broad-based improvement, but this effect had disappeared at the completion of treatment. At posttreatment, the CBGT and phenelzine groups showed an equal number of responders, and both groups had significantly better results than the two placebo control groups. Finally, following a 6-month maintenance phase, the CBGT group again had almost the same percentage of responders as the medication group. However, when follow-up assessments were conducted 6 months after termination of the maintenance phase, the individuals who had received CBGT showed a trend of sustained treatment

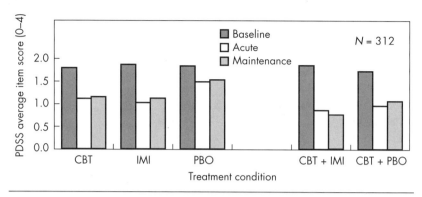

FIGURE 10–1   Comparison of baseline, acute, and maintenance treatments for intent-to-treat sample.

CBT = cognitive-behavioral therapy, IMI = imipramine, PBO = placebo, PDSS = Panic Disorder Severity Scale.

Source.   Adapted from Barlow et al. 2000.

gains over those who had received medication ($P < 0.09$). These data are presented in Figure 10–2. These results suggest that although CBT may take slightly longer to achieve its effects, over time these successes seem more durable than gains made with medication.

These large multisite studies are representative of a number of studies showing efficacy of psychological treatments, particularly CBT, for each of the anxiety disorders. This evidence, developed utilizing the most sophisticated methodological tools available, although widely reported, has not proved to be the panacea that some hoped for.

Problems With Current CBT Treatments

A number of significant limitations to CBT currently exist, and future research must continue to address these issues. Obviously, there are still a considerable number of patients who do not respond well to this type of remedy, and the reasons for their lack of response remain somewhat of a mystery. Thus, although this treatment is effective for many people, there is plenty of room for improvement.

Another problem that has become apparent with CBT manualized treatments is that there are simply too many of them. Clinicians must use separate handbooks, workbooks, and protocols for each disorder. Not only can this be quite costly, but it can take a significant amount of training to become adequately familiar with each of the distinct protocols. Finally, because the protocols are somewhat complex, dissemination of treatments to

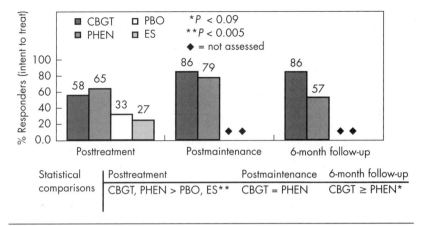

FIGURE 10–2   Placebo-controlled comparison of cognitive-behavioral group treatment (CBGT) and other treatments for social phobia.

ES = educational-supportive group therapy, PBO = pill placebo, PHEN = phenelzine.
Source.   Adapted with permission from 1) Heimberg RG, Liebowitz MR, Hope DA, et al.: "Cognitive Behavioral Group Therapy vs Phenelzine Therapy for Social Phobia: 12-Week Outcome." *Archives of General Psychiatry* 55:1133–1141, 1998. Copyright ©1998, American Medical Association. All rights reserved. 2) Liebowitz MR, Heimberg RG, Schneier FR, et al.: "Cognitive-Behavioral Group Therapy Versus Phenelzine in Social Phobia: Long Term Outcome." *Depression and Anxiety* 10:89–98, 1999. Copyright ©1999, Wiley-Liss, Inc., a subsidiary of John Wiley & Sons, Inc.

providers becomes an obstacle (Barlow et al. 1999). Many clinicians are still unaware of the theoretical underpinnings and specific applications of the different strategies. More important, there is a lack of awareness of the success of these approaches. Unless these treatments become more "user friendly," it is unlikely that nonresearch clinicians will have a sufficient understanding of and access to empirically supported techniques.

PROLOGUE TO THE FUTURE

Modern Learning Theory and Cognitive Neuroscience

In an effort to gain a more complete understanding of anxiety, particularly in psychopathological form, investigators are taking a fresh look at the basic processes involved in theories of classical conditioning, and the findings illustrate a very different process from the salivating dog of introductory textbooks. In an article exploring theoretical conceptualizations of the etiology of panic disorder, Bouton et al. (2001) suggest that early panic attacks result in conditioned associations between the attack and a variety of interoceptive and exteroceptive cues. When these cues are elicited in a non-panic situation, a constellation of behavioral and physiological responses arise, which we collectively call "anxiety." Thus, anxiety is a state of relatively low-level arousal preparing us for possible future danger. Panic, on the other hand, is a surge in autonomic arousal produced in the actual presence of an extremely dangerous situation. These mechanisms are not necessarily mutually exclusive. In fact, modern learning theory suggests that anxiety may initiate panic because anxiety too can become a conditioned stimulus. It seems that small physiological, behavioral, and emotional changes can become associated with an extreme fear reaction (such as panic) with or without conscious knowledge of the cues. These conditioned events can begin to influence behavior at a subconscious level, such that strengthening of the association between physical and emotional cues and panic begins to occur (LeDoux 1996). Brain imaging techniques have offered support for this interpretation, even indicating differences in the neurobiological bases of conscious and unconscious conditioning processes (Öhman 1999). Future work in understanding the actual functional brain changes in anxiety disorders continues, and researchers are now using imaging strategies to examine changes in brain function after cognitive-behavioral treatments for anxiety (Furmark et al. 2002). Thus, the future investigation of anxiety will involve a comprehensive study of the psychological, emotional, and neurobiological correlates of emotion-based conditioning procedures.

Emotion Regulation

A particularly important concept for understanding emotional disorders is that of emotion regulation. This refers to the strategies individuals use to influence the occurrence, experience, intensity, and expression of a wide range of emotions (e.g., Richards and Gross 2000). Emotion regulation and dysregulation seem to play an important role in anxiety disorders and other psychopathology, and levels of positive and negative emotions as well as their functional relationships often differ depending on the particular disorder (Gross and Levenson 1997). Emotion disorders seem characterized to some degree by attempts to control both positive and negative emotions (affect) in a variety of contexts. Individuals concerned about the expression and experience of their feelings may attempt to suppress, hide, or ignore them, with unintended consequences (Gross and Levenson 1997). This is because excessive attempts to control emotional experience often lead to an increase in the very feelings the individual is attempting to regulate, as demonstrated by attempts to control emotions after initial panic attacks (Craske et al. 1990). Furthermore, the degree to which one attempts to control emotions is somewhat related to the degree of intensity with which an individual experiences negative emotions, which can quickly become overwhelming (Lynch et al. 2001). These overpowering experiences often lead to attempts at thought suppression as a convenient and accessible way to reduce emotional responsiveness. This pattern may erupt in a vicious cycle of increased physiological and emotional arousal leading to more unsuccessful attempts at suppression, which in turn contribute to growing psychological distress. It seems that emotional inhibition (including emotional thought suppression) mediates the relationship between high levels of intensity of negative affect and degree of psychological distress (Lynch et al. 2001). In other words, intense negative affect leads to general psychological distress, but this relationship is much stronger when individuals attempt to suppress or hide their emotions. Thus, it is clear that future treatments for psychological disorders must focus on this issue and develop treatments specifically targeted at emotional dysregulation.

THE FUTURE

Decades of research on the nature, development, and treatment of anxiety disorders have begun to illuminate the complexity of the emotional, behavioral, and neurobiological components of these disorders. For example, anxiety and mood disorders seem to have much more in common than previously thought. Thus, forthcoming models will represent a blurring of theoretical approaches, as CBT treatments will be conceptualized from a single theoretical understanding with only the specific application of the techniques varying for each disorder (Brown and Barlow 2002). Undoubtedly, increased knowledge of psychopathology will lead to more finely targeted treatments for anxiety, which will benefit both clients and clinicians. Instead of having to learn and apply numerous (and possibly unnecessary) strategies, clinicians will be able to learn a single, more precise technique. As a result, clients will benefit significantly from highly trained therapists administering only those intensively focused procedures necessary for change.

Given this new perspective, it is apparent that a number of crucial strategies should be included in developing new treatment paradigms. First, most would agree that encouraging exposure or contact with the feared stimulus or stimuli is fundamental. Of course, this contact can be created through either situational or imaginal exposure—as long as the individual is experiencing significant anxiety as a result of the exposure. Second, much research has demonstrated that an inherent aspect of almost all anxiety disorders is the client's sense of uncontrollability or unpredictability

(Barlow 1988). Successful treatments must challenge these beliefs either through cognitive restructuring or exposure-based work. Although seemingly similar to Bandura's (1977) notion of self-efficacy, control and predictability actually have more to do with feeling actively involved in creating one's environment. Encouraging clients to "take back the reins" of their lives is a powerful component in enhancing treatment outcome. Finally, shifting attention from an internal, evaluative self-focus to a more external, situationally based focus is also important in treatment. The extreme intensity with which patients focus on and evaluate their own thoughts and sensations prevents them from understanding the objective dangerousness of the situation. However, less internalized attention does not mean distraction, because this strategy also prevents emotional processing. Therapies should aim to help patients process their emotions and reactions to the specific stressors without negative evaluation.

Treatment development in our center is now focused on creating a single, unified approach to emotional disorders. This process begins by incorporating emotion regulation strategies into the four general components of cognitive-behavioral treatment. The psychoeducational aspect of treatment addresses the nature and purpose of emotions—how and why we experience them and how it is possible for them to become "disordered." Heritability of emotional tendencies, early learning experiences, and specific emotional learning experiences as a result of trauma or modeling are included as important parts of this portion of treatment; it is necessary that patients understand the origin of their emotions and why they are interpreted as dangerous. Cognitive restructuring examines both probability overestimation and decatastrophizing, with an emphasis on the probability and catastrophic interpretation of negative *affect*. This aspect will help individuals realize how subtle avoidance of these feelings inhibits emotional processing. The unified treatment also addresses common experiential avoidance in anxiety disorders while relating the avoidance behaviors to each specific individual. The final phase of an integrative CBT approach focuses on modifying action tendencies (MAT). Patients are encouraged to behave in a way that blocks the action tendencies associated with fear and anxiety. This includes situational exposure, combating thought suppression, encouraging emotion recognition, and facilitating acceptance of thoughts, feelings, and emotions. For instance, MAT for generalized anxiety disorder will focus on emotional arousal, whereas MAT for major depressive disorder will include behavioral activation to prevent withdrawal. On the other hand, MAT for panic disorder will encourage emotional and somatic activation. These concepts can easily be related to each specific anxiety disorder without causing one to lose sight of the "big picture"–that anxiety and mood disorders have a common background.

These "future directions" are beginning to be realized. Recently, preliminary data from an intensive treatment for patients with moderate to severe agoraphobia suggest that the unification of therapeutic modalities into a straightforward, emotion-focused protocol is quite successful. In fact, effect sizes for this new treatment for panic disorder severity and disability associated with panic disorder are substantially larger compared with the standard 12-week CBT treatment protocol for panic disorder and agoraphobia. Although this is only the beginning, it provides sufficient groundwork for forthcoming research on the success of treating anxiety from an emotional dysregulation perspective.

Thus, in the journey from Wolpe's systematic desensitization experiments to current manualized cognitive-behavioral treatment we have learned much about the nature of fear and anxiety. Biological and psychological research have come together to enrich the way we conceptualize anxiety. This research in turn is contributing to the goal of producing an integrated treatment that is applicable to a variety of disorders. However, only by uncovering the remaining facets of psychopathology in the context of translational research will we be able to understand and treat fear and anxiety from a unified conceptual basis.

REFERENCES

Agras WS, Leitenberg H, Barlow DH: Social reinforcement in the modification of agoraphobia. Arch Gen Psychiatry 19:423–427, 1968

Bandura A: Self-efficacy: toward a unifying theory of behavioral change. Psychol Rev 84:191–215, 1977

Barlow DH: New perspectives on panic: review of RH Hallan's Anxiety: Psychological Perspectives on Panic and Agoraphobia. Behav Res Ther 24:693–696, 1986a

Barlow DH: Behavioral conception and treatment of panic. Psychopharmacol Bull 22:802–806, 1986b

Barlow DH: Anxiety and Its Disorders: The Nature and Treatment of Anxiety and Panic. New York, Guilford, 1988

Barlow DH: Effectiveness of behavior treatment for panic disorder with and without agoraphobia, in Treatment of Panic Disorder: A Consensus Development Conference. Edited by Wolfe BE, Maser JD. Washington, DC, American Psychiatric Press, 1994, pp 105–120

Barlow DH: Unraveling the mysteries of anxiety and its disorders from the perspective of emotion theory. Am Psychol 55:1247–1263, 2000

Barlow DH: Anxiety and Its Disorders: The Nature and Treatment of Anxiety and Panic, 2nd Edition. New York, Guilford, 2002

Barlow DH, Cerny JA: Psychological Treatment of Panic. New York, Guilford, 1988

Barlow DH, Leitenberg H, Agras WS, et al: The transfer gap in systematic desensitization: an analogue study. Behav Res Ther 7:191–197, 1969

Barlow DH, Levitt JT, Bufka LF: The dissemination of empirically supported treatments: a view to the future. Behav Res Ther 37 (suppl):147–162, 1999

Barlow DH, Gorman JM, Shear MK, et al: Cognitive-behavioral therapy, imipramine, or their combination for panic disorder: a randomized controlled trial. JAMA 283:2529–2536, 2000

Beck AT: Depression: Clinical, Experimental, and Theoretical Aspects. New York, Harper & Row, 1967 (republished as Depression: Causes and Treatment. Philadelphia, University of Pennsylvania Press, 1972)

Bouton ME, Mineka S, Barlow DH: A modern learning theory perspective on the etiology of panic disorder. Psychol Rev 108:4–32, 2001

Brown TA, Barlow DH: Classification of anxiety and mood disorders, in Anxiety and Its Disorders: The Nature and Treatment of Anxiety and Panic, 2nd Edition. New York, Guilford, 2002, pp 292–327

Craske MG, Rachman SJ: Return of fear: perceived skill and heart rate responsivity. Br J Clin Psychol 26:187–199, 1987

Craske MG, Miller PP, Rotunda R, et al: A descriptive report of features of initial unexpected panic attacks in minimal and extensive avoiders. Behav Res Ther 28:395–400, 1990

Emmelkamp PMG: Phobic and Obsessive-Compulsive Disorders: Theory, Research, and Practice. New York, Plenum, 1982

Foa E, Kozak M: Emotional processing of fear: exposure to corrective information. Psychol Bull 99:20–35, 1986

Furmark T, Tillfors M, Marteinsdottir I, et al: Common changes in cerebral blood flow in patients with social phobia treated with citalopram or cognitive-behavioral therapy. Arch Gen Psychiatry 59:425–433, 2002

Grey S, Rachman SJ, Sartory G: Return of fear: the role of inhibition. Behav Res Ther 10:124–133, 1981

Gross JJ, Levenson RW: Hiding feelings: the acute effects of inhibiting negative and positive emotion. J Abnorm Psychol 106:95–103, 1997

Heimberg RG, Liebowitz MR, Hope DA, et al: Cognitive behavioral group therapy vs phenelzine therapy for social phobia: 12-week outcome. Arch Gen Psychiatry 55:1133–1141, 1998

Jansson L, Öst LG: Behavioral treatments for agoraphobia: an evaluative review. Clin Psychol Rev 2:311–336, 1982

Lang AJ, Craske MG: Manipulations of exposure-based therapy to reduce return of fear: a replication. Behav Res Ther 38:1–12, 2000

Lang AJ, Craske MG, Bjork RA: Implications of a new theory of disuse for the treatment of emotional disorders. Clinical Psychology: Science and Practice 6:80–94, 1999

Lang PJ: Imagery in therapy: an information processing analysis of fear. Behav Ther 8:862–886, 1977a

Lang PJ: Physiological assessment of anxiety and fear, in Behavioral Assessment: New Directions in Clinical Psychology. Edited by Cone JD, Hawkins RA. New York, Brunner/Mazel, 1977b

Lang PJ: A bio-informational theory of emotional imagery. Psychophysiology 16:495–512, 1979

Lang PJ: The cognitive psychophysiology of emotion: fear and anxiety, in Anxiety and the Anxiety Disorders. Edited by Tuma AH, Maser JD. Hillsdale, NJ, Lawrence Erlbaum, 1985, pp 131–170

LeDoux JE: The Emotional Brain: The Mysterious Underpinnings of Emotional Life. New York, Simon & Schuster, 1996

Liebowitz MR, Heimberg RG, Schneier FR, et al: Cognitive-behavioral group therapy versus phenelzine in social phobia: long term outcome. Depress Anxiety 10:89–98, 1999

Lynch TR, Robins CJ, Morse JQ, et al: A mediational model relating affect intensity, emotion inhibition, and psychological distress. Behav Ther 32:519–536, 2001

Marks IM: Phobic disorders four years after treatment: a prospective follow-up. Br J Psychiatry 118:683–686, 1971

Öhman A: Distinguishing unconscious from conscious emotional processes: methodological considerations and theoretical implications, in Handbook of Cognition and Emotion. Edited by Dalgleish T, Power M. Chichester, England, Wiley, 1999, pp 321–352

Öhman A, Mineka S: Fears, phobias, and preparedness: toward an evolved module of fear and fear learning. Psychol Rev 108:483–522, 2001

Rescorla RA: Conditioned inhibition and extinction, in Mechanisms of Learning and Motivation. Edited by Dickenson A, Boakes RA. Hillsdale, NJ, Lawrence Erlbaum, 1979

Richards JM, Gross JJ: Emotion regulation and memory: the cognitive costs of keeping one's cool. J Pers Soc Psychol 79:410–424, 2000

Watson JP, Marks IM: Relevant and irrelevant fear in flooding: a crossover study of phobic patients. Behav Ther 2:275–293, 1971

White KS, Barlow DH: Panic disorder and agoraphobia, in Anxiety and Its Disorders: The Nature and Treatment of Anxiety and Panic, 2nd Edition. New York, Guilford, 2002, pp 328–379

Wolpe J: Psychotherapy by Reciprocal Inhibition. Stanford, CA, Stanford University Press, 1958

Wolpe J: The Practice of Behavior Therapy, 2nd Edition. Elmsford, NY, Pergamon, 1973

Young JE, Weinberger AD, Beck AT: Cognitive therapy for depression, in Clinical Handbook for Psychological Disorders: A Step-by-Step Treatment Manual. Edited by Barlow DH. New York, Guilford, 2001, pp 264–302

11

New Molecular Targets for Antianxiety Interventions

Jack M. Gorman, M.D.
Justine M. Kent, M.D.

From the late 1950s through the 1970s, a series of medications were introduced to treat psychiatric disorders of almost every category, including depression, psychosis, bipolar illness, and anxiety disorder. This wave of activity is now commonly referred to as the "psychopharmacology revolution" because it established for the first time that medications could be used to treat psychiatric syndromes and suggested that these syndromes might have a basis in aberrant brain function.

It is important to remember, however, that most of these new medications, including benzodiazepines, monoamine oxidase inhibitors, tricyclics, phenothiazines, and lithium, were discovered by serendipity. No rational plan based on an understanding of the brain circuits involved in psychiatric illness could be used to develop psychiatric drugs. Even more recent developments, such as the introduction of atypical antipsychotics, anticonvulsants for bipolar illness, and selective serotonin reuptake inhibitors (SSRIs), are essentially derivative copies of these earlier drugs, so that only a modicum of scientific direction has been added to accidental discovery.

Two important developments now promise to change our agenda for discovering medications to treat psychiatric illness. First, for the first time we have animal models of some illnesses, or at least for parts of those illnesses, so that the molecular and cellular bases for disorders of mood, emotion, cognition, and behavior can be located in some cases. Second, powerful new techniques of neuroimaging are delineating the brain circuitry involved in many psychological abnormalities. As a result of these developments taken together, we are now poised to discover new interventions for psychiatric illness based on a rational scientific approach and knowledge of basic pathophysiology.

The anxiety disorders are a prime example of this progress. Although it is difficult to conceive of a clear animal model for schizophrenia or mania, it is relatively easy to do so for the fear and avoidant behaviors characteristic of humans with anxiety disorders. Consequently, we now have a series of animal models that have great appeal for studying the neural basis of both normal and pathological anxiety in humans. This has already resulted in the identification of several molecular targets that promise to be useful in the search for better ways to treat anxiety disorders. Furthermore, because anxiety and fear are fundamental components of almost all psychiatric illnesses, the work done to enhance our understanding of anxiety disorders will almost surely help us treat many other conditions as well.

BEYOND BENZODIAZEPINES

The first widely prescribed antianxiety medications were the benzodiazepines. These medications were shown to be rapidly anxiolytic and to have a much better safety margin in terms of overdose and addiction potential than previously used antianxiety drugs such as meprobamate and barbiturates. However, it quickly became apparent that benzodiazepines have a number of serious shortcomings: They are sedating, they potentiate the effects of alcohol, they produce significant cognitive and motor impairment, and they are difficult for patients to discontinue because of physical dependency. The judicious use of benzodiazepines remains an important component of treating patients with anxiety problems, but they are problematic for treating patients with anxiety disorders, who may require long-term intervention and relatively high doses. One solution to this may come through understanding better how benzodiazepines work and thereby creating effective but less burdensome analogues.

All benzodiazepines operate by potentiating the effects of the brain's main inhibitory neurotransmitter, gamma-aminobutyric acid (GABA) (Tecott 2000). They do so by binding to a receptor that is part of the $GABA_A$ receptor complex. When GABA binds to a $GABA_A$ receptor, a chloride ion channel is gated such that there is an increase in movement of negatively charged chloride ions from the extracellular to the intracellular compartment. This hyperpolarizes the postsynaptic neuron, making it relatively refractory to further stimulation by excitatory postsynaptic potentials (EPSPs). Benzodiazepines potentiate these GABA effects, opening the chloride ion channel wider and longer and thus maximizing the hyperpolarization of the neuron. Because $GABA_A$-benzodiazepine receptors are ubiquitously expressed throughout most of the central nervous system (CNS), the result of benzodiazepine administration is to reduce neural transmission in most of the brain. Hence, benzodiazepines are not only anxiolytic, but also hypnotic and anticonvulsant.

These effects of benzodiazepines explain a number of their shortcomings. For example, their interaction with alcohol is probably mediated by a binding site on the $GABA_A$ receptor complex for alcohol itself. Dependency on benzodiazepines probably arises when, after continuous use, GABA becomes inadequate to gate the chloride ion channel by itself. Sudden withdrawal of the benzodiazepine then results in a "snapping shut" of the channel, restricting chloride ion influx and resulting in a maximally depolarized neuron that is more excitable than normal.

Recently, it has been shown that the $GABA_A$ receptor is composed of five protein subunits (Rudolph et al. 1999). These subunits consist of various combinations of several different proteins, designated alpha, beta, and gamma. A genetically altered mouse with the gene encoding the alpha-1 subunit deleted has been generated (McKernan et al. 2000). The mouse demonstrates complete anxiolytic response to benzodiazepines on a number of tests but is less subject to sedation than the wild-type animal. From this rodent knockout model, it is now understood that the alpha-1 subtype of the $GABA_A$ receptor mediates the sedative properties of benzodiazepines. Molecules have subsequently been generated that bind to benzodiazepine receptors except for those $GABA_A$ receptors that include an alpha-1 subunit. Preliminary evidence suggests that such compounds may have antianxiety effects in humans but lack the troubling hypnotic properties of ordinary benzodiazepines.

Such molecular engineering may not yet create the "perfect" benzodiazepine. For example, it is unknown whether the development of drugs with little or no affinity for the alpha-1 subtype $GABA_A$ receptor will reduce the dependency problems inherent in prescribing benzodiazepines. Nevertheless, this approach combines sophisticated molecular biology with animal modeling to introduce a whole new strategy for designing antianxiety medications on a rational basis.

The exploration for better benzodiazepines has opened another avenue of research: possible abnormalities in the GABA system itself. Goddard et al. (2001) showed using magnetic resonance spectroscopy that GABA levels are lower in the occipital lobe of patients with panic disorder than in psychiatrically healthy control subjects. Several medications that enhance GABA neurotransmission, such as the selective GABA reuptake inhibitor tiagabine, are now under investigation for the treatment of anxiety disorders.

ANTIDEPRESSANTS TO TREAT ANXIETY

In the 1990s, antidepressants began replacing benzodiazepines as the pharmacological treatment of choice for anxiety disorders. It had been known for a number of years that tricyclic antidepressants are more effective than benzodiazepines for treating obsessive-compulsive disorder (OCD) and at least as effective for treating panic disorder. It was believed, however, that generalized anxiety disorder (GAD) responded only to benzodiazepines. A number of studies now dispute that assertion. For example, Rocca and colleagues (1997) compared the SSRI paroxetine, the tricyclic imipramine, and a benzodiazepine for treatment of GAD patients. As expected, the benzodiazepine showed effects more quickly than the antidepressants. However, by the end of the 8-week study, both antidepressants showed significantly better antianxiety effects than the benzodiazepine. This observation has been made in other studies as well (Rickels et al. 1993). Interestingly, antidepressants seem more effective than benzodiazepines for the so-called psychic aspects of anxiety, including worry and psychic tension, whereas benzodiazepines may be more effective for the "somatic" aspects, such as insomnia, muscle tension, and gastrointestinal complaints.

Currently, two antidepressants are approved for the treatment of GAD by the U.S. Food and Drug Administration (FDA), extended-release venlafaxine and paroxetine. The SSRIs have been shown to be effective treatments for most of the anxiety disorders, including OCD, GAD, panic disorder, social anxiety disorder (SAD), and posttraumatic stress disorder (PTSD). This has stimulated great interest in the role that serotonin neurotransmission may play in the pathogenesis of anxiety disorder.

Serotonin-synthesizing neurons are contained in relatively restricted areas of the brainstem, designated as the dorsal and ventral raphe regions. SSRIs block the presynaptic neuronal reuptake of serotonin, thus increasing synaptic levels of the neurotransmitter. Positron emission tomography (PET) imaging studies utilizing radioligands that selectively label the serotonin transporter protein necessary for serotonin reuptake have shown that relatively low doses of SSRI result in high levels of serotonin reuptake inhibition even before the drugs usually have had time to exert a therapeutic effect (Kent et al. 2002). Because the serotonin-containing neurons in the raphe send afferent projections to almost every other part of the CNS and also down the spinal cord to the periphery, this powerful enhancement of synaptic serotonin levels by SSRIs profoundly affects brain function. Thus, SSRIs have a broad spectrum of therapeutic applications, including depression, anxiety disorders, and eating disorders, but they also produce important adverse effects, most notably sexual side effects. As is the case with benzo-diazepines, the limitation of SSRIs is that their effects cannot be targeted at systems known to be involved in the generation of fear and avoidance, but rather affect almost all brain systems.

A potential solution to these problems may again come from the use of molecular genetic strategies. The laboratory of Rene Hen at Columbia University has shown that the anxiolytic effects of SSRIs are at least in part mediated by stimulation of a subset of postsynaptic serotonin receptors, the 5-hydroxytryptamine type 1A (5-HT_{1A}) receptor, specifically in fore-brain regions (Gross et al. 2002; Ramboz et al. 1998; Zhuang et al. 1999). The studies suggest that specifically targeting the postsynaptic 5-HT_{1A} re-ceptor in the forebrain may be a way to obtain the full antianxiety benefits of SSRIs without many of the adverse side effects.

The success of the SSRIs in treating anxiety disorders has created a pre-occupation with serotonin among psychiatric investigators, but it must be remembered that drugs that are selective norepinephrine (or noradrener-gic) reuptake inhibitors work just as well as SSRIs for some anxiety condi-tions, including panic disorder. A number of groups, including that of Dennis Charney at Yale University, showed in the 1980s that stimulation of the noradrenergic system with probes such as yohimbine produced panic attacks in patients with panic disorder but not in psychiatrically healthy volunteers (Charney et al. 1987). Our group at Columbia Univer-sity showed that clonidine, a drug that decreases brain noradrenergic ac-tivity, but not the beta-adrenergic blocker propranolol or the benzodiaz-epine diazepam, reduces anxiety levels in panic disorder patients during sodium lactate infusion (Coplan et al. 1992; Gorman et al. 1983; Liebowitz et al. 1995). We also showed that patients with panic disorder have ele-vated plasma levels of the first metabolite of noradrenaline, 3-methoxy-4-hydroxyphenylglycol (MHPG), compared with psychiatrically healthy control subjects (Coplan et al. 1997). All of these findings implicate hyper-activity of the noradrenergic neurotransmission system in anxiety disor-der. Recently, a nontricyclic selective noradrenergic reuptake inhibitor, reboxetine, was shown to be superior to placebo in treating panic disorder patients (Versiani et al. 2002).

There has been a tendency to view the involvement of serotonin and noradrenaline in anxiety disorders as representing two parallel, noninter-acting systems. In fact, there is abundant preclinical evidence, both ana-tomical and physiological, documenting robust interactions between the two systems. For example, Pierre Blier's group (Szabo et al. 2000) has shown that the SSRI citalopram has the same effect, albeit slower, in re-ducing the firing rate of noradrenergic neurons in the locus ceruleus as the selective noradrenergic reuptake inhibitor desipramine. Similarly, our group showed that fluoxetine, an SSRI, nevertheless reduces plasma MHPG levels in successfully treated patients with panic disorder (Coplan et al. 1997). Thus, interactions between serotonergic and noradrenergic systems exist on multiple levels. There is now controversy about whether medications that have direct effects on both the serotonergic and noradrenergic systems, such as venlafaxine, mirtazapine, milnacipram, and possibly paroxetine, are superior in efficacy and speed of onset of action compared with SSRIs or selective noradrenergic reuptake inhibitors for treatment of mood and anxiety disorders. It is clear that understanding the interactions between these systems puts the field in a better position to exploit both in finding more effective therapies.

NEW LEADS FROM THE FEAR CONDITIONING REALM

DSM-III (American Psychiatric Association 1980) created a new system of psychiatric diagnosis by offering operationalized criteria for all listed conditions. Published in 1980, it has since been revised on several occasions, but the essential features remain untouched. Anxiety disorders, for example, are subdivided into several subcategories, all with specific criteria for diagnosis. The implication is that these different types of anxiety disorders, such as panic disorder, SAD, OCD, GAD, and PTSD, are fundamentally different from each other.

Yet little evidence supports such distinctions. We know that anxiety disorders are highly comorbid with each other and with depression, and family studies show substantial overlap in heritability. Fearful, shy, and avoidant children have a high risk of later developing anxiety disorders, but no specific type of childhood anxiety predicts a specific adult anxiety disorder. Hence, the notion results that adult anxiety disorders arise from some common substrate and that the distinctions among the subcategories may not reflect important underlying biologically based abnormalities.

An interesting example of the change in viewpoint can be seen in our own work with patients with panic disorder. Several years ago, before neuroimaging techniques were sophisticated enough to help psychiatric researchers to any real extent, we became interested in the possibility that studying respiratory changes in panic disorder patients might give us a "window" into brain function. We observed that patients with panic disorder hyperventilate during panic attacks (Goetz et al. 1993) and that inhalation of small amounts (5%) of carbon dioxide mixed in room air provoked greater ventilatory response and more panic attacks in patients with panic disorder than in psychiatrically healthy control subjects (Gorman et al. 1988). The findings suggested at first that panic disorder patients might suffer from an inherited abnormality in respiratory physiology, possibly at the level of the chemoreceptor zone in the ventral medulla.

However, more recently we noted that although patients with panic disorder are significantly more likely to experience panic attacks when given carbon dioxide, psychiatrically healthy volunteers, patients with depression, and patients with premenstrual dysphoric disorder also sometimes experience a panic attack (Kent et al. 2001). Furthermore, regardless of diagnosis, individuals experiencing a panic attack during carbon dioxide inhalation demonstrate the same exaggerated ventilatory response as the panic patient having a panic attack (Gorman et al. 2001). Thus, the physiological response to carbon dioxide inhalation appears to be a function of having a panic attack, not of having a diagnosis of panic disorder.

What, then, determines why patients with panic disorder are more likely to panic during carbon dioxide inhalation than other subjects? We have argued that the discriminating factor is the level of fear. Carbon dioxide inhalation produces a sense of air hunger. Psychiatrically healthy volunteers notice that they need to breathe faster and deeper, but patients with panic disorder catastrophize the situation, are reminded of the sensations common to their naturally occurring panic attacks, and insist that the experiment be terminated (which is done immediately). The possibility that anxiety disorders represent an abnormality in brain systems mediating fear responses opens a whole world of preclinical neuroscience on which to draw. One of the most compelling resources is the literature on fear conditioning.

As described in detail elsewhere in this volume, a number of investigators have shown that conditioned fear in rodents requires the activity of a well-defined circuit in the brain that involves the sensory thalamus, the lateral and central nuclei of the amygdala, and several effector sites in the brain, including the locus ceruleus, parabrachial nucleus, periaqueductal gray region, and the hypothalamus (Gorman et al. 2000). Conditioning to the explicit fear cue, such as a loud tone previously paired with a mild foot shock, produces characteristic behaviors and responses, including freezing; increased heart rate, blood pressure, and respiration; and increased release of adrenal glucocorticoids. This requires the normal activity of the amygdala. Conditioning to the context in which the pairing of tone and shock was conducted requires the normal activity of the hippocampus. Fear conditioning is now known to involve a type of neural plasticity in the amygdala called long-term potentiation (Rogan et al. 1997), and both the acquisition and extinction of conditioned fear require protein synthesis

(Nader et al. 2000). Conditioned fear acquisition and extinction can be blocked by a number of pharmacological interventions, including administration of glutamate antagonists (Maren et al. 1996).

We recently completed a series of experiments that we believe demonstrate the analogy of conditioned fear in rodents to panic anxiety in humans. We used the respiratory stimulant doxapram, which we and others have shown is one of the most reliable ways to elicit a panic attack in patients with panic disorder but has much less effect in psychiatrically healthy volunteers (Gutman et al., in preparation; Lee et al. 1993). We showed that doxapram not only increases anxiety levels and breathlessness in patients with panic disorder compared with psychiatrically healthy volunteers, but also increases freezing responses in fear-conditioned rats compared with injection of isotonic saline (Sullivan et al. 2003). Doxapram also increased fear responses relative to vehicle in a number of other anxiety models in rodents, including the open field test and the social interaction test. Finally, we observed that doxapram administration increased the expression of the early immediate gene *c-fos* in the central nucleus of the amygdala (Sullivan et al. 2003). Taken together, this series of studies documents that the same procedure that produces anxiety attacks in vulnerable humans has a significant effect in increasing fear responses in experimental animals and activates a part of the brain, the amygdala, known to be critical for the acquisition and expression of fear behaviors.

Many neuroimaging studies, using both PET and functional magnetic resonance imaging (fMRI) techniques, have now shown that the amygdala is activated in psychiatrically healthy persons during fear responses. For example, brief exposure to masked "fearful" faces produces selective activation of the amygdala in healthy volunteers compared with masked "neutral" faces (Whalen et al. 1998). Patients with anxiety disorder appear to activate the amygdala at lower thresholds than nonanxious volunteers. Patients with PTSD showed more amygdala activation when read scripts depicting scenarios reminiscent of the original trauma that caused the anxiety disorder compared with healthy volunteers read similarly frightening scripts (Rauch et al. 1996). Patients with SAD activated the amygdala with greater intensity in response to being shown pictures of neutral faces paired with an aversive odor compared with healthy, nonanxious subjects (Birbaumer et al. 1998). There are many other examples in the neuroimaging literature involving both psychiatrically healthy subjects and patients with anxiety disorder, but the overall impression is that the amygdala is a critical part of the brain for the expression of fear in humans as well as in experimental animals.

EXPLORING THE NEUROCHEMICAL ENVIRONMENT OF THE AMYGDALA

Given that the amygdala, including its inputs and outputs, is a crucial brain structure for the mediation of fear and avoidance behavior, the next step is to examine the neurotransmitters involved in amygdala activity. Manipulation of these neurochemical systems should provide a means to affect anxiety.

One such neurotransmitter of great interest is corticotrophin-releasing factor (CRF). This 41–amino acid peptide is released by the hypothalamus and enters the portal circulation. It then stimulates pituitary release of adrencorticotropic hormone (ACTH), which enters the systemic circulation and ultimately results in adrenal release of glucocorticoids such as corticosterone in the rat and cortisol in humans. It is well known that increases in adrenal glucocorticoids occur in peripheral blood during almost all forms of stress and fear responses in all mammalian species. Thus, increased glucocorticoid level is a sensitive marker of the fear level of an organism.

In addition to its hypothalamic origin, CRF is released by extrahypothalamic sites in the brain, most notably the amygdala. CRF released by the amygdala mediates many of the manifestations of the conditioned fear response in experimental animals, in part by directly stimulating the locus ceruleus and increasing brain noradrenergic activity (Butler et al. 1990). CRF is known to be an anxiogenic molecule. When injected directly into brain of experimental animals, it increases fear responses and avoidance (Linthorst et al. 1997). This is also seen in transgenic mice that overexpress the gene for the CRF type 1 (CRF_1) receptor (Stenzel-Poore et al. 1994). By contrast, fear responses and locus ceruleus firing rate are reduced in animals given CRF receptor antagonists (Keck and Holsboer 2001; Skutella et al. 1994) and in mice with deletion of the gene for the CRF_1 receptor (Smith et al. 1998). Benzodiazepines, SSRIs, and noradrenergic reuptake inhibitors all decrease the release of CRF in the brain. Hence, there is abundant evidence that CRF is an important neurotransmitter in fear responding in experimental animals.

In humans, there is also evidence that CRF plays a role in anxiety. We have shown that cortisol levels are elevated in panic disorder patients immediately prior to experiencing a panic attack in the laboratory (Coplan et al. 1998), and Bandelow et al. (2000) recently showed increased salivary cortisol levels in panic patients experiencing naturally occurring panic attacks. CRF levels are also elevated in the cerebrospinal fluid of patients with PTSD (Bremner et al. 1997a). Elevations of CRF and cortisol have also been shown in patients with depression (Behan et al. 1996). There is evidence that overexposure to glucocorticoids can produce atrophy of the hippocampus in experimental animals (Sapolsky 2000). In humans, several studies have now shown decreased hippocampal volume in patients with depression (Sheline et al. 1996) and in patients with PTSD (Bremner et al. 1997b).

It seems important, therefore, to develop agents that block the anxiogenic effects of CRF. A number of such agents have been developed for animal studies, but only one has been reported to date in a trial involving humans. Zobel et al. (2000) administered a nonpeptide CRF_1 receptor antagonist to patients with major depression in an uncontrolled study. The CRF_1 antagonist reduced both depression and anxiety levels and was remarkably well tolerated by the patients. Unfortunately, this particular compound was associated with liver toxicity in another study and is not currently in clinical development. Other CRF antagonists are now available, however, for clinical testing, and many predict that these will prove to be important antianxiety agents in the future.

In a similar vein, receptors for the brain peptide substance P are highly localized in areas of the brain involved in fear behaviors, such as the amygdala and hippocampus (Kramer et al. 1998). Substance P antagonists (SPAs) decrease fear behaviors, such as ultrasonic distress vocalizations, in experimental animals (Kramer et al. 1998). One clinical trial involving a SPA has been reported (Kramer et al. 1998); in this placebo-controlled trial MK-869 produced antidepressant effects that were equivalent to those of paroxetine and superior to those of placebo in patients with major depression. Only the SPA MK-869 produced antianxiety effects that were superior to placebo in this trial. Furthermore, MK-869 was better tolerated than the SSRI. Thus, targeting molecules that are specifically located within known "fear circuits" in the brain holds the promise of finding effective antianxiety agents that, by virtue of more restricted CNS effects, may have reduced adverse side effect potential.

POTENTIAL ROLE OF PROMOTING NEUROGENESIS

The startling discovery has recently been made that, contrary to long-held beliefs, the mammalian brain is capable of generating new neurons during adult life (Eriksson et al. 1998; Gould et al. 1999a; van Praag et al. 2002). This has been demonstrated to most reviewers' satisfaction within the hippocampus of species as diverse as rodents, nonhuman primates, and humans. There is debate about whether prefrontal cortex is also a site for neurogenesis in adult mammals. Within the hippocampus it has now been shown that newly formed neurons mature to the point that they show fully developed axons and dendrites, make synaptic connections, and can yield electrophysiological recordings characteristic of mature neurons (van Praag 2002). At least within the hippocampus there appears to be an ongoing balance between programmed cell death, known as apoptosis, and neurogenesis.

Several animal studies have now shown that stress limits hippocampal neurogenesis (Gould et al. 1998). This is also the case for CRF and glucocorticoids, reinforcing the rationale for developing CRF antagonists (Duman et al. 2001). Another interesting impediment to neurogenesis is the brain's major excitatory neurotransmitter, glutamate (Cameron et al. 1995).

Many synapses that convey sensory information to the amygdala and that convey information downstream from the amygdala are glutamatergic. As mentioned earlier, glutamate antagonists reduce the acquisition of conditioned fear. Blocking the N-methyl-D-aspartate (NMDA)–type glutamate receptor produces an anxiolytic effect and an antidepressant effect according to preclinical studies (Berman et al. 2000). Skolnick (1999) has argued that antidepressants also block the NMDA receptor. For example, Rosenberg et al. (2000) treated children with OCD with the SSRI paroxetine and measured glutamate levels in the brain using magnetic resonance spectroscopy before and after treatment. They found that paroxetine reduced OCD symptoms, as expected, but also reduced brain glutamate concentration. Hence, there is now reason to believe that decreasing glutamate activity may reduce anxiety and promote neurogenesis.

We and others have explored the use of a metabotropic glutamate receptor agonist, LY354740. Metabotropic glutamate receptor (mGLUr) agonists activate a presynaptic receptor that triggers a negative feedback signal to the neuron and decreases release of glutamate into the synapse. We showed that LY354740 reduces the cortisol response to the anxiogenic agent yohimbine in nonhuman primates (Coplan et al. 2001). Levine et al. (in press) showed that LY354740 decreases the anxiety response to carbon dioxide inhalation in human subjects. Other strategies are now being developed that may reduce anxiety by modulating the glutamate neurotransmission system.

ROLE OF NEUROTROPHIC FACTORS

If we accept the notion that promotion of neurogenesis may be associated with an antistress or antifear effect, then identifying methods for directly increasing the development of new neurons may be even more beneficial than blocking the effects of agents that impede neurogenesis. Neuro-trophic factors are molecules in the nervous system that regulate neuronal survival, development, orientation, and plasticity. Of these agents, brain-derived neurotrophic factor (BDNF) is one of the most abundant in the brain (McAllister et al. 1999). Duman and colleagues have shown that all currently available antidepressant treatments increase BDNF expression when given chronically, but not acutely (Duman et al. 1997). Even elec-troshock, the animal analogue of electroconvulsive therapy, increases neurogenesis and BDNF expression. Stress has been shown to decrease hippocampal levels of BDNF, whereas local infusion of BDNF into the brain has antidepressant effects in animal models (Shirayama et al. 2002). Chen et al. (2001) recently compared postmortem samples from de-pressed patients who at the time of death were taking antidepressants with samples from depressed patients who were not. They found higher BDNF levels in all brain regions examined in samples from patients who had taken antidepressant medications.

The implication is that drugs that are effective in treating anxiety and de-pression may do so in part by stimulating the activity of neurotrophic factors such as BDNF and thereby enhancing neurogenesis. At the present time, no neurotrophic agent is available for direct human administration, but this promises to be an interesting avenue for future antianxiety intervention.

IS PSYCHOTHERAPY A TYPE OF ANTIANXIETY MEDICATION?

Animal models of anxiety focus mainly on the areas of the brain that are most highly developed in rodents, such as the amygdala and hippocam-pus. Although there is evidence that the medial prefrontal cortex (mPFC) suppresses amygdala activity and that lesions of the mPFC impair extinc-tion of conditioned fear (Morgan et al. 1993), it is clear that the rodent pre-frontal cortex is a poor reflection of the primate's. Aspects of anxiety disorders that are probably uniquely human, such as catastrophic cogni-tions and excessive worry about the future, most likely involve brain struc-tures such as the prefrontal cortex that are not easily modeled in rodents.

Furthermore, there is evidence that learning affects neurogenesis. A number of studies have shown that learning and novelty enhance hippoc-ampal neurogenesis in experimental animals (Gould et al. 1999b). So far, we have discussed interventions for anxiety that involve medications that affect the activity of the amygdala. However, there is reason to suspect that interventions that affect prefrontal cortical control over the amygdala and hippocampus may also be effective in treating anxiety.

Several studies indicate that reduced prefrontal activity is a component of anxious responses in humans. In healthy volunteers, for example, Hariri et al. (2000) found that a fear-inducing stimulus activated the amygdala, but when the subjects were simultaneously exposed to the fearful stimulus and asked to perform a task requiring prefrontal activation, there was less amygdala activation. Shin et al. (2001) and others have shown that patients with PTSD demonstrate reduced activation of the anterior cingulate during fear-inducing stimuli exposure compared with psychiatrically healthy volunteers. Recently, we found that subjects about to experience a panic attack showed significantly less activation of the orbitofrontal gyrus compared with subjects who did not have a panic attack (Kent et al., submitted). All of these findings suggest that a reduction in prefrontal activity, perhaps representing an inability to use cognitive skills and reason to modify limbic fear responses, plays an important role in anxiety.

These findings also suggest that interventions aimed at increasing prefrontal governance over limbic activity might be successful in reducing anxiety and fear in humans. Psychotherapy is presently the best candidate for such an intervention. Cognitive-behavioral–type psychotherapies have been shown to be at least as effective as medications in the treatment of OCD, GAD, PTSD, SAD, and panic disorder. Moreover, several studies suggest that response to cognitive-behavioral therapy is more durable than response to medication (Barlow et al. 2000). We speculate that such focused psychotherapies operate by stimulating prefrontal cortical activity, essentially bringing reason to bear on potentially anxiogenic situations. Hence, at least in the case of cognitive-behavioral types of interventions, psychotherapy for anxiety disorders may function in exactly the same way as medication. In both cases, the intervention ameliorates abnormal brain circuitry and thereby lessens fear.

CONCLUSIONS

By now it should be clear that the main grounds for excitement in the search for better antianxiety treatments lies in the belief that we understand something about the basic substrate that subserves fear and avoidant behavior. By borrowing from animal models and using neuroimaging to study the human brain, we have learned that a conserved brain circuitry, which we have called the "fear network" (Gorman et al. 2000), underlies anxiety in humans. The fear network, which includes the amygdala and its projections, the hippocampus, and the prefrontal cortex, among other brain sites, appears to be overly sensitive in patients with anxiety. This heightened sensitivity may represent the aspect of vulnerability to anxiety disorders that is controlled by heritable factors.

We have focused on a few examples in which knowledge of the anatomy of fear directs an understanding of pharmacological interventions for anxiety. Some involve treatments already available to us, including benzodiazepines and drugs that affect reuptake of serotonin and noradrenaline. These drugs, among many other actions, decrease activity in the amygdala. Other interventions involve treatments that are in the experimental stages at the present time. These include medications that block the activity of CRF, substance P, and glutamate or that enhance neurogenesis by stimulating neurotrophic factors such as BDNF. These interventions, because they target molecules and receptors that are highly localized within the fear network but not in other regions of brain, have the potential to treat anxiety with fewer adverse side effects than current treatments. Finally, we have speculated that focused psychosocial treatments, such as cognitive-behavioral therapy, may function in many respects like a pharmacological agent.

It is too early to know if and exactly when antianxiety treatments that are rationally based on anatomical and physiological knowledge will be successful in treating anxiety disorders in patients. We do know, however, that progress in other medical specialties has always been enhanced by a firm grasp of fundamental pathophysiology. For many years psychiatric researchers have been frustrated by an inability to explore the organ of interest to us, the brain. Now, for the first time we have translatable basic neuroscience and sophisticated neuroimaging techniques that permit us to look directly into the living brain and study human emotion in detail. The next decade should be one of enormous progress in identifying new molecular targets for the treatment of anxiety disorders.

REFERENCES

American Psychiatric Association: Diagnostic and Statistical Manual of Mental Disorders, 3rd Edition. Washington, DC, American Psychiatric Association, 1980

Bandelow B, Wedeking D, Pauls J, et al: Salivary cortisol in panic attacks. Am J Psychiatry 157:454–456, 2000

Barlow DH, Gorman JM, Shear MK, et al: Cognitive-behavioral therapy, imipramine, or their combination for panic disorder: a randomized controlled trial: JAMA 283:2529–2536, 2000

Behan DP, Grigoriadis DE, Lovenberg T, et al: Neurobiology of corticotrophin releasing factor (CRF) receptors and CRF-binding protein: implications for the treatment of CNS disorders. Mol Psychiatry 1:265–277, 1996

Berman RM, Cappiello A, Anand A, et al: Antidepressant effects of ketamine in depressed patients. Biol Psychiatry 47:351–354, 2000

Birbaumer N, Grodd W, Diedrich O, et al: fMRI reveals amygdala activation to human faces in social phobics. Neuroreport 9:1223–1226, 1998

Bremner JD, Licinio J, Darnell A, et al: Elevated CSF corticotrophin-releasing factor concentrations in posttraumatic stress disorder. Am J Psychiatry 154:624–629, 1997a

Bremner JD, Randall P, Vermetten E, et al: Magnetic resonance imaging–based measurement of hippocampal volume in posttraumatic stress disorder related to childhood physical and sexual abuse: a preliminary report. Biol Psychiatry 41:23–32, 1997b

Butler PD, Weiss JM, Stout JC, et al: Corticotropin-releasing factor produces fear-enhancing and behavioral activating effects following infusion into the locus coeruleus. J Neurosci 10:176–183, 1990

Cameron HA, McEwen BS, Gould E: Regulation of adult neurogenesis by excitatory input and NMDA receptor activation in the dentate gyrus. J Neurosci 15:4687–4692, 1995

Charney DS, Woods SW, Goodman WK, et al: Neurobiological mechanisms of panic anxiety: biochemical and behavioral correlates of yohimbine-induced panic attacks. Am J Psychiatry 144:1030–1036, 1987

Chen BD, Dowlatshahi D, MacQueen GM, et al: Increased hippocampal DBNF immunoreactivity in subjects treated with antidepressant medication. Biol Psychiatry 50:260–265, 2001

Coplan JD, Liebowitz MR, Gorman JM, et al: Noradrenergic function in panic disorder: effects of intravenous clonidine pretreatment on lactate induced panic. Biol Psychiatry 31:135–46, 1992

Coplan JD, Papp LA, Pine D, et al: Clinical improvement with fluoxetine therapy and noradrenergic function in patients with panic disorder. Arch Gen Psychiatry 54:643–648, 1997

Coplan JD, Goetz R, Klein DF, et al: Plasma cortisol concentrations preceding lactate-induced panic: psychological, biochemical, and physiological correlates. Arch Gen Psychiatry 55:130–136, 1998

Coplan JD, Mathew SJ, Smith ELP, et al: Effects of LY354740, a novel glutamatergic metabotropic agonist, on nonhuman primate hypothalamic-pituitary-adrenal axis and noradrenergic function. CNS Spectr 6:607–617, 2001

Duman RS, Heninger GR, Nestler EJ: Molecular and cellular theory of depression. Arch Gen Psychiatry 54:597–606, 1997

Duman RS, Malberg J, Nakagawa S: Regulation of adult neurogenesis by psychotropic drugs and stress. J Pharmacol Exp Ther 299:401–407, 2001

Eriksson PS, Perfilieva E, Bjork-Eriksson T, et al: Neurogenesis in the adult human hippocampus. Nat Med 4:1313–1317, 1998

Goddard AW, Mason GF, Almai A, et al: Reductions in occipital cortex GABA levels in panic disorder detected with 1H–magnetic resonance spectroscopy. Arch Gen Psychiatry 58:556–561, 2001

Goetz RR, Klein DF, Gully R, et al: Panic attacks during placebo procedures in the laboratory: physiology and symptomatology. Arch Gen Psychiatry 50:280–285, 1993

Gorman JM, Levy GF, Liebowitz MR, et al: Effect of acute beta-adrenergic blockade on lactate-induced panic. Arch Gen Psychiatry, 40:1079–1083, 1983

Gorman JM, Fyer MR, Goetz R, et al: Ventilatory physiology of patients with panic disorder. Arch Gen Psychiatry 45:31–39, 1988

Gorman JM, Sullivan GM, Kent JM, et al: A neuroanatomical hypothesis of panic disorder: revised. Am J Psychiatry 157:493–505, 2000

Gorman JM, Kent J, Martinez JM, et al: Physiologic changes during carbon dioxide inhalation in patients with panic disorder, major depression and premenstrual dysphoric disorder: evidence for a central fear mechanism. Arch Gen Psychiatry 58:125–131, 2001

Gould E, Tanapat P, McEwen BS, et al: Proliferation of granule cell precursors in the dentate gyrus of adult monkeys is diminished by stress. Proc Natl Acad Sci U S A 95:3168–3171,1998

Gould E, Reeves AJ, Graziano MSA, et al: Neurogenesis in the neocortex of adult primates. Science 286:548, 1999a

Gould E, Beylin A, Tanapat P, et al: Learning enhances adult neurogenesis in the hippocampal formation. Nat Neurosci 2:260–265, 1999b

Gross C, Zhuang X, Stark K, et al: Serotonin 1a receptor acts during development to establish normal anxiety-like behavior in the adult. Nature 416:396–400, 2002

Gutman D, Coplan J, Papp L, et al: Doxapram induced panic attacks and cortisol elevation. (in preparation)

Hariri AR, Bookheimer SY, Mazziotta JC: Modulating emotional responses: effects of a neocortical network on the limbic system. Neuroreport 11:43–48, 2000

Keck ME, Holsboer F: Hyperactivity of CRH neuronal circuits as a target for therapeutic interventions in affective disorders. Peptides 22:835–844, 2001

Kent JM, Papp LA, Martinez JM, et al: Specificity of panic response to CO_2 inhalation in panic disorder: a comparison with major depression and premenstrual dysphoric disorder. Am J Psychiatry 158:58–67, 2001

Kent JM, Coplan JD, Lombardo I, et al: Occupancy of brain serotonin transporters during treatment with paroxetine in patients with social phobia: a positron emission tomography study with [^{11}C] McN 5652. Psychopharmacology (Berl) 164:341–348, 2002

Kent JM, Coplan JD, Laruelle M, et al: Reduced orbitofrontal CBF predicts panic response to a respiratory stimulant in panic disorder (submitted)

Kramer MS, Cutler N, Feighner J, et al: Distinct mechanism for antidepressant activity by blockade of central substance P receptors. Science 281:1640–1645, 1998

Lee YJ, Curtis GC, Weg JG, et al: Panic attacks induced by doxapram. Biol Psychiatry 33:295–297, 1993

Levine LR, Gaydos BL, Sheehan DV, et al: The mGlu2/3 receptor agonist, LY354740, reduces panic anxiety induced by a CO_2 challenge in patients diagnosed with panic disorder. Neuropharmacology (in press)

Liebowitz MR, Coplan JD, Martinez JM, et al: Effects of intravenous diazepam pretreatment on lactate-induced panic. Psychiatry Res 58:127–138, 1995

Linthorst ACE, Flachskamm C, Hopkins SH, et al: Long-term intracerebroventricular infusion of corticotrophin-releasing hormone alters neuroendocrine, neurochemical, autonomic, behavioral, and cytokine responses to a systemic inflammatory challenge. J Neurosci 17:4448–4460, 1997

Maren S, Aharonov G, Stote DL, et al: *N*-Methyl-D-aspartate receptors in the basolateral amygdala are required for both acquisition and expression of conditioned fear in rats. Behav Neurosci 10:1365–1374,1996

McAllister AK, Katz LC, Lo DC: Neurotrophins and synaptic plasticity. Neuroscience 22:295–318, 1999

McKernan RM, Rosahl TW, Reynolds DS, et al: Sedative but not anxiolytic properties of benzodiazepines are mediated by the $GABA_A$ receptor alpha-1 subtype. Nat Neurosci 3:587–592, 2000

Morgan RA, Romanski LM, LeDoux JE: Extinction of emotional learning: contribution of medical prefrontal cortex. Neurosci Lett 163:109–113, 1993

Nader K, Schafe GE, LeDoux JE: Fear memories require protein synthesis in the amygdala for reconsolidation after retrieval. Nature 406:722–726, 2000

Ramboz S, Oostring R, Amara DA, et al: Serotonin receptor 1A knockout: an animal model of anxiety-related disorder. Proc Natl Acad Sci U S A 95:14476–14481, 1998

Rauch SL, van der Kolk BA, Fisler RE, et al: A symptom provocation study of posttraumatic stress disorder using positron emission tomography and script-driven imagery. Arch Gen Psychiatry 53:380–387, 1996

Rickels K, Downing R, Schweizer E, et al: Antidepressants for the treatment of generalized anxiety disorder. Arch Gen Psychiatry 50:884–895, 1993

Rocca P, Fonzo V, Scotta M, et al: Paroxetine efficacy in the treatment of generalized anxiety disorder. Acta Psychiatr Scand 95:444–450, 1997

Rogan MT, Staubli UV, LeDoux LE: Fear conditioning induces associative long-term potentiation in the amygdala. Nature 390:604–607, 1997

Rosenberg DR, MacMaster FP, Keshavan MS, et al: Decrease in caudate glutamatergic concentrations in pediatric obsessive-compulsive disorder patients taking paroxetine. J Am Acad Child Adolesc Psychiatry 39:1096–1103, 2000

Rudolph U, Crestain F, Benke D, et al: Benzodiazepine actions mediated by specific γ-aminobutyric acid A receptor subtypes. Nature 401:796–800, 1999

Sapolsky RM: Glucocorticoids and hippocampal atrophy in neuropsychiatric disorders. Arch Gen Psychiatry 57:925–935, 2000

Sheline Y, Wany P, Gado MH, et al: Hippocampal atrophy in recurrent major depression. Proc Natl Acad Sci U S A 93:3908–3913, 1996

Shin LM, Whalen PJ, Pitman RK, et al: An fMRI study of anterior cingulate function in posttraumatic stress disorder. Biol Psychiatry 50:932–942, 2001

Shirayama Y, Chen AC, Nakagawa S, et al: Brain-derived neurotrophic factor produces antidepressant effects in behavioral models of depression. J Neurosci 22:3251–3261, 2002

Skolnick P: Antidepressants for the new millennium. Eur J Pharmacol 375:31–40, 1999

Skutella T, Probst JC, Criswell H, et al: Antisense oligodeoxynucleotide complementary to corticotrophin-releasing hormone mRNA reduces anxiety in shuttle-box performance. Neuroreport 5:2181–2185, 1994

Smith GW, Aubry JM, Dellu F, et al: Corticotropin-releasing factor receptor 1–deficient mice display decreased anxiety, impaired stress response, and aberrant neuroendocrine development. Neuron 20:1093–1102, 1998

Stenzel-Poore MP, Heinrichs SC, Rivest S, et al: Overproduction of corticotrophin-releasing factor in transgenic mice: a genetic model of anxiogenic behavior. J Neurosci 14:2579–2584, 1994

Sullivan GM, Apergis J, Gorman JM, et al: Rodent doxapram model of panic: behavioral effects and c-fos immunoreactivity in the amygdala. Biol Psychiatry 53:863–870, 2003

Szabo ST, de Montigny C, Blier P: Progressive attenuation of the firing activity of locus coeruleus noradrenergic neurons by sustained administration of selective serotonin reuptake inhibitors. Int J Neuropsychopharmacol 3:1–11, 2000

Tecott LH: Designer genes and anti-anxiety drugs. Nat Neurosci 3:529–530, 2000

van Praag H, Schinder AF, Christie BR, et al: Functional neurogenesis in the adult hippocampus. Nature 415:1030–1034, 2002

Versiani M, Cassano G, Perugi G, et al: Reboxetine, a selective norepinephrine reuptake inhibitor, is an effective and well-tolerated treatment for panic disorder. J Clin Psychiatry 63:31–37, 2002

Whalen PJ, Rauch SL, Etcoff NL, et al: Masked presentations of emotional facial expressions modulate amygdala activity without explicit knowledge. J Neurosci 18:411–418, 1998

Zhuang X, Gross C, Sanarelli L, et al: Altered emotional states in knockout mice lacking 5-HT$_{1A}$ or 5-HT$_{1B}$ receptors. Neuropsychopharmacology 21 (suppl 2):52S–60S, 1999

Zobel AW, Nickel T, Künzel HE, et al: Effects of the high-affinity corticotropin-releasing hormone receptor 1 antagonist R121919 in major depression: the first 20 patients treated. J Psychiatr Res 34:171–181, 2000

12

Dissociating Components of Anxious Behavior in Young Rhesus Monkeys

A Precursor to Genetic Studies

Judy L. Cameron, Ph.D.
Silviu Bacanu, Ph.D.
Kristine D. Coleman, Ph.D.
Ronald E. Dahl, M.D.
Bernard J. Devlin, Ph.D.
Jeffrey A. Rogers, Ph.D.
Neal D. Ryan, M.D.
Douglas E. Williamson, Ph.D.

The research reviewed in this chapter was supported by grant MH41712 from the National Institute of Mental Health, grant RR00163 from the National Institute of Research Resources, and funds from the John D. and Catherine T. MacArthur Foundation and the James S. McDonnell Foundation Research Network on "Early Experience and Brain Development."

We thank Dr. Hill Goldsmith for his helpful assistance in translating Lab-TAB protocols designed for temperament assessment in young children into comparable tests for young monkeys, and we express appreciation for the helpful discussions with the members of the Network on Early Experience and Brain Development, and with Dr. Jerome Kagan, on strategies for dissecting the various aspects of anxious behavior. We are grateful for the excellent technical assistance provided in behavioral phenotyping by R. Clark, T. Owenby, W. Zhang, and E. Gorenson and to W. Shelledy, R. Garcia, A. Panga, and A. Vinson for their expert analysis of paternity and other pedigree relationships among the study animals. The authors are also indebted to the staff of the Division of Animal Resources at Oregon National Primate Research Center (ONPRC) for their excellent care of the monkeys used in this study.

Childhood anxiety disorders adversely affect millions of individuals, leading to substantial morbidity and mortality, and often persisting into adulthood (Black 1993; Kashani et al. 1991; Kotsopoulos 1989; Pine 1999; Pine et al. 1998; Pollack 2001). Childhood anxiety disorders are often comorbid with depression; moreover, these disorders co-occur within families (Angold and Costello 1993; Kovacs et al. 1989; Ryan et al. 1987), and the younger the affected proband, the greater the risk for the disorders in other family members (Kupfer et al. 1989; Neuman et al. 1997; Weissman et al. 1988). Twin studies suggest that familial clustering of anxiety disorders (e.g., generalized anxiety disorder [Kendler et al. 1987, 1992]; phobias such as agoraphobia and social, animal, and situational phobias [Kendler et al. 1993]; and panic disorder [Kendler et al. 1995]) is due predominantly to genetic factors.

Anxiety and depressive disorders are complex, and a number of personality and temperamental traits have been identified that appear to underlie or predate these disorders. Many of these behavioral traits also demonstrate substantial heritability. For example, anxiety sensitivity, which is the fear of anxiety-related sensations, has an estimated heritability of 45% (Stein et al. 1999) and is a critical risk factor for panic disorder, itself highly heritable (Kendler et al. 1995). Fearfulness, denoting the ease with which an individual becomes frightened, is closely associated with all forms of anxiety disorders (Rosen and Schulkin 1998) and also shows substantial heritability (Stevenson et al. 1992). Increased neuroticism appears to be a risk factor for depression (Duggan et al. 1995), and levels of neuroticism and extroversion may differentiate individuals with seasonal affective disorder from those with bipolar disorder (Jain et al. 1999). Normal developmental and temperament studies have provided evidence for a predisposition toward behavioral inhibition, defined as withdrawal from or timidity toward the unfamiliar (Garcia Coll et al. 1984; Kagan et al. 1988; Reznick et al. 1992), as a temperament trait that is associated with increased rates of anxiety disorders later in life (Biederman et al. 1993; Hirshfeld et al. 1992; Kagan and Snidman 1999; Merikangas et al. 1998) and is heritable (Cyphers et al. 1990). Behavioral inhibition emerges as a stable trait early in infancy (Kagan et al. 1988) and is associated with behavioral withdrawal or inhibition in the face of novel or threatening stimuli, as well as with a lowered threshold of arousal in response to uncertain or novel stimuli (Kagan et al. 1988). It is similar to the temperamental category of harm avoidance, defined by Cloninger and colleagues as a tendency to respond intensely to aversive stimuli and to inhibit behavior and avoid punishment (Cloninger 1987). These investigators have shown that the integrated assessment of temperamental traits has strong predictive value for antidepressant responses in depressed patients (Joyce et al. 1994; Nelson and Cloninger 1995). As a group, personality and temperament traits show substantial heritabilities that range from 30% to 60% (Bouchard 1994; Loehlin 1992).

Recently investigators have begun to recognize that efforts to identify genes underlying the development of anxiety disorders benefit from a broadening of research scope to include assessment of temperamental and personality traits that are precursors to anxiety disorders (Blangero et al. 2000; Gershenfeld and Paul 1998; Merikangas et al. 2002; Moldin 1997). Some studies are also incorporating information concerning subclinical levels of anxiety symptoms (Legrand et al. 1999; Stein et al. 1999; Topolski et al. 1997). This strategy increases power, and it has been argued that behavioral traits may represent phenotypes that show more homogeneity than complex anxiety disorders and thus may be more strongly related to expression of particular genes, facilitating gene discovery (Gershenfeld and Paul 1998; Moldin 1997). A key aspect of this strategy is the identification of robust, dissectable phenotypes for genetic analysis. In children, the development of standardized laboratory assessments to supplement parent questionnaires has aided significantly in the definition of temperamental traits (Calkins et al. 1996; Fox et al. 1995; Goldsmith and Campos 1990; Goldsmith and Rieser-Danner 1990; Goldsmith et al. 1999; Kagan 1989; Kagan et al. 1984).

USE OF ANIMAL MODELS TO STUDY THE GENETICS OF ANXIOUS BEHAVIOR

Another strategy that could aid substantially in the detailed understanding of the genetic mechanisms underlying complex behavioral traits is the use of model organisms (Gershenfeld and Paul 1998; Moldin 1997). Studies of laboratory animals contribute directly to our understanding of the brain mechanisms involved in the production of the complex forms of behavior characteristic of individuals with anxiety disorders (see reviews by Davis 1998; Mathew et al. 2001; Rosen and Schulkin 1998). Animal models have been particularly useful for examining the influence of various experiential factors on the development of anxious behaviors (Coplan et al. 1996; Davis 1998; Kalin et al. 1995; LeDoux et al. 1988, 1990; Rosenblum and Paully 1984) and for identifying the roles of specific anatomical regions and neural circuits in mediating anxious behaviors (Amaral 2002; Davis 1998; LeDoux et al. 1988, 1990). Far fewer studies have utilized animal models to help elucidate the genetic underpinnings of anxious behavior.

Most of these studies have identified strains or breeds of animals that show increased rates of anxious behavior and then characterized physiological and central nervous system differences in these animals (Boissy 1995; Gershenfeld and Paul 1998). For the most part, differences in gene expression linked to differences in anxious behavior have not been identified, although more recent studies, using knockout or transgenic approaches, are beginning to demonstrate how changes in the expression of specific genes lead to changes in anxious behavior (Gross et al. 2000).

One disadvantage of many animal models for the study of complex behaviors is the relatively large behavioral and evolutionary distance between organisms traditionally used for genetic studies (e.g., *Drosophila*, mice) and humans. In this regard, various species of nonhuman primates are more useful for modeling human behavior; they have similar brain structure, complex forms of behavior including social interactions, and close evolutionary relationships to humans (Fleagle 1999). Moreover, there appear to be related causes for the display of anxious and depressive behaviors in monkeys and humans (Harris 1989; Rosenblum and Paully 1987; Suomi 1997), evidence of similar behavioral reactions to environmental stimuli (Harlow and Novak 1973; Rosenblum and Paully 1987), and evidence for similar underlying neural regulation of these behaviors (Coplan et al. 1995; Kalin et al. 1987; Kraemer and McKinney 1979).

For example, in a situation such as separation from the primary caregiver, infant monkeys behave in ways that are very similar to the way a child might behave under the same conditions, showing both anxious and depression-like behaviors (Table 12–1). Bowlby (1960) and Spitz (1946) observed that when human infants and children are removed from their mothers, they initially react with increased movement and crying. After a few weeks, some children develop specific behaviors associated with anxiety or depression, such as lack of interest in play and loss of appetite (Bowlby 1960; Spitz 1946). Similar behaviors have been described for monkeys that have been separated from their mothers (Boccia et al. 1994; Harlow and Suomi 1974; Hinde et al. 1966; Kaufman and Rosenblum 1967; Rosenblum and Paully 1987). The initial reaction of young monkeys is often characterized by an increase in movement and cooing (a distress vocalization), followed by decreases in exploratory behavior, decreases in social play, and increases in self-directed behaviors such as huddling (Boccia et al. 1994; Harlow and Suomi 1974; Kaufman and Rosenblum 1967; Rosenblum and Paully 1987), which have been termed despair behaviors. As is the case with humans, not every monkey develops behavioral abnormalities after separation from the mother (Boccia et al. 1994; Kraemer and McKinney 1979; Suomi et al. 1978). It is interesting to note that approximately

TABLE 12–1 Behaviors commonly associated with depression and/or anxiety in children[a] and despair behaviors in young monkeys occurring consequent to maternal separation[b]

Children	Monkeys
Crying	Increased cooing
Listlessness	Decreased exploratory behavior
Increased solitude	Decreased social play
Loss of energy	Increased self-directed behavior (including huddling)

Source.   [a]Kotsopoulos 1989. [b]Boccia et al. 1994; Rosenblum and Paully 1987.

25% of monkeys develop psychological disturbances when separated from their mothers, which is the same percentage reported in humans (Boccia et al. 1994).

Monkeys also respond to pharmacological agents similarly to humans. Medications that have anxiolytic effects in humans have been shown to abate the expression of related behavioral abnormalities in monkeys. For example, imipramine, an antidepressant that can decrease anxious behavior in children (Harris 1989), can also reduce the incidence of huddling and distress vocalizations in young monkeys recently separated from their mothers (Harris and Newman 1987; Suomi et al. 1978). The drug begins to have an affect in approximately 14 days in both children and monkeys (Suomi et al. 1978). Diazepam, which has known anxiolytic effects in human anxiety disorders (Hollister 1984), decreases distress vocalizations in young monkeys separated from their mothers (Kalin et al. 1987).

REFINING AND SUBDIVIDING "ANXIOUS BEHAVIOR" IN MONKEYS

Unlike assessment in children, where information regarding anxious behavior can come from unstructured or structured interviews with the child, parents, and caregivers, from administration of standardized inventories, or from direct behavioral observations, assessments in animals rely exclusively on direct behavioral observations. Behaviors that are commonly used to assess "level of anxiety" in an animal include propensity to inspect or explore a novel object or environment (File 2001; Kabbaj and Akil 2001), and reactivity (via vocalizations or facial expressions) to a threatening social or nonsocial stimulus (Belzung et al. 2001; Kalin and Shelton 1989; Kalin et al. 1991; Roy et al. 2001). How these measures of anxious behavior are related to each other has received little study, and thus a number of questions regarding the identification of anxious animals remain unanswered at this time. Specifically, it is difficult to predict whether a given animal that is identified as anxious in one test will also be identified as anxious in another test. Further, we do not know whether different individuals may be identified as anxious depending on the test utilized or the specific behavior (e.g., vocalization, level of exploration, production of fearful facial expression) assessed.

Refinement of the "anxious" phenotype in this way is critical to successful genetic analysis, because different genes may influence different components of the phenotype. As a first step in our long-term goal of utilizing a nonhuman primate model to dissect the genetics of anxious behavior, we have undertaken a series of studies (Coleman et al. 2003; Williamson et al. 2003) to examine how different testing paradigms (involving exposure to novel objects or environments, and to threatening social and nonsocial stimuli) influence the display of various behaviors (e.g., inspection of novelty, production of vocalizations and fear grimaces) that have been classified as forms of anxious behavior in infant rhesus macaques (*Macaca mulatta*). These studies have provided the basis for future analysis of genetic "risk" for anxiety among rhesus infants. We have performed preliminary heritability analyses to identify specific behaviors that appear to be heritable in our macaque population (Williamson et al. 2003).

Assessment of Anxious Behaviors in Young Monkeys

For these studies we used four different testing paradigms commonly used to assess anxious, fearful, and/or inhibited behavior in young children and other species (File 2001; Goldsmith and Rieser-Danner 1990; Kalin and Shelton 1989). Three of the four tests (the Free Play, Remote-Controlled Car, and Human Intruder tests, to be described) were based on tests designed by Dr. Hill Goldsmith and collaborators as part of the Laboratory Temperament Assessment Battery (Lab-TAB), Locomotor version 3.0 (Goldsmith and Rothbart 1991). This battery was designed to allow standardization of temperament and behavior testing in young children, and to provide a quantitative and repeatable assessment of behavior in various conditions. The fourth test (Novel Fruit test) was designed to examine the propensity of young monkeys to approach a novel, rewarding stimulus when placed in an unfamiliar environment.

Eighty-five rhesus monkeys approximately 4 months of age (mean 115 ± 3 days; 37 males, 48 females) were used for these studies. Monkeys were reared either indoors in single cages with their mothers as part of the time-mated breeding colony (mother-reared, $n=40$) or in large (1 acre) outdoor corral breeding groups of approximately 100–150 animals (socially reared, $n=45$) at the Oregon National Primate Research Center

(ONPRC), in Beaverton, Oregon. In preparation for behavioral testing, the socially reared infants and their mothers were transferred into single cages in a holding area adjacent to the corral 1 to 2 days prior to testing. Use of the holding area occurs several times a year when monkeys receive health checks; thus, the mothers had experience with this procedure.

Approximately 10 minutes prior to the initiation of behavioral testing, the mother of the infant to be tested was sedated with 5 μg/kg ketamine HCl, given as an intramuscular injection. Once the sedative took effect, both mother and infant were placed in a transfer box and brought to the behavioral testing facility. The transfer from home cage to testing facility took approximately 5 minutes. When the mother-infant pair arrived at the testing facility, they were placed together in a playroom (described subsequently) and the Free Play and Remote-Controlled Car tests were performed. The infant was then separated from the mother and placed in a novel cage in a different room, for the Human Intruder and Novel Fruit tests. The Free Play and Remote-Controlled Car tests were videotaped through a one-way window in the playroom. The Human Intruder and Novel Fruit tests were videotaped from behind a blind. Behavior recorded on videotapes was scored using a computer program (Observer Video Pro version 4.0, Noldus Information Technology, The Netherlands) in which both behavioral states (behavioral patterns measurable by duration, with a distinct start and end [e.g., movement]) and behavioral events (behavioral patterns without a measurable duration [e.g., vocalizations]) could be assessed (see Table 12–2 for a list of the behaviors assessed).

Free Play Test

The Free Play test was designed to test the infant's propensity to explore an unfamiliar environment. This test was based on the Free Play episode in the Child Lab-TAB manual, which was designed for 12-month-old infants. The playroom (2.4 m × 3.0 m) contained a climbing structure (127 cm × 61 cm × 198 cm) and nine novel toys arranged in a semicircle. A one-way window in the door to the room allowed observation and videotaping. When the infant and mother arrived at the testing room, they were immediately placed in an infant car seat, where the mother was strapped in a sitting position and given a second dose of sedative (10 μg/kg ketamine HCl) to ensure that she remained sedated throughout the test. The mother was kept present to avoid the confounder of separation anxiety, but sedation prevented her from interfering with the infant's behavior. The infant was videotaped for the first 5 minutes after its arrival in the playroom (Free Play 1) to allow assessment of its initial reaction to the novel environment, and again after a half-hour acclimation period (Free Play 2).

TABLE 12–2   Behaviors scored in four temperament tests

Behavior	Description of behavior	Test
Vocalization	Coos and shrieks	FP 1
		FP 2
		RC
		HI Alone1
		HI Alone2
		HI Profile
		HI Stare
Fear grimace	Overt fearful facial expression (lips pulled back, baring teeth) directed toward car or intruder	RC
		HI Stare
Inspection of novelty: toy play	Infant intentionally touched or displaced novel object (including toys and car seat) with hands or mouth	FP 1
		FP 2
Inspection of novelty: cage explore	Intentional exploration of environment; including touching or biting cage	HI Alone1
		HI Alone2
		HI Profile
Inspection of novelty: inspect fruit	Infant approached within 3 cm of the fruit and appeared to be looking at it	NF
Inspection of novelty: touch fruit	Intentional contact with food	NF

Note. FP = Free Play test, HI = Human Intruder test, NF = Novel Fruit test, RC = Remote-Controlled Car test.

Remote-Controlled Car Test

The Remote-Controlled Car test was used to examine the responsiveness of infants to a frightening, nonsocial stimulus (a bright remote-controlled car that entered the room unexpectedly and approached the infant). The test was modeled after the Remote-Controlled Spider episode in the Loco-motor 3.0 version of the Child Lab-TAB manual. This test consisted of five epochs. The first epoch involved the car entering the room through a small doorway and pausing for 10 seconds. In the next epoch the car approached to within 0.3 m of the infant and paused for 10 seconds. The car then retreated slightly (1 m) and paused for 10 seconds. The car again approached the infant (stopping 0.3 m from the infant) and paused for 10 seconds. The final epoch consisted of the car leaving the room.

Human Intruder Test

The Human Intruder test was a modification of the test originally developed by Kalin and colleagues (Kalin and Shelton 1989; Kalin et al. 1991) for use in monkeys, and was utilized to assess behavioral responsiveness to both nonthreatening and threatening social stimuli. A similar test (Stranger Approach) has been used by Dr. Goldsmith and colleagues in

Child Lab-TAB Locomotor version 3.0. This test measured behavioral response in three situations: being alone in a novel cage, being in the presence of a human stranger whose gaze was diverted from the monkey (nonthreatening social stimulus), and being in the presence of a human stranger making direct eye contact with the monkey (threatening social stimulus).

Following the Remote-Controlled Car test, the infant was brought from the playroom and placed alone in a standard monkey cage located in a novel room. The infant was allowed 10 minutes to adapt, after which the monkey was videotaped from behind a blind for four 2-minute periods (8 minutes total). Testing began with a 2-minute control period with no human present (Alone1). In the second period (Profile), a human intruder who had never been in contact with the monkey entered the room and stood about 0.3 m from the cage with facial profile presented to the monkey. The intruder left the room, and the infant was alone for the third period (Alone2). In the fourth period (Stare), the human intruder reentered the room and stood 0.3 m from the cage, making continuous direct eye contact with the infant. Direct eye contact is generally considered a threatening facial expression for monkeys.

Novel Fruit Test

The Novel Fruit test was designed to test the infant's inclination to explore an ecologically relevant novel object (pieces of unfamiliar fruit and familiar fruit). Two minutes after completion of the Human Intruder test, the intruder entered the room and placed a slice of kiwi, a fruit that is novel to the monkeys, in the cage. The intruder left the room, and the infant was videotaped for 5 minutes. The intruder reentered the room and placed a piece of apple, a fruit the monkeys had seen previously, in the cage, and the infant was videotaped for an additional 5 minutes. Latency to inspection and touching of each of the fruits was measured.

Factor Analysis of Behaviors

To examine the intercorrelations of the behaviors and how they cluster into common factors, factor analyses were performed on all measured behaviors (Williamson et al. 2003). Only items with a minimum factor loading of 0.50 were considered significant. To limit the number of factors identified, only those factors with eigenvalues greater than 1.95 were examined in detail. The correlation matrix factor analysis revealed that seven factors explained a total of 56.7% of the overall variability within the behaviors. The eigenvalues were 3.59, 2.69, 2.57, 2.39, 2.23, 2.00, and 1.97

for factors 1 through 7, respectively. The overall variance explained by each of the factors was 11.6%, 8.7%, 8.3%, 7.7%, 7.5%, 6.5%, and 6.4% for factors 1 through 7, respectively. A summary of the seven factors and their corresponding behaviors is given in Table 12–3.

Factor 1 consisted of vocalizations across all four conditions of the Human Intruder test. Factor 2 consisted of movement behavior during the Alone1, Profile, and Alone2 conditions of the Human Intruder test. Factor 3 comprised vocalizations during period 1 and period 2 of the Free Play test, plus teeth grinding during the Profile and Stare conditions of the Human Intruder test. Factor 4 was made up of time spent away from the mother, activity level, and toy play during period 2 of the Free Play test. Latency to leave the mother during the Free Play test, as well as time away and activity during period 1 of the Free Play test, loaded on factor 5. Exploratory behavior during the Alone1, Profile, and Alone2 conditions of the Human Intruder test loaded on factor 6. Finally, factor 7 consisted of latency to inspect and touch the kiwi fruit during the Novel Fruit test.

The results of these analyses support the hypothesis that *vocalizations* and *exploration of novelty* are prominent behaviors displayed by monkeys in conditions that can promote anxiety. Fear grimacing, which we predicted would be another common reaction in these tests, was displayed by only a small proportion of monkeys, and only in the Stare condition of the Human Intruder test and in the Remote-Controlled Car test. Moreover, there was no correlation in the production of fear grimaces between these two tests. Fear grimacing did not appear in any of the factors explaining the majority of the variance in these tests.

Surprisingly, none of the factors contained both vocalizations and exploration. Additionally, for each of these variables, the behavior in different tests generally aggregated in different factors (see Table 12–3). Vocalizations aggregated in two factors. Factor 1 had vocalizations in all epochs of the Human Intruder test, whereas factor 3 had vocalizations in the two periods of the Free Play test. Exploration of novelty aggregated in five factors, none of which included exploratory behaviors from more than one test. Thus, certain attributes that we associate with anxious behavior appear to be essentially uncorrelated and this lack of correlation could have a dramatic impact on which animals are categorized as anxious.

Preliminary Genetic Analyses of the Seven Factors

Only one of the factors showed statistically significant heritability with the available sample size. Factor 2 (movement during Alone1, Profile, and Alone2 of the Human Intruder test) showed an estimated heritability of

TABLE 12–3   Summary of factor analysis for behaviors displayed across the four tests

Identified factor	Behavior	Variance explained
Factor 1	**Distress vocalizations**	11.6%
	HI Alone1: vocalizations	
	HI Profile: vocalizations	
	HI Alone2: vocalizations	
	HI Stare: vocalizations	
Factor 2	**Movement**	8.7%
	HI Alone1: movement	
	HI Profile: movement	
	HI Alone2: movement	
Factor 3	**Distress cues**	8.3%
	HI Profile: teeth grinding	
	HI Stare: teeth grinding	
	FP 1 and 2: vocalizations	
Factor 4	**Delayed independence**	7.7%
	FP 2: time away from mother	
	FP 2: movement	
	FP 2: toy play	
Factor 5	**Early independence**	7.5%
	FP 1: latency to leave mother	
	FP 1: time away from mother	
	FP 1: movement	
	FP 2: latency to leave mother	
Factor 6	**Explore familiar environment**	6.5%
	HI Alone1: explore	
	HI Profile: explore	
	HI Alone2: explore	
Factor 7	**Explore novelty**	6.4%
	NF: inspect kiwi	
	NF: touch kiwi	

Note.   FP = Free Play test, HI = Human Intruder test, NF = Novel Fruit test.

1.0 $(P \leq 0.01)$. Although it is unlikely that the true heritability is 1.0, these data do indicate that this behavior is influenced by genetic variation among the study subjects. Three factors showed indications of possible heritability but did not reach statistical significance. The estimated heritability for factor 3 was $h^2 = 0.58$ $(P \leq 0.10)$, whereas factor 5 exhibited a heritability of $h^2 = 0.83$ $(P \leq 0.10)$ and factor 7 produced an estimate of $h^2 = 1.0$ but did not reach significance $(P \leq 0.10)$. It is possible that some or all of these three factors will show significant heritabilities once a larger number of animals can be included in the analysis.

CONCLUSIONS

The interpretation of these findings for the genetics of anxious behavior in our population of rhesus monkeys remains unresolved. One possible explanation is that different genetic variants underlie the different forms of anxious behavior, and their impact could also differ according to the context (e.g., with or without the presence of a threatening stimulus, in the presence of a social threat versus a nonsocial threat). Our preliminary heritability analysis, although revealing some substantial differences in the heritabilities of behaviors across tests, cannot yet weigh in on the genetic correlations among these traits (for more detail, see Williamson et al. 2003). We anticipate having sufficient data to perform such analyses in the near future.

The notion that specific types of anxious behavior are separable from each other, have different etiologies, and may lead to different outcomes is supported by findings from several other groups of investigators. Kalin et al. (1991) have speculated that overly intense but context-appropriate responses to situations such as the Human Intruder test may be a risk factor for the development of social phobia, but not generalized anxiety. Mick and Telch (1998) reported that behavioral inhibition is not a general risk factor for the development of anxiety, but rather is associated specifically with social anxiety.

It is important to keep in mind that these are preliminary results, based on a small sample size. Further work is needed to completely define how the measurement of various behaviors in different tests influence the identification of an individual as anxious, and especially to understand how such assessments may be influenced by developmental processes. However, this work is adding to a small but growing number of investigators (e.g., Belzung et al. 2001; Carola et al. 2002) who are looking at behavior across multiple standardized tests, to further our understanding of behaviors that may influence the assessment of anxiety.

REFERENCES

Amaral DG: The primate amygdala and the neurobiology of social behavior: implications for understanding social anxiety. Biol Psychiatry 51:11–17, 2002
Angold A, Costello EJ: Depressive comorbidity in children and adolescents: empirical, theoretical, and methodological issues. Am J Psychiatry 150:1779–1791, 1993
Belzung C, El Hage W, Moindrot N, et al: Behavioral and neurochemical changes following predatory stress in mice. Neuropharmacology 41:400–408, 2001
Biederman J, Rosenbaum JF, Bolduc-Murphy EA, et al: A 3-year follow-up of children with and without behavioral inhibition (see comments). J Am Acad Child Adolesc Psychiatry 32:814–821, 1993

Black B: Neurobiology of anxiety disorders. Child Adolesc Psychiatr Clin N Am 4:749–762, 1993

Blangero J, Williams JT, Almasy L: Quantitative trait locus mapping using human pedigrees. Hum Biol 72:35–62, 2000

Boccia ML, Laudenslager ML, Reite ML: Intrinsic and extrinsic factors affect infant responses to maternal separation. Psychiatry 57:43–50, 1994

Boissy A: Fear and fearfulness in animals. Q Rev Biol 70:165–191, 1995

Bouchard TJJ: Genes, environment, and personality. Science 264:1700–1701, 1994

Bowlby J: Grief and mourning in infancy and early childhood. Psychoanal Study Child 15:9–52, 1960

Calkins SD, Fox NA, Marshall TR: Behavioral and physiological antecedents of inhibited and uninhibited behavior. Child Dev 67:523–540, 1996

Carola V, D'Olimpio F, Brunamonti E, et al: Evaluation of the elevated plus-maze and open-field tests for the assessment of anxiety-related behaviour in inbred mice. Behav Brain Res 134:49–57, 2002

Cloninger CR: A systematic method for clinical description and classification of personality variants. Arch Gen Psychiatry 44:266–273, 1987

Coleman K, Dahl RE, Ryan ND, et al: Growth hormone response to growth hormone-releasing hormone and clonidine in young monkeys: correlation with behavioral characteristics. J Child Adolesc Psychopharmacol 13:211–225, 2003

Coplan JD, Rosenblum LA, Gorman JM: Primate models of anxiety: longitudinal perspectives. Psychiatr Clin North Am 18:727–743, 1995

Coplan JD, Andrews MW, Rosenblum LA, et al: Persistent elevations of cerebrospinal fluid concentrations of corticotropin-releasing factor in adult non-human primates exposed to early life stressors: implications for the pathophysiology of mood and anxiety disorders. Proc Natl Acad Sci U S A 93:1619–1623, 1996

Cyphers LH, Phillips K, Fulker DW, et al: Twin temperament during the transition from infancy to early childhood. J Am Acad Child Adolesc Psychiatry 29:392–397, 1990

Davis M: Are different parts of the extended amygdala involved in fear versus anxiety? Biol Psychiatry 44:1239–1247, 1998

Duggan C, Sham P, Lee A, et al: Neuroticism: a vulnerability marker for depression evidence from a family study. J Affect Disord 35:139–143, 1995

File SE: Factors controlling measures of anxiety and responses to novelty in the mouse. Behav Brain Res 125:151–157, 2001

Fleagle JG: Primate Adaptation and Evolution. New York, Academic Press, 1999

Fox NA, Rubin KH, Calkins SD, et al: Frontal activation asymmetry and social competence at four years of age. Child Dev 66:1770–1784, 1995

Garcia Coll C, Kagan J, Reznick JS: Behavioral inhibition in young children. Child Dev 55:1005–1019, 1984

Gershenfeld HK, Paul SM: Towards a genetics of anxious temperament: from mice to men. Acta Psychiatr Scand Suppl 393:56–65, 1998

Goldsmith HH, Campos JJ: The structure of temperamental fear and pleasure in infants: a psychometric perspective. Child Dev 61:1944–1964, 1990

Goldsmith HH, Rieser-Danner L: Assessing early temperament, in Handbook of Psychological and Educational Assessment of Children, Vol 2: Personality, Behavior, and Context. Edited by Reynolds CR, Kamphaus R. New York, Guilford, 1990, pp 345–378

Goldsmith HH, Rothbart MK: Contemporary instruments for assessing early temperament by questionnaire and in the laboratory, in Explorations in Temperament: International Perspectives on Theory and Measurement. Edited by Strelau J, Angleitner A. New York, Plenum, 1991, pp 249–272

Goldsmith HH, Lemery KS, Buss KA, et al: Genetic analyses of focal aspects of infant temperament. Dev Psychol 35:972–985, 1999

Gross C, Santarelli L, Brunner D, et al: Altered fear circuits in 5-HT(1A) receptor KO mice. Biol Psychiatry 48:1157–1163, 2000

Harlow HF, Novak MA: Psychopathological perspectives. Perspect Biol Med 16:461–478, 1973

Harlow HF, Suomi SJ: Induced depression in monkeys. Behav Biology 12:273–296, 1974

Harris JC: Experimental animal modeling of depression and anxiety. Psychiatr Clin North Am 12:815–836, 1989

Harris JC, Newman JD: Mediation of separation distress by alpha 2–adrenergic mechanisms in a non-human primate. Brain Res 410:353–356, 1987

Hinde RA, Spencer-Booth Y, Bruce M: Effects of 6-day maternal deprivation on rhesus monkey infants. Nature 210:1021–1033, 1966

Hirshfeld DR, Rosenbaum JF, Biederman J, et al: Stable behavioral inhibition and its association with anxiety disorder. J Am Acad Child Adolesc Psychiatry 31:103–111, 1992

Hollister LO: Clinical aspects of anti-anxiety agents, in Anxiolytics: Neurochemical, Behavioral, and Clinical Perspectives. Edited by Burrows G, Norman TR, Davies B. Amsterdam, Elsevier, 1984, pp 106–126

Jain U, Blais MA, Otto MW, et al: Five-factor personality traits in patients with seasonal depression: treatment effects and comparisons with bipolar patients. J Affect Disord 55:51–54, 1999

Joyce PR, Mulder RT, Cloninger CR: Temperament predicts clomipramine and desipramine response in major depression. J Affect Disord 30:35–46, 1994

Kabbaj M, Akil H: Individual differences in novelty-seeking behavior in rats: a *c-fos* study. Neuroscience 106:535–545, 2001

Kagan J: The concept of behavioral inhibition to the unfamiliar, in Perspective on Behavioral Inhibition. Edited by Reznick JS. Chicago, IL, University of Chicago Press, 1989, pp 1–23

Kagan J, Snidman N: Early childhood predictors of adult anxiety disorders. Biol Psychiatry 46:1536–1541, 1999

Kagan J, Reznick JS, Clarke C, et al: Behavioral inhibition to the unfamiliar. Child Dev 55:2212–2225, 1984

Kagan J, Reznick JS, Snidman N: Biological bases of childhood shyness. Science 240:167–171, 1988

Kalin NH, Shelton SE: Defensive behaviors in infant rhesus monkeys: environmental cues and neurochemical regulation. Science 243:1718–1721, 1989

Kalin NH, Dawson G, Tariot P, et al: Function of the adrenal cortex in patients with major depression. Psychiatry Res 22:117–125, 1987

Kalin NH, Shelton SE, Takahashi LK: Defensive behaviors in infant rhesus monkeys: ontogeny and context-dependent selective expression. Child Dev 62:1175–1183, 1991

Kalin NH, Shelton SE, Lynn DE: Opiate systems in mother and infant primates coordinate intimate contact during reunion. Psychoneuroendocrinology 20:735–742, 1995

Kashani JH, Dandoy AC, Orvaschel H: Current perspectives on anxiety disorders in children and adolescents: an overview. Compr Psychiatry 32:481–95, 1991

Kaufman IC, Rosenblum LA: Depression in infant monkeys separated from their mothers. Science 155:1030–1031, 1967

Kendler KS, Heath AC, Martin NG, et al: Symptoms of anxiety and symptoms of depression: same genes, different environments? Arch Gen Psychiatry 44:451–457, 1987

Kendler KS, Neale MC, Kessler RC, et al: Major depression and generalized anxiety disorder: same genes, (partly) different environments? Arch Gen Psychiatry 49:716–722, 1992

Kendler KS, Neale MC, Kessler RC, et al: Major depression and phobias: the genetic and environmental sources of comorbidity. Psychol Med 23:361–371, 1993

Kendler KS, Walters EE, Neale MC, et al: The structure of the genetic and environmental risk factors for six major psychiatric disorders in women: phobia, generalized anxiety disorder, panic disorder, bulimia, major depression and alcoholism. Arch Gen Psychiatry 52:374–383, 1995

Kotsopoulos S: Phenomenology of anxiety and depressive disorders in children and adolescents. Psychiatr Clin North Am 12:803–814, 1989

Kovacs M, Gatsonis C, Paulauskas SL, et al: Depressive disorders in childhood, IV: a longitudinal study of comorbidity with and risk for anxiety disorders. Arch Gen Psychiatry 46:776–782, 1989

Kraemer GW, McKinney WT: Interactions of pharmacological agents which alter biogenic amine metabolism and depression: an analysis of contributing factors within a primate model of depression. J Affect Disord 1:33–54, 1979

Kupfer DJ, Frank E, Carpenter LL, et al: Family history in recurrent depression. J Affect Disord 17:113–119, 1989

LeDoux JE, Iwata J, Cicchetti P, et al: Different projections of the central amygdaloid nucleus mediate autonomic and behavioral correlates of conditioned fear. J Neurosci 8:2517–2529, 1988

LeDoux JE, Cicchetti P, Xagoraris A, et al: The lateral amygdaloid nucleus: sensory interface of the amygdala in fear conditioning. J Neurosci 10:1062–1069, 1990

Legrand LN, McGue M, Iacono WG: A twin study of state and trait anxiety in childhood and adolescence. J Child Psychol Psychiatry 40:953–958, 1999

Loehlin JC: Genes and Environment in Personality Development. Newbury Park, CA, Sage, 1992

Mathew SJ, Coplan JD, Gorman JM: Neurobiological mechanisms of social anxiety disorder. Am J Psychiatry 158:1558–1567, 2001

Merikangas KR, Swendsen JD, Preisig MA, et al: Psychopathology and temperament in parents and offspring: results of a family study. J Affect Disord 51:63–74, 1998

Merikangas KR, Avenevoli S, Acharyya S, et al: The spectrum of social phobia in the Zurich cohort study of young adults. Biol Psychiatry 51:81–91, 2002

Mick MA, Telch MJ: Social anxiety and history of behavioral inhibition in young adults. J Anxiety Disord 12:1–20, 1998

Moldin SO: The maddening hunt for madness genes. Nat Genet 17:127–129, 1997

Nelson EC, Cloninger CR: The tridimensional personality questionnaire as a predictor of response to nefazodone treatment of depression. J Affect Disord 35:31–35, 1995

Neuman RJ, Geller B, Rice JP, et al: Increased prevalence and earlier onset of mood disorders among relatives of prepubertal versus adult probands. J Am Acad Child Adolesc Psychiatry 36:466–473, 1997

Pine DS: Pathophysiology of childhood anxiety disorders. Biol Psychiatry 46:1555–1566, 1999

Pine DS, Cohen P, Gurley D, et al: The risk for early adulthood anxiety and depressive disorders in adolescents with anxiety and depressive disorders. Arch Gen Psychiatry 55:56–64, 1998

Pollack MH: Comorbidity, neurobiology, and pharmacotherapy of social anxiety disorder. J Clin Psychiatry 62:24–29, 2001

Reznick JS, Hegeman IM, Kaufman ER, et al: Retrospective and concurrent self-report of behavioral inhibition and their relation to adult mental health. Dev Psychopathol 4:301–302, 1992

Rosen JB, Schulkin J: From normal fear to pathological anxiety. Psychol Rev 105:325–350, 1998

Rosenblum LA, Paully GS: The effects of varying environmental demands on maternal and infant behavior. Child Dev 55:305–314, 1984

Rosenblum LA, Paully GS: Primate models of separation-induced depression. Psychiatr Clin North Am 10:437–447, 1987

Roy V, Belzung C, Delarue C, et al: Environmental enrichment in BALB/c mice: effects in classical tests of anxiety and exposure to a predatory odor. Physiol Behav 74:313–320, 2001

Ryan ND, Puig-Antich J, Ambrosini P, et al: The clinical picture of major depression in children and adolescents. Arch Gen Psychiatry 44:854–861, 1987

Spitz RA: Anaclitic depression: an inquiry into the genesis of psychiatric conditions in early childhood. Psychoanal Study Child 2:313–347, 1946

Stein MB, Jang KL, Livesley WJ: Heritability of anxiety sensitivity: a twin study. Am J Psychiatry 156:246–251, 1999

Stevenson J, Batten N, Cherner M: Fears and fearfulness in children and adolescents: a genetic analysis of twin data. J Child Psychol Psychiatry 33:977–985, 1992

Suomi SJ: Early determinants of behaviour: evidence from primate studies. Br Med Bull 53:170–184, 1997

Suomi SJ, Seaman SF, Lewis JK, et al: Effects of imipramine treatment of separation-induced social disorders in rhesus monkeys. Arch Gen Psychiatry 35:321–325, 1978

Topolski TD, Hewitt JK, Eaves LJ, et al: Genetic and environmental influences on child reports of manifest anxiety and symptoms of separation anxiety and overanxious disorders: a community-based twin study. Behav Genet 27:15–28, 1997

Weissman MM, Warner V, Wickramaratne P, et al: Early onset major depression in parents and their children. J Affect Disord 15:269–277, 1988

Williamson DE, Coleman K, Devlin BJ, et al: Heritability of fearful/anxious endophenotypes in infant rhesus macaques: a preliminary report. Biol Psychiatry 53:284–291, 2003

13

The Anatomy of Fear

Microcircuits of the Lateral Amygdala

Luke R. Johnson, Ph.D.
Joseph E. LeDoux, Ph.D.

More than a century ago, Kraepelin argued that different components of dementia praecox are due to disruptions in different brain circuits. In particular, he proposed that disorders of reasoning could be localized to the frontal lobes and disorders of delusions to the temporal lobes (McCarley et al. 1993; Shenton et al. 1992). Ever since, the identification of pathological changes in the brain that might underlie mental disorders has been a goal of neuropsychiatry. Although much research has been performed, and progress has been made, a detailed understanding of the neural basis of psychiatric disorders remains a hope rather than an achievement.

The discovery that drugs that alter the levels of monoamine neuromodulators in the brain relieve symptoms in several psychiatric disorders led to a massive effort to understand the effects of such drugs on the brain. One outcome of this research has been the realization that the therapeutic effects of drugs are not due to a single, universal action of the drug, but to actions in specific circuits. For example, the finding that schizophrenia could be treated by altering levels of dopamine in the brain was a major therapeutic breakthrough. However, the more recent discovery that dopamine function is altered only in certain parts of the brain has led to a major shift in the way mental disorders are conceptualized. They are no longer

The work of L.R.J. is supported by a NARSAD Young Investigator Award.

thought of in terms of a global chemical imbalance in the brain but instead are viewed in terms of changes in the role of a chemical within specific brain systems.

Until drugs can be developed that target the specific circuits altered in the disorder, they will continue to produce incomplete symptom relief and side effects. But this goal cannot be achieved without an understanding of the circuits that are altered.

Recent progress in uncovering the neural basis of conditioned fear offers hope for new approaches to understanding and treating fear-related disorders, such as anxiety disorders (panic, posttraumatic stress disorder [PTSD], phobias, generalized anxiety) and paranoia. Conditioned fear is a procedure in which a neutral stimulus is transformed into a fear-arousing event when paired with an aversive stimulus. Using this procedure in studies of rats, specific brain nuclei have been identified that are necessary for the conditioning to occur. Further, cellular changes associated with the learning occur in these same nuclei, and disruption of this activity prevents the learning from taking place (Davis and Whalen 2001; LeDoux 2000; Maren 2001). It seems reasonable, as a working hypothesis, to propose that fear-related disorders involve alterations in the brain networks that normally process fearful events. If so, then studies of the neural basis of fear conditioning might be an important step toward understanding fear pathology.

A key region in the fear-processing network is the lateral nucleus of the amygdala (LA). In this chapter we review the neuronal organization of the LA and begin to ask how its fear learning and expression are encoded in its microcircuitry. It is not our intent to suggest that psychopathology is necessarily localizable to specific nuclei of the amygdala. Rather, we argue that understanding the specifics of how microcircuits within the amygdala underlie fear-related behavior can help us understand how alterations in these circuits might account for fear pathology.

FEAR

The term *fear* refers to both subjective states (the feeling of fear) and bodily responses (behavioral, autonomic, and endocrine changes) elicited by threatening stimuli. In this chapter, we use the term mainly in reference to the bodily responses. That is, we discuss the brain circuits that produce bodily responses in reaction to threatening stimuli. The behavioral and physiological responses to fear include activation of the hypothalamic-pituitary-adrenal (HPA) axis, reduced tolerance to pain, activation of the autonomic nervous system, and defensive behaviors (freezing and then fight or flight) (LeDoux 2000).

The detection of threats and the production of protective bodily responses is a vital part of biological survival. The brain has circuits that are "prewired" to respond to certain stimuli (ancestral threats) and to learn about novel stimuli that occur in association with prewired dangers. In this way, individuals can use information from past situations to avoid potentially dangerous organisms, objects, and situations.

Pathological fear occurs when the fear response elicited is inappropriate to the stimulus. This inappropriate identification and response to fear-provoking stimuli, leading to distressing and debilitating symptoms, characterize fear-related disorders, including panic, PTSD, generalized anxiety, phobias, and paranoia (including paranoid psychosis). Moreover, fear and psychopathology appear to interact throughout development; recent work shows that early expression of fear-based anxiety attacks in development is highly correlated with later development of psychosis and suicide (Goodwin and Hamilton 2002).

FEAR CONDITIONING

The aforementioned constellation of fear responses can be evoked by stimuli that have gained emotional significance through classical conditioning. Classical conditioning of fear-provoking stimuli (fear conditioning) is inducible in all organisms studied to date, including fruit flies, fish, birds, rats, dogs, and humans (LeDoux 2000).

Fear conditioning requires the coordinated presentation or pairing of two sensory inputs. One input is an initially neutral stimulus (which becomes the conditioned stimulus [CS]), and the other input is a biologically significant event (the unconditioned stimulus [US]). The pairing of these stimuli results in a conditioned response (CR) such that the initially neutral stimulus (CS) now elicits the same behavioral response as the US. In the behavioral model of auditory fear conditioning, in both humans and animals, a neutral auditory tone stimulus is paired with an electric shock such that presentation of the auditory tone comes to elicit fear responses (see Figure 13–1).

FEAR CONDITIONING AND THE AMYGDALA

The auditory CS and nociceptive US converge in the LA (Romanski and LeDoux 1992; Romanski et al. 1993). Fear conditioning is dependent on nociceptive inputs from the spinothalamic tract that terminate in the amygdala either directly from the thalamus or via the cortex (Shi and

Davis 1999). Although nociceptive inputs also terminate in the central amygdala directly from the spinal cord and the parabrachial area (Bernard and Besson 1990; Bernard et al. 1990; Burstein and Potrebic 1993), evidence suggests that the convergent input in the LA is most likely the initial site of US-CS convergence and learning (LeDoux 2000; Muller et al. 1997).

Considerable evidence also demonstrates convergent acoustic input to the LA. The acoustic signal conveying the tone CS enters the LA via the auditory thalamus and the auditory association cortex (Romanski and LeDoux 1992; Romanski et al. 1993). Both of these pathways enter the LA, where they converge with US signals (Figure 13–1). The two auditory routes may provide different aspects of the CS to the LA, with the thalamic input providing a basic schema of the CS and the cortical input providing more specific details. Either of these pathways is sufficient for conditioning to simple auditory stimuli, but the cortical pathway seems to be required for learning about more complex stimuli (LeDoux 2000; Romanski and LeDoux 1992).

Activation of the bodily responses is controlled via the central nucleus of the amygdala, which receives direct projections from the LA (Figure 13–1). The central nucleus in turn projects to the various brainstem areas that control the different responses (Davis and Whalen 2001). The brain's fear system thus appears to require a series of sequentially connected nuclei, with the apex for sensory convergence and motor activation located in the LA.

The LA has been shown to be capable of considerable plasticity during fear conditioning. The firing rates of cells in the LA increase before, during, and following conditioning trials (Quirk et al. 1995; Repa et al. 2001). These changes precede the expression of fear responses, suggesting that plastic changes in LA neurons drive fear behavior.

Recent studies have revealed heterogeneity in the learning behavior of LA neurons (Repa et al. 2001). One population of LA neurons showed transient increases in firing rates during learning. These rapid changes were extinguished rapidly when the CS was presented without the US. A second population of neurons required more training trials of CS-US pairings before firing rates increased, but following learning these plastic changes endured through extinction trials (Repa et al. 2001). The transiently plastic neurons were located dorsally in the dorsal LA whereas long-term plastic cells were in a more ventral part of the dorsal LA (the LA has a dorsal nucleus [LAd], and cells were distributed dorsally and ventrally within the LAd).

The finding of heterogeneity of cell learning behavior and anatomical distribution suggests a complex network within the LA, such that dorsally located cells may act as "trigger cells" for longer-term learning in ventral

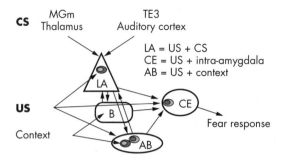

FIGURE 13–1   Schematic representation of the auditory fear conditioning circuit.

Auditory and nociceptive sensory pathways converge in the lateral amygdala (LA). The LA has projections to the central amygdala (CE) by which the amygdala is able to elicit a fear response, which includes activation of the autonomic nervous system, activation of the HPA axis, and freezing responses. Auditory signals reach the LA from the auditory cortex (TE3) and also directly from the auditory thalamus (medial geniculate, medial division [MGm]). In addition, some nociceptive signals reach the LA via the thalamus. AB = accessory basal nucleus of the amygdala, B = basal nucleus of the amygdala, CS = conditioned stimulus (auditory signal), US = unconditioned stimulus (nociceptive signal).

cells (Repa et al. 2001). To understand the anatomy of fear behavior, we must begin to understand the microanatomy and behavior of the circuits that form and store learned fear memories.

The amygdala has been extensively implicated in the neurobiology of fear, in both animal studies (Fanselow and LeDoux 1999; LeDoux 2000) and recent functional imaging studies in humans (Isenberg et al. 1999; Morris et al. 1996). For example, conditioned fear stimuli activate the amygdala when presented freely or subliminally (LaBar et al. 1995, 1998; Morris et al. 1996, 1998). Fearful faces and threatening words also activate the amygdala in humans. The activation from fearful faces exceeds that from happy faces, and the presentation of subliminal fearful stimuli is also detectable by the amygdala (Isenberg et al. 1999; LaBar et al. 1995, 1998; Morris et al. 1996). Unilateral human amygdala lesions result in fear conditioning deficits (LaBar et al. 1995, 1998). Further implicating the involvement of the human amygdala in fear conditioning are recent functional magnetic resonance imaging (fMRI) studies that reveal potentiated amygdala activation following fear conditioning in humans (LaBar et al. 1995, 1998).

Human amygdala involvement is found in a constellation of anxiety and paranoid disorders. These include individuals with paranoid delusions, who show increased amygdala and mesotemporal activation and reduced frontal activation in response to both threatening and neutral stimuli (Aggleton 1993; Epstein et al. 1999; Isenberg et al. 1999). In addition, the left amygdala has been shown to be disproportionately activated in familial depressive disorder (Drevets et al. 1992). The apparent involvement of the amygdala in these psychopathologies presumably arises from the amygdala's role as a neural structure mediating fear learning and fear responses.

AMYGDALA CELLS AND MICROCIRCUITS

Establishing how the LA senses, encodes, and responds to fearful stimuli ultimately requires an intimate knowledge of the LA's cellular structure, network organization, and function. One notable observation about LA neurons is that they are usually quiescent in either anesthetized or awake animals (Bordi and LeDoux 1992; Clugnet et al. 1990; Gaudreau and Pare 1996). In contrast imaging studies in human and animals, single-unit recording studies reveal that the amygdala becomes highly active in response to conditioned and unconditioned threats. Thus, an understanding of how LA neurons respond to synaptic input and what their properties are when activated is essential to understanding the role of the LA in fear and fear conditioning.

Earlier work reported up to seven unique populations of LA neurons based on firing characteristics and morphology (Faulkner and Brown 1999). This classification was reduced by several authors to three unique populations: pyramidal projection neurons, which use glutamate as a transmitter; stellate (starlike) projection neurons, which also use glutamate as a transmitter; and interneurons, whose axons ramify only within the LA and which use gamma-aminobutyric acid (GABA) as a transmitter (Rainnie et al. 1991a, 1991b). Sugita et al. (1993) also reported three types of LA neurons based on differences in the action potential afterpotential and response to neurotransmitters. LA pyramidal neurons were found to have a depolarizing afterpotential, and two populations of nonpyramidal neurons were found to have long- or short-lasting hyperpolarizing afterpotentials.

More recent and detailed studies have reduced the classification of LA neurons to just two populations: principal (projection) neurons and GABA interneurons (Faber et al. 2001; Pare and Gaudreau 1996; Rosenkranz and Grace 1999). These authors found that only one population of principal neurons could be identified morphologically. Cells differed physiologically only in their spike adaptations, driven by underlying potassium conductances. The differences suggested that a continuum of responses was possible, so they may be driven by a preparation (in vitro brain slice) artifact. Alternatively, they could represent subtle differences between LA principal neurons that could have a significant effect on LA network properties.

In summary, the LA contains at least two major groups of neurons: 1) pyramidal projection neurons that use glutamate as a transmitter and can be identified by action potential accommodation in response to depolarizing current injection, broad action potentials, and a depolarized resting membrane potential (in vitro <70 mV) (Figure 13–2A); and 2) interneurons, whose axons presumably ramify only within the LA, which use GABA as a neurotransmitter, and which can be identified electrophysiologically by the absence of action potential accommodation in response to depolarizing current injection, by narrow action potentials, and by a less depolarized resting membrane potential (in vitro >70 mV) (Figure 13–2B).

Another important distinction between principal and GABA interneurons is their spontaneous and maximal firing rates. Principal neurons tend to be quiescent in vivo and in vitro unless activated by a US or CS in vivo or a current injection in vitro. Following synaptic activation LA principal neurons can fire action potentials up to 20 Hz. In contrast, presumed GABAergic interneurons are often spontaneously firing both in vivo and in vitro, and in vitro can be induced to fire up to 100 Hz. In addition, intercalated neurons are a population of small soma neurons positioned both laterally and medially to the LA that also use GABA as a neurotransmitter and anatomically may be considered part of the LA. These neurons are not included in our microcircuit analysis of the LA.

Although recent progress has been made in understanding aspects of the LA's cellular structure, understanding of its network organization is in its infancy. The classification of neurons as principal neurons is based on the observation that these neurons are the most numerous and they project their axons from the LA. To establish the cellular foundation of the LA neuronal microcircuitry, recent data from our laboratory have quantified these neurons and their extensive neuronal processes for the first time.

The LA of the rat contains $60,322 \pm 408$ neurons in each hemisphere (Hou and LeDoux, unpublished). Of these, $16,917 \pm 471$, or 27%, are GABAergic neurons (excluding the intercalated nuclei). Thus, 73% of the LA consists of glutamatergic principal/projection neurons. Further preliminary quantification reveals that the LA contains 488 m (5%–95% confidence interval 352–517 m) of principal neuron dendrites on which 95 million dendritic spines (5%–95% confidence interval 63–147 million) are located (Johnson et al. 2001). Dendritic spines form the major postsynap-

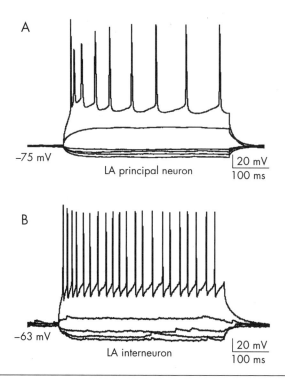

FIGURE 13–2   Electrophysiological profile of lateral amygdala neurons in vitro.

Lateral amygdala (LA) neurons can be divided into principal (projection) neurons, which usually have a pyramidal morphology with spiny dendrites, and interneurons (presumed to be GABAergic), which usually have a rounded soma and smooth, sparsely spiny dendrites.

A: Response of a principal neuron to depolarizing and hyperpolarizing current injection (traces are overlaid). In response to depolarizing currents, principal neurons responded with active sodium spikes that show robust adaptation.

B: Response of a presumably GABAergic interneuron to depolarizing and hyperpolarizing current injection (traces are overlaid). In response to depolarizing currents, interneurons respond with active sodium spikes that, in contrast to principal neurons, show no spike adaptation. Interneurons fire at a very high frequency whereas principal neurons rapidly become quiescent. (Neurons recorded in vitro from the rat LA.)

tic sites for incoming CS afferents from thalamus and cortex, and may also be postsynaptic sites for US and intra-LA communication.

The presynaptic side of LA principal/projection neurons possesses extensive intra-LA axons. In the LA, our preliminary quantification reveals 372 m

(5%–95% confidence interval 213–524 m) of presynaptic axons. These axons possess 20 million boutons (5%–95% confidence interval 15–26 million). Axonic boutons generally form synaptic specializations with various postsynaptic targets, including dendritic spines. Each individual principal neuron can possess up to 18 mm of axon within the LA (Johnson et al. 2001, 2002a, 2002b). The extent of these axons and boutons indicates an extensive excitatory microcircuit within the LA (Johnson et al. 2001).

To further understand how this extensive excitatory LA microcircuit processes and encodes fear memories, we have sought to understand principles of excitatory axon organization within the LA. Using anatomical and electrophysiological techniques, we have examined both the spatial and the temporal organization of principal neuron excitatory axon organization in the LA. Individual LA principal neurons, identified electrophysiologically and reconstructed in three dimensions, were observed to have a single axon, with the axon hillock located at the soma or primary dendrite. This axon branches and ramifies multidirectionally and extensively throughout the LA (Figure 13–3). Local axon branches can be observed, from some neurons, dorsally, ventrally, medially, and laterally from the principal neuron soma. Axon distributions are weighted toward projecting ventrally. However, not all neurons have axons that project in all the other directions. The direction of the axons appears to be determined, at least in part, by the lateral to medial location of the soma (Figure 13–4) (Johnson et al. 2002a, 2002b).

In the medial to lateral axis, axons are organized along a gradient such that neurons located medially have a weighted projection laterally and ventrally, and laterally located neurons have the opposite projection—lateral neurons project medially and ventrally (Figure 13–4) (Johnson et al. 2002a, 2002b). This arrangement allows LA principal neurons to excite adjacent neurons while simultaneously sending signals to LA output targets. Moreover, many neurons also project dorsally in the LA to where the majority of thalamic and cortical afferents enter the amygdala. These transverse and reciprocal connections may provide a circuit for reciprocal and reverberating excitation (Figure 13–4) (Johnson et al. 2002a, 2002b). Furthermore, propagating depolarizing waves have been demonstrated within the LA (Johnson et al. 2002b) that may reverberate.

Principal neurons are by definition projection neurons—neurons that project efferents from their nucleus. Thus, in addition to local axons, they send their axons out of the LA to adjacent nuclei. The most common targets identified from our single-neuron studies are the basal and central nucleus of the amygdala. In addition, axons were observed to project medially into the ventral caudate and laterally into adjacent cortex (data not shown).

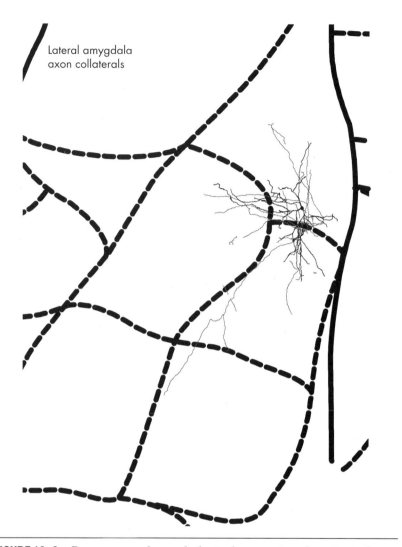

Lateral amygdala axon collaterals

FIGURE 13–3 Reconstructed morphological properties of a principal neuron of the lateral amygdala.

The neuron is shown to scale against a brain atlas of the lateral amygdala (LA). Soma, dendrites, and dendritic spines are shown in *black*. Axon and axonal boutons are shown in *red*. (Neuron recorded and labeled in vitro from the rat LA.) Axon can be seen projecting ventrally into the basal nucleus of the amygdala. In addition, extensive axon collaterals can be seen ramifying within the LA. Individual LA neurons can possess up to 18 mm of axon. The LA contains approximately 488 m of principal neuron dendrites and 372 m of principal neuron local axons. **For a color version of this figure, please see the color insert at the back of this book.**

Source. Atlas outline adapted from Paxinos and Watson 1998.

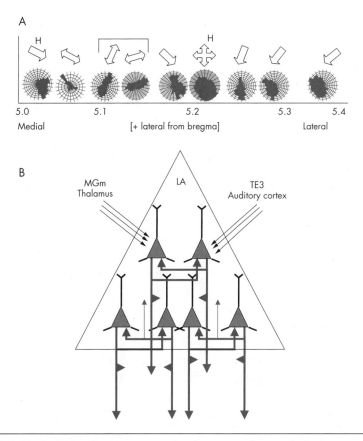

FIGURE 13–4   Polar histograms and schematic of intra–lateral amygdala local axon projection patterns.

A: Polar histograms of axon projection patterns from individual lateral amygdala (LA) projection neurons. LA principal neurons send their major projection in a ventral direction, with some collateral projections dorsally. Histograms are arranged in order along a medial to lateral axis according to the location of their soma, where an organization can be seen. In addition to ventral and dorsal axon projections, neurons located laterally send a major projection in a medial direction toward the center of the LA. Neurons located medially send a major projection in the opposite direction, laterally toward the center of the LA. (Neurons in bracket do not appear to fit this organization.) H = neurons recovered from horizontal slices; all others are coronal.

B: Schematic of axon projection patterns in the LA. Axon collaterals are arranged such that most neurons send axons ventrally and toward the center of the LA. Many also possess a component of dorsally projecting neurons. All LA principal neurons are potentially extensively interconnected. MGm = medial geniculate, medial division.

For a color version of this figure, please see the color insert at the back of this book.

These data demonstrate the relative complexity of the key cellular machinery underlying mammalian conditioned fear, but also begin to approach it as both finite and tractable microcircuitry. Because LA principal cells have a largely homogeneous electrophysiological and dendritic morphological profile, axonal organizational heterogeneity and potential reverberating interconnectivity provide a mechanism by which heterogeneous plastic and learning responses may be derived. The recent findings of Repa et al. (2001), that dorsally located LA principal neurons are rapid and transiently plastic whereas more ventrally located cells are slow and long-term plastic (even beyond extinction), may be achieved by a reverberating circuit that provides increased temporal coincidence to ventral cells (Johnson et al. 2002b).

This extensive excitatory microcircuit in the LA is countered by a significant population of GABAergic interneurons. These neurons make up 27% of neurons in the lateral amygdala and therefore exert significant control of LA microcircuits. The ability to modulate this GABAergic control confers direct modulation of LA microcircuits. As described earlier, LA principal neurons are usually quiescent in vivo and in vitro; thus, they are under considerable GABAergic tone until activated by CS and US. The control of this GABA circuitry enables control of the balance between CS and US activation of excitatory reverberating circuits. Thus, adjustment of tonic GABA regulation of LA microcircuits could have profound effects on the storage and retrieval of fear memories. How neuromodulators control LA microcircuits is discussed in the next section.

MODULATORS OF FEAR MICROCIRCUITS: THE DOPAMINE-SEROTONIN PARADOX

The major pharmacological therapies for fear disorders available today, and used over modern psychopharmacological history, target the monoaminergic systems of brain: norepinephrine, dopamine, and serotonin. The exceptions are benzodiazepines and barbiturates that target GABA receptors. All systemically administered drugs that act on the central nervous system presumably bind to receptors throughout the brain's nuclei and circuits. Data on how these drugs act on the brain's fear systems, especially microcircuits of the lateral amygdala, are only beginning to emerge. In this section we focus on recent data suggesting a microcircuit-specific mode of action of serotonin and dopamine in the lateral amygdala.

Serotonin (5-hydroxytryptamine [5-HT]) reuptake inhibitors act at the serotonin transporter to reduce reabsorption of synaptically released serotonin and thus effectively increase the serotonin available to postsynaptic receptors. Increasing evidence suggests a dysfunction of serotonergic functions in persons with the fear disorder anxiety (Ressler and Nemeroff 2000). Both serotonergic hypo- and hyperfunction have been suggested, with the majority of evidence indicating hypofunction (Ressler and Nemeroff 2000). Even within the healthy population, the presence of the short-allele (less efficient) form of the serotonin transporter gene has been associated with anxiety-like traits (Lesch et al. 1996). Moreover, recent evidence shows that this same polymorphism is associated with differential activation of the amygdala in response to fearful stimuli (Hariri et al. 2002). Persons carrying the short allele of the serotonin transporter gene (associated with more anxious behaviors) have increased amygdala activation (fMRI measure), suggesting hyper- or overactivation of the amygdala in response to "relevant environmental stimuli" (Hariri et al. 2002). The increased amygdala response to fear in the short-allele population apparently suggests serotonergic hyperfunction. The authors suggested that the blood oxygen level–dependent (BOLD) fMRI signal may reflect excitation of LA neurons via excitatory 5-HT receptors or alternatively via desensitization of inhibitory 5-HT$_{1A}$ receptors (Hariri et al. 2002). Because LA microcircuits coexist with extensive GABAergic (inhibitory) interneurons, any hyperresponsiveness of the LA is likely to occur in concert with modified GABA tone.

Dopamine has been extensively implicated in disorders of fear, including the paranoid disorders amphetamine-induced paranoia and paranoid delusions of schizophrenia. The amygdala as a key temporolimbic structure was one of the first consistently identified structures showing changes in the schizophrenia disease process, including elevated dopamine levels (Reynolds 1983). Amphetamine promotes the release of dopamine through action on dopamine storage and transport at the synapse. Amphetamine-induced psychosis is characterized by frightening paranoid hallucinations and is often associated with ongoing flashbacks. These flashbacks have been shown to be triggered by mild fear of other people (Yui et al. 1998). In rat models both acute administration of amphetamine and the D1 agonist SKF 38393 produced an enhanced fear using the acoustic startle reflex. Moreover, infusion of the D1 antagonist SCH 23390 into the basal amygdala and LA reduced fear using conditioned freezing (Nader and LeDoux 1999).

The aforementioned studies indicate a functional role for serotonin and dopamine in the amygdala as modulators of fear and also indicate their involvement, but not necessarily causation, in fear psychopathology. The evidence to date, broadly defined, suggests that serotonin hypofunction and dopamine hyperfunction can generate fear-associated behavior. LA principal neurons are activated strongly by unconditioned noxious stimuli and also by sensory inputs directly (conditioned stimuli) from the sensory thalami (medial geniculate for auditory stimuli). Following conditioning, the CS alone elicits a strong (potentiated) response from LA principal neurons (LeDoux 2000; Quirk et al. 1995; Repa et al. 2001). Much data indicate that to achieve this increased CS activation of amygdala neurons requires potentiation of synaptic strength at thalamic input synapses to the LA (LeDoux 2000). In addition, LA principal neurons are under tonic GABAergic inhibition by local GABAergic interneurons; thus, any modification of GABA tone in the LA is likely to have a profound effect on LA neuron excitability.

Although our knowledge of the neurobiology of dopamine systems has progressed tremendously, especially its role in the prefrontal cortex (Goldman-Rakic 1995; Williams and Goldman-Rakic 1995), our knowledge of the physiology and anatomy of dopamine systems in the amygdala is comparatively incomplete. Goldman-Rakic and colleagues working in the primate prefrontal cortex have determined that D1 receptor agonists enhance working memory performance by promoting pyramidal neuron firing. Furthermore, this D1 enhancement is dose and temporally dependent, because activation of GABAergic interneurons by dopamine eventually leads to inhibition of pyramidal neurons and with it the enhancement of working memory. Anatomical analysis of the prefrontal cortex reveals that pyramidal neurons are more likely to be postsynaptic to dopamine afferents than interneuron populations (Goldman-Rakic 1995; Krimer et al. 1997; Williams and Goldman-Rakic 1995). Recent milestone work by Rosenkranz and Grace has begun to address the role of dopamine in the basal amygdala and LA. Using both extra- and intracellular recording in vivo, they have identified an afferent-specific modulation by dopamine. Their work has shown that although auditory sensory afferents (medial geniculate, medial division [MGm] and auditory cortex [TE3]) drive LA principal neurons, input from prelimbic and infralimbic prefrontal cortex (also glutamatergic) inhibits LA principal neurons (Rosenkranz and Grace 1999, 2001, 2002). Afferents from infralimbic cortex have been associated with the extinction of conditioned fear (Quirk et al. 2000).

Comparing the effects of dopamine on the firing rates of two populations of LA neurons, Rosenkranz and Grace (1999) found that LA principal neurons were inhibited whereas GABA interneurons were excited. Coadministration of dopamine or dopamine pharmacological agents showed amygdala afferents to be differentially regulated by dopamine. Prefrontal cortical and thalamic afferents (MGm) are inhibited by dopamine whereas TE3 afferents are potentiated (Rosenkranz and Grace 1999, 2001, 2002). From working in vitro with the whole-cell patch clamp technique, our data indicate that dopamine can act via the D1 receptor to potentiate the amplitude of GABAA potentials in the LA. However, we found this effect on both cortical and subcortical sensory afferents; the D1 agonist SKF 38393 potentiates the inhibitory postsynaptic potential (IPSP) component of the excitatory postsynaptic potential (EPSP)/IPSP sequence induced in principal neurons (Figure 13–5) (Johnson et al. 2000).

These data indicate that dopamine may act in the LA microcircuit, via D1 receptors, directly on GABA interneurons. Further evidence shows an anatomical framework for this microcircuit organization. Dopamine afferent terminals make synaptic contact with GABA neurons in the LA (Johnson et al. 2000). Dopaminergic effects may not be limited to GABA neurons in the LA, as some workers have reported direct effects on EPSPs (Rosenkranz and Grace 2002). However, these effects may be network specific; our data indicate that principal neurons found to be both in a feedforward GABA local network and having these GABA neurons postsynaptic to the D1 receptor form a subpopulation within the LA of 30% of neurons identified. Moreover, these neurons with a dopamine-modulated GABA input did not also show modulation of their EPSPs by D1 agonists when tested directly (Figure 13–6) (Johnson et al. 2000).

Recent data also indicate serotonin to have similar modes of action in the LA. Two studies using in vivo extracellular and in vitro whole-cell path clamp recordings have also associated LA GABA neuron networks with the action of serotonin (Rainnie 1999; Stutzmann and LeDoux 1999). LA principal neurons are potently activated by stimulation of sensory inputs from the thalamus and cortex, and also by direct application of glutamate. This activation can be inhibited by local co-administration of serotonin (Stutzmann and LeDoux 1999; Stutzmann et al. 1998). The serotonergic inhibition can be blocked by the additional local administration of GABA antagonists (Stutzmann and LeDoux 1999). This suggests that serotonin, like dopamine, mediates its effects via local GABA neurons. Addressing this issue in vitro, Rainnie (1999) found that serotonin, acting at 5-HT_2 receptors, can excite presumed GABA interneurons of the basolateral amygdala complex (BLA).

Serotonin can modulate network excitability in the BLA by increasing GABA inhibition. In addition, serotonin, like dopamine, can modulate the amplitude of synaptic mediated excitatory potentials (and currents, EPSP/EPSC) as a second mode to regulate excitation. Serotonin dose-dependently reduced EPSC amplitude on both BLA projection neurons and interneurons (Rainnie 1999). These data indicate that at lower concentrations, serotonin (acting at 5-HT_2 receptors) regulates excitability by activating GABA networks; then at higher concentrations, serotonin shunts excitatory synaptic

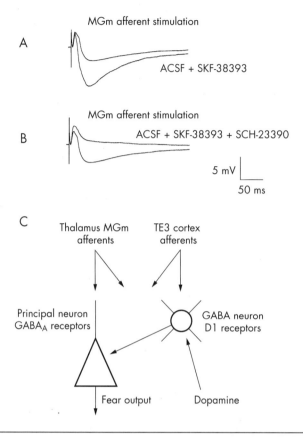

FIGURE 13–5 Effects of the neuromodulator dopamine acting at D1 receptors on lateral amygdala principal neurons.

A, B: Voltage traces of lateral amygdala (LA) principal neurons with an evoked excitatory followed by inhibitory postsynaptic potential (EPSP/IPSP). In this example EPSP/IPSPs were evoked following stimulation of afferents, which arise in the auditory thalamus (MGm) and project to the LA. *(A)* The dopamine D1 receptor SKF-38393 increases the amplitude of the IPSP but not the EPSP. *(B)* The dopamine D1 receptor antagonist SCH-23390 both reverses the effect of the agonist and further reduces the amplitude of the IPSP. ACSF = artificial cerebrospinal fluid.

C: Schematic of the LA network and its modulation by dopamine acting at D1 receptors. Both LA principal and GABA interneurons receive input from the two major auditory inputs (MGm and TE3), creating a feedforward inhibitory network. Dopamine acting at D1 receptors on a subpopulation of GABA interneurons can modulate feedforward, presumably by increasing GABA neuron firing. This subpopulation of GABA neurons can inhibit or disinhibit the output of components of the LA fear circuit. TE3 = auditory cortex.

input to the BLA (Rainnie 1999). Although not tested as directly, dopamine appears to have the same network regulation. At lower concentrations, dopamine (acting at D1 receptors) regulates excitability by activating GABA networks; then at higher concentrations, dopamine shunts excitatory synaptic input to the BLA.

Given the mounting neuropsychiatric evidence suggesting that fear may be potentiated by hyposerotonergic function (Hariri et al. 2002; Ressler and Nemeroff 2000) and the animal evidence that fear can be potentiated by hyperdopaminergic function (Greba and Kokkinidis 2000; Guarraci et al. 1999a, 1999b; Nader and LeDoux 1999), both acting in the LA, these data present a paradox, because their cellular modes of action in the LA are strikingly similar. One possible explanation not yet explored is differential LA microcircuit regulation. Thus, because the LA is a center for disparate US and CS convergence, and the subsequent storage and retrieval of conditioned fear, it remains a possibility that different aspects of fear are encoded over the wider LA microcircuit and that dopamine and serotonin can modulate independent aspects.

CONCLUSIONS

The amygdala is a key structure in the neurobiology of fear. Moreover, the LA has been shown to be the site of convergence and memory storage of CS and US associations in the formation of conditioned fear memories (LeDoux 2000). The LA contains at least two populations of neurons: 1) GABA neurons, which regulate excitation in 2) principal glutamatergic neurons. We have shown that these principal neurons form an excitatory network of interconnected neurons (Johnson et al. 2002). We are only beginning to understand the organization of this network and how it likely contributes to the formation and storage of long-term fear memories.

Several lines of evidence suggest that LA networks may play a significant role in fear memories. These include network models that provide a framework that may account for aspects of LA microcircuit design and function. In the 1949 Hebbian postulate, transiently reverberating cellular ensembles can sustain activity to facilitate temporal coincidence detection (Sejnowski 1999). We have demonstrated that the unilateral LA contains approximately 372 m of presynaptic local axons (Johnson et al. 2001). In addition, these axons project in all directions in the LA, including the feedback direction (Figures 13–3 and 13–4) (Johnson et al. 2002a, 2002b). Moreover, we have detected multiple-component polysynaptic field potentials in the LA in response to both thalamic and cortical afferent stimulation (Johnson et al.

2002b). Taken together, these data suggest that incoming CS (and US) information could reverberate and facilitate aspects of coincidence detection throughout the LA (Figure 13–6A), as predicted by Hebb.

The landmark auto-associative network design proposed by Hopfield (1982) provides a system whereby a network can complete pattern recognition. This network allows the retrieval of an entire memory trace from partial memory cues; any disruption of pattern recognition during storage and retrieval of conditioned fear could theoretically lead to fear pathology. The key component of this network is a recurrent excitatory feedback. The network based on the additive power of simple components (single neurons) is designed such that a first array of interconnected neurons receive specific synaptic input from an information source (in the lateral amygdala, CS and US sources). Then a second array of neurons receives synaptic input only from the first array and not from the outside source. Thus, each secondary neuron is interconnected with and feeds back to each primary neuron. This arrangement (simplified here) allows for the formation of a "content-addressable memory" that can be obtained from any of the subparts of the network (Hopfield 1982). In terms of a fear microcircuit of the LA, every second-tier neuron would store aspects of a fear memory. Activation of any one neuron (by a CS) would enable complete recall of the entire memory via the network (Figure 13–6A). A similar arrangement has been proposed and demonstrated in hippocampal spatial memory networks (Nakazawa et al. 2002). We have provided data to support some aspects of this proposed arrangement in LA microcircuits (Johnson et al. 2002b).

We have discussed in this chapter how the key working properties of LA principal neurons differ only by their connectivity. However, in their functional response to learning CS-US associations, principal neurons can be divided into dorsal (transiently plastic) and ventral (long-term plastic) subsets (Repa et al. 2001). Transiently plastic neurons were found to be located in the dorsal portion of the dorsolateral subdivision of the LA. These neurons rapidly increased their firing rates after CS-US pairing trials (i.e., formation of a memory), but upon presentation of the CS alone, which began the extinction trials, the neurons rapidly lost the potentiated CS response. On the other hand, principal neurons located ventrally, but still in the dorsolateral subdivision of the LA, were slow to acquire a potentiated response, requiring more CS-US pairings. However, once the CS was acquired, neurons maintained their potentiated response to the CS for long periods during extinction trials, even beyond the point where the animal no longer displayed a behavioral response to the CS (i.e., freezing). This suggests the possibility that reverberatory interconnectivity between the neuron populations occurs such that plasticity in ventral neurons is dependent on plasticity in the dorsal neurons, and that different aspects of fear memories are encoded between the two populations. It also raises the possibility that feedback to the dorsal neurons from the ventral neurons signals a transfer of memory and enables the dorsal neurons to be available for the acquisition of new fear memories. Ventral (long-term plastic) cells may maintain aspects of the entire fear memory as a content-addressable memory that requires triggering from the dorsal (transiently plastic) neurons.

Errors in LA microcircuit content-addressable memory may account for anxiety or even fear memory flashbacks. Perturbation of the LA fear network is possible during monoamine activation, which occurs under periods of stress and hypervigilance. The actions of serotonin and dopamine within the LA suggest that LA microcircuits are key components for the storage and retrieval of fear memories. Dopamine (at D1 receptors) and serotonin (at $5\text{-}HT_2$ receptors) excite GABAergic interneurons, leading to potentiated inhibition of LA principal neurons. Neuropsychiatric pathological evidence, however, suggests that serotonin hypofunction and dopamine hyperfunction occur in fear disorders of anxiety and paranoia, respectively. We propose that dopamine and serotonin act on different components of the LA microcircuit. First, different populations of GABAergic neurons containing dopamine or serotonin receptors provide feedforward inhibitory control over different LA principal neurons. These principal neurons are located in the second array of long-term plastic neurons as described previously in reference to the auto-associative model (Figure 13–6). This arrangement would allow different aspects of memory to be distributed, stored, and retrieved in a content-addressable manner. Thus, different components of the circuit would be utilized under periods of increased serotonergic and dopaminergic control.

In our model we propose that LA principal neurons in the dopamine/GABA inhibition subcircuit may receive additional CS (auditory) input from the cortex. Thus, under periods of stress and arousal, dopamine may synchronize LA principal neuron firing and streamline the LA (inhibiting cortical input). Under such conditions, the circuit can distribute, store, and retrieve memories from a restricted synaptic range, utilizing only rudimentary thalamic sensory inputs. This arrangement would maximize fear learning and attentional processing under periods of stress and arousal. However, excessive dopamine-derived vigilance could potentially create a state of exaggerated fear as defined by paranoid disorders. Conversely, hyposerotonergic function within the LA microcircuit could lead an individual to have a non-gated (by inhibitory GABA interneurons) or open fear circuit whereby all sensory input, including low-threshold or background activity, is liable to potential CS-US pairing and the creation of a state of anxiety.

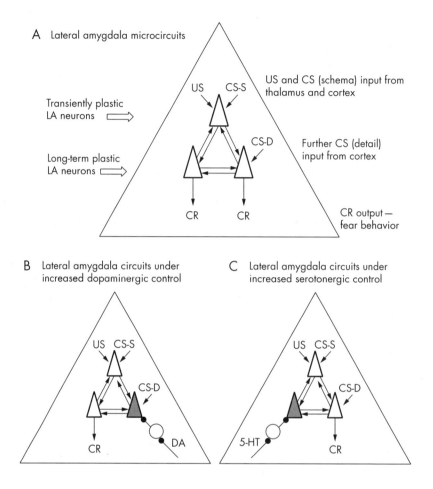

A   Lateral amygdala microcircuits

Transiently plastic
LA neurons

US   CS-S   US and CS (schema) input from
thalamus and cortex

Long-term plastic
LA neurons

CS-D   Further CS (detail)
input from cortex

CR   CR   CR output —
fear behavior

B   Lateral amygdala circuits under
increased dopaminergic control

US CS-S

CS-D

CR   DA

C   Lateral amygdala circuits under
increased serotonergic control

US CS-S

CS-D

5-HT   CR

In summary, LA microcircuits are extensive information processors.
Within these microcircuits fear memories are distributed, stored, and recalled. Fully understanding these networks and understanding how to adjust the balance of modulation, both pharmacologically and with behavioral therapy, will provide more precisely targeted treatment for fear
disorders. These data provide a mechanism by which psychopharmacological agents acting on different transmitter systems (e.g., GABA, serotonin, and dopamine) may act co-dependently within the context of a microcircuit for fear. It is hoped that with continued emphasis on translational
research, the basic science of the anatomy of fear will be able to identify
the precise determinants of conditioned fear and thus greatly improve our
ability to treat those with pathological disorders of fear.

FIGURE 13–6   Schematic of known and proposed components of the lateral amygdala microcircuit for fear *(opposite).*
The lateral amygdala (LA) is shown as a *large triangle; small triangles* represent the soma of pyramidal principal/projection neurons; *circles* represent the soma of GABAergic interneurons. Principal neurons of the LA display plasticity to fear learning.

A: A network of interconnected principal neurons. Dorsally located neurons receive convergent unconditioned stimulus (US) and conditioned stimulus (CS) inputs (from auditory thalamus and cortex). The auditory thalamus is known to project to these neurons, where it provides a basic precortically processed auditory stimulus (schema) to the LA. More ventrally located inputs may receive aspects of direct CS and US inputs and in addition will receive intra-LA excitatory synaptic connections that will store and encode aspects of conditioned fear. Dorsally located neurons learn rapidly and are transiently plastic in response to learned fear, whereas more ventrally located neurons show increased latency to learn and are long-term plastic. Aspects of both a Hebbian reverberating network and a Hopfield auto-associative network exist within the LA. LA principal neurons are connected in a network possessing feedback and topographically organized lateral excitation. Reverberating intra-LA networks may sustain temporal coordination of CS and US and other LA inputs. Aspects of a Hopfield net may allow distributed storage of fear memories such that the network can allow generalization of fear and recall from partial cues. Pathology in this microcircuit could be manifested as disorders of fear generalization and distorted fear cue responses. CR = conditioned response.

B, C: Models of dopamine (DA) and serotonin (5-HT) modulation of the LA fear microcircuit via GABAergic interneurons. *(B)* Increased dopamine transmission or responsivity may cause increased generalization to CS cues during fear learning and recall by inhibiting a sub-LA network that receives additional cortical input. The LA microcircuit response to increased dopamine transmission would promote increased fear learning and recall under periods of arousal and stress. *(C)* Increased serotonin transmission may focus the LA fear microcircuit. Inhibition of a subnetwork that processes precortical stimuli would allow only cortically processed sensory inputs and fear cues to activate the LA, thus decreasing generalization cues to fear and anxiety.

REFERENCES

Aggleton JP: The contribution of the amygdala to normal and abnormal emotional states. Trends Neurosci 16:328–333, 1993

Bernard JF, Besson JM: The spino(trigemino)pontoamygdaloid pathway: electrophysiological evidence for an involvement in pain processes. J Neurophysiol 63:473–490, 1990

Bernard JF, Huang GF, Besson JM: Effect of noxious somesthetic stimulation on the activity of neurons of the nucleus centralis of the amygdala. Brain Res 523:347–350, 1990

Bordi F, LeDoux J: Sensory tuning beyond the sensory system: an initial analysis of auditory response properties of neurons in the lateral amygdaloid nucleus and overlying areas of the striatum. J Neurosci 12:2493–2503, 1992

Burstein R, Potrebic S: Retrograde labeling of neurons in the spinal cord that project directly to the amygdala or the orbital cortex in the rat. J Comp Neurol 335:469–485, 1993

Clugnet MC, LeDoux JE, Morrison SF: Unit responses evoked in the amygdala and striatum by electrical stimulation of the medial geniculate body. J Neurosci 10:1055–1061, 1990

Davis M, Whalen PJ: The amygdala: vigilance and emotion. Mol Psychiatry 6:13–34, 2001

Drevets WC, Videen TO, Price JL, et al: A functional anatomical study of unipolar depression. J Neurosci 12:3628–3641, 1992

Epstein J, Stern E, Silbersweig D: Mesolimbic activity associated with psychosis in schizophrenia: symptom-specific PET studies. Ann N Y Acad Sci 877:562–574, 1999

Faber ES, Callister RJ, Sah P: Morphological and electrophysiological properties of principal neurons in the rat lateral amygdala in vitro. J Neurophysiol 85:714–723, 2001

Fanselow MS, LeDoux JE: Why we think plasticity underlying Pavlovian fear conditioning occurs in the basolateral amygdala. Neuron 23:229–232, 1999

Faulkner B, Brown TH: Morphology and physiology of neurons in the rat perirhinal-lateral amygdala area. J Comp Neurol 411:613–642, 1999

Gaudreau H, Pare D: Projection neurons of the lateral amygdaloid nucleus are virtually silent throughout the sleep–waking cycle. J Neurophysiol 75:1301–1305, 1996

Goldman-Rakic PS: Cellular basis of working memory. Neuron 14:477–485, 1995

Goodwin RD, Hamilton SP: The early onset panic attack as a predictor of severe psychopathology. Psychiatry Res 109:71–79, 2002

Greba Q, Kokkinidis L: Peripheral and intraamygdalar administration of the dopamine D1 receptor antagonist SCH 23390 blocks fear-potentiated startle but not shock reactivity or the shock sensitization of acoustic startle. Behav Neurosci 114:262–272, 2000

Guarraci FA, Frohardt RJ, Kapp BS: Amygdaloid D1 dopamine receptor involvement in Pavlovian fear conditioning. Brain Res 827:28–40, 1999a

Guarraci FA, Frohardt RJ, Young SL, et al: A functional role for dopamine transmission in the amygdala during conditioned fear. Ann N Y Acad Sci 877:732–736, 1999b

Hariri AR, Mattay VS, Tessitore A, et al: Serotonin transporter genetic variation and the response of the human amygdala. Science 297:400–403, 2002

Hopfield JJ: Neural networks and physical systems with emergent collective computational abilities. Proc Natl Acad Sci U S A 79:2554–2558, 1982

Isenberg N, Silbersweig D, Engelien A, et al: Linguistic threat activates the human amygdala. Proc Natl Acad Sci U S A 96:10456–10459, 1999

Johnson LR, Farb CR, LeDoux JE: GABAergic inhibition in the fear conditioning circuit of the lateral amygdala is potentiated by dopamine D1 agonists. Society for Neuroscience Abstracts 26, Program No. 466.1, 2000

Johnson LR, Hou M, Albert L, et al: Quantification of the neuronal structure of the fear conditioning circuit of the lateral amygdala. Society for Neuroscience Abstracts 27, Program No. 187.11, 2001

Johnson LR, Alphs HA, Albert L, et al: Microcircuits of the lateral amygdala revealed by single neuron axon reconstruction and quantification. Paper presented at the NYAS Meeting on the Amygdala, Galveston, TX, 2002a

Johnson LR, Doyere V, Alphs HA, et al: Propagating excitatory potentials within the fear conditioning circuit of the lateral amygdala. Society for Neuroscience Abstracts 28, Program No. 85.16, 2002b

Krimer LS, Jakab RL, Goldman-Rakic PS: Quantitative three-dimensional analysis of the catecholaminergic innervation of identified neurons in the macaque prefrontal cortex. J Neurosci 17:7450–7461, 1997

LaBar KS, LeDoux JE, Spencer DD, et al: Impaired fear conditioning following unilateral temporal lobectomy in humans. J Neurosci 15:6846–6855, 1995

LaBar KS, Gatenby JC, Gore JC, et al: Human amygdala activation during conditioned fear acquisition and extinction: a mixed-trial fMRI study. Neuron 20:937–945, 1998

LeDoux JE: Emotion circuits in the brain. Annu Rev Neurosci 23:155–184, 2000

Lesch KP, Bengel D, Heils A, et al: Association of anxiety-related traits with a polymorphism in the serotonin transporter gene regulatory region. Science 274:1527–1531, 1996

Maren S: Neurobiology of Pavlovian fear conditioning. Annu Rev Neurosci 24:897–931, 2001

McCarley RW, Shenton ME, O'Donnell BF, et al: Uniting Kraepelin and Bleuler: the psychology of schizophrenia and the biology of temporal lobe abnormalities. Harv Rev Psychiatry 1:36–56, 1993

Morris JS, Frith CD, Perrett DI, et al: A differential neural response in the human amygdala to fearful and happy facial expressions. Nature 383:812–815, 1996

Morris JS, Ohman A, Dolan RJ: Conscious and unconscious emotional learning in the human amygdala (see comments). Nature 393:467–470, 1998

Muller J, Corodimas KP, Fridel Z, et al: Functional inactivation of the lateral and basal nuclei of the amygdala by muscimol infusion prevents fear conditioning to an explicit conditioned stimulus and to contextual stimuli. Behav Neurosci 111:683–691, 1997

Nader K, LeDoux JE: Inhibition of the mesoamygdala dopaminergic pathway impairs the retrieval of conditioned fear associations. Behav Neurosci 113:891–901, 1999

Nakazawa K, Quirk MC, Chitwood RA, et al: Requirement for hippocampal CA3 NMDA receptors in associative memory recall. Science 297:211–218, 2002

Pare D, Gaudreau H: Projection cells and interneurons of the lateral and basolateral amygdala: distinct firing patterns and differential relation to theta and delta rhythms in conscious cats. J Neurosci 16:3334–3350, 1996

Paxinos G, Watson C: The Rat Brain in Stereotaxic Coordinates, 4th Edition. Sydney, Australia, Academic Press, 1998

Quirk GJ, Repa C, LeDoux JE: Fear conditioning enhances short-latency auditory responses of lateral amygdala neurons: parallel recordings in the freely behaving rat. Neuron 15:1029–1039, 1995

Quirk GJ, Russo GK, Barron JL, et al: The role of ventromedial prefrontal cortex in the recovery of extinguished fear. J Neurosci 20:6225–6231, 2000

Rainnie DG: Serotonergic modulation of neurotransmission in the rat basolateral amygdala. J Neurophysiol 82:69–85, 1999

Rainnie DG, Asprodini EK, Shinnick-Gallagher P: Excitatory transmission in the basolateral amygdala. J Neurophysiol 66:986–998, 1991a

Rainnie DG, Asprodini EK, Shinnick-Gallagher P: Inhibitory transmission in the basolateral amygdala. J Neurophysiol 66:999–1009, 1991b

Repa JC, Muller J, Apergis J, et al: Two different lateral amygdala cell populations contribute to the initiation and storage of memory. Nat Neurosci 4:724–731, 2001

Ressler KJ, Nemeroff CB: Role of serotonergic and noradrenergic systems in the pathophysiology of depression and anxiety disorders. Depress Anxiety 12 (suppl 1):2–19, 2000

Reynolds GP: Increased concentrations and lateral asymmetry of amygdala dopamine in schizophrenia. Nature 305:527–529, 1983

Rogan MT, Staubli UV, LeDoux JE: Fear conditioning induces associative long-term potentiation in the amygdala. Nature 390:604–607, 1997

Romanski LM, LeDoux JE: Equipotentiality of thalamo-amygdala and thalamo-cortico-amygdala circuits in auditory fear conditioning. J Neurosci 12:4501–4509, 1992

Romanski LM, Clugnet MC, Bordi F, et al: Somatosensory and auditory convergence in the lateral nucleus of the amygdala. Behav Neurosci 107:444–450, 1993

Rosenkranz JA, Grace AA: Modulation of basolateral amygdala neuronal firing and afferent drive by dopamine receptor activation in vivo. J Neurosci 19:11027–11039, 1999

Rosenkranz JA, Grace AA: Dopamine attenuates prefrontal cortical suppression of sensory inputs to the basolateral amygdala of rats. J Neurosci 21:4090–4103, 2001

Rosenkranz JA, Grace AA: Cellular mechanisms of infralimbic and prelimbic prefrontal cortical inhibition and dopaminergic modulation of basolateral amygdala neurons in vivo. J Neurosci 22:324–337, 2002

Sejnowski TJ: The book of Hebb. Neuron 24:773–776, 1999

Shenton ME, Kikinis R, Jolesz FA, et al: Abnormalities of the left temporal lobe and thought disorder in schizophrenia: a quantitative magnetic resonance imaging study. N Engl J Med 327:604–612, 1992

Shi C, Davis M: Pain pathways involved in fear conditioning measured with fear-potentiated startle: lesion studies. J Neurosci 19:420–430, 1999

Stutzmann GE, LeDoux JE: GABAergic antagonists block the inhibitory effects of serotonin in the lateral amygdala: a mechanism for modulation of sensory inputs related to fear conditioning. J Neurosci 19:RC8, 1999

Stutzmann GE, McEwen BS, LeDoux JE: Serotonin modulation of sensory inputs to the lateral amygdala: dependency on corticosterone. J Neurosci 18:9529–9538, 1998

Sugita S, Tanaka E, North RA: Membrane properties and synaptic potentials of three types of neurone in rat lateral amygdala. J Physiol 460:705–718, 1993

Williams GV, Goldman-Rakic PS: Modulation of memory fields by dopamine D1 receptors in prefrontal cortex (see comments). Nature 376:572–575, 1995

Yui K, Ishiguro T, Goto K, et al: Factors affecting the development of spontaneous recurrence of methamphetamine psychosis. Acta Psychiatr Scand 97:220–227, 1998

14

The Amygdala and Social Behavior

What's Fear Got to Do With It?

David G. Amaral, Ph.D.

     Most brain regions are undoubtedly involved in multiple biological and behavioral functions. Interestingly, research directed at one of these functions often generates a literature that has little or no overlap with research on other functions. The hippocampal formation, for example, has generated a large literature demonstrating that it plays a prominent role in spatial or declarative memory (Morris and Frey 1997; Squire and Zola 1996; Squire and Zola-Morgan 1991). There is a smaller, although still substantial, literature indicating that the hippocampal formation plays a negative-feedback role in the hypothalamic-pituitary-adrenal axis (Baram et al. 1997; Herman et al. 1998; Sapolsky et al. 1991; van Haarst et al. 1997). However, it is rare that stress and memory are dealt with in the same publication, with the notable exception of papers on stress-induced memory deficits (Bremner and Narayan 1998).

    Work on the amygdaloid complex has also followed several parallel pathways. Work beginning with the reports of Kluver and Bucy (1938) indicated that damage to the amygdala and surrounding temporal lobe produced myriad effects but most prominently decreased emotional reactivity. Aggleton and colleagues (Aggleton and Passingham 1981) confirmed this with more selective lesions confined to the amygdala and suggested that it takes near total, bilateral lesions to achieve the hypoemotionality described by Kluver and Bucy. The most exhaustive analysis of the role of the amygdala in emotionality, and fear in particular, has been carried out in the rodent (Davis and Whalen 2001; LeDoux 1995), in which an enormous literature has been generated. With the notable exception of Kalin and colleagues (Kalin 1993; Kalin et al. 2001), relatively little modern work has been carried out in the nonhuman primate on the relationship between the amygdala and emotional behavior. In contrast, there has been a long and rich literature that relates the nonhuman primate amygdala to mediation of social communication.

An early study by Rosvold et al. (1954) explicitly investigated the role of the amygdala in nonhuman primate social behavior. The researchers took previously unfamiliar macaque monkeys and formed artificial social groups. Once stable dominance hierarchies had been established, they removed the most dominant individual in the group and subjected it to a bilateral lesion of the amygdala. The animal was then returned to the social troop. The researchers found that these high-ranking and previously aggressive rhesus monkeys fell in the dominance hierarchy and became extremely submissive following the bilateral amygdalectomy.

The most extensive analysis of the amygdala and primate social behavior was conducted by Kling and colleagues (Dicks et al. 1968; Kling 1972; Kling and Brothers 1992; Kling et al. 1970). These studies were carried out using free-ranging vervet and rhesus monkeys as well as laboratory-housed animals. In studies carried out in Cayo Santiago (a "monkey island" just off the coast of Puerto Rico), macaque monkeys were prepared with bilateral damage of the amygdala and anterior temporal lobe and released back into their natal social groups. These animals did not reestablish contact with other group members, did not engage in social interactions, and usually remained socially isolated. In most cases, the amygdala-lesioned monkeys were attacked and died either from their wounds, from predation, or from malnutrition. When caged, amygdalectomized stump-tailed macaques were observed in a social group, they generally displayed a decrease in aggression and a reduction in positive social behaviors, such as huddling and grooming (Kling and Cornell 1971). Although results from studies such as these suggest that the amygdala is important for social behavior, they also show that the consequences of amygdala lesions may be dependent on the environment in which the animals' social interactions are recorded, the size of the social groups, the particular species under study, and in some cases, the sex of the animal receiving the amygdala lesion (Kling 1972).

Although emotional responsivity and social communication are certainly related functions, much of the literature on emotional behavior, which is heavily focused on fear conditioning, is devoid of a social context. And at least some of the literature on social communication is not explicitly related to emotionality. The latter point is particularly apparent in certain human imaging studies. The amygdala has been associated with the perception of angle of eye gaze, which conveys social interest or intent but can be devoid of emotional context (Emery 2000; Haxby et al. 2002; Young et al. 1995). Although it appears that the amygdala is preferentially activated by faces conveying negative emotion (Adolphs et al. 1995; Morris et al. 1996), it remains controversial whether positive emotions are also salient signals for the amygdala (Gorno-Tempini et al. 2001; Killgore and Yurgelun-Todd 2001; Morris et al. 1996). So intimately has the amygdala become associated with social communication that a number of investigators have suggested that pathology of the amygdala may be responsible for the core social deficits of autism (Baron-Cohen et al. 2000; Sweeten et al. 2002).

The conclusion from this short introduction is that there is a substantial literature to support the contention that the amygdala is highly involved in the mediation of species-typical social behavior as well as emotional responsivity, both within and outside of a social context. We began our program of studies on the neurobiology of primate social behavior with the intention of further specifying the role of the amygdala in macaque monkey social behavior. The long-term goal was to investigate the roles of many of the subnuclei of the amygdala in particular component processes of social behavior. However, we were also interested in evaluating the effects of amygdala lesions on emotional responsivity in order to compare our studies with those in the literature as well as to calibrate our lesion and behavioral approaches. Thus far, we have carried out extensive behavioral and physiological analyses of both mature and infant rhesus monkeys following complete, bilateral ibotenic acid lesions of the amygdaloid complex.

WHY STUDY THE EFFECTS OF AMYGDALA LESIONS ON PRIMATE SOCIAL BEHAVIOR?

Given the substantial literature that exists on the role of the amygdala in social behavior, one might wonder what prompted us to reexamine this topic. A number of technical issues related to the previous lesion studies have proven to be problematic in other areas of neuroscience research. For example, until recently, all lesions in the nonhuman primate were made using either radiofrequency or suction ablation techniques. These destructive techniques suffer from the "fiber of passage" problem: they not only remove or destroy cell bodies in the lesioned nucleus, but also damage axons that travel through the targeted brain area. We know from our neuroanatomical studies that there are pathways from temporal lobe structures such as the entorhinal cortex that pass through the amygdala en route to other brain regions. Thus, it is impossible to determine whether behavioral changes resulting from a destructive lesion of the amygdala is due to the elimination of its neurons and projections or to inadvertent damage to projections that run through it. Moreover, most previous destructive lesions were not adequately selective in their targets, often destroying neighboring brain regions. Many of the early lesion studies, for example, employed the suction ablation technique, which damaged the surrounding perirhinal cortex en route to the amygdala. The perirhinal cortex plays important roles in high-level visual processing and other cognitive functions (Buckley and Gaffan 1997; Erickson and Desimone 1999; Miyashita et al. 1998). Consequently, one can reasonably ask whether the changes in social behavior observed in the earlier studies were the result of damage to the amygdala, to the fibers of passage, or to areas adjacent to the amygdala, such as the perirhinal and entorhinal cortices. This question is further complicated by the fact that histological analysis often was not carried out, and certainly not carried out in a quantitative fashion.

Finally, earlier studies used some behavioral data collection methods that were subjective and resulted in little actual data that could be analyzed statistically. Often the investigators did not use an established ethogram or catalogue of social behavior. There were no direct comparisons between lesion and control groups; subjects were usually chosen at random from an established social group, and their behavior was recorded before and after placement of the lesions. The subjects used were commonly of mixed age and sex, and there was virtually no effort to control for neuroendocrine differences among subjects due to reproductive status or gender.

Rather than employing suction ablation or other destructive lesion techniques, we have used the selective neurotoxin ibotenic acid, which is injected stereotaxically into the brain, causing minimal damage to adjacent areas. This toxin has the advantage of destroying only cell bodies and leaving fibers of passage through the amygdala intact (Jarrard 2002). In addition to use of the more selective neurotoxin approach, the stereotaxic placement of every lesion was made more accurate by using an individual magnetic resonance imaging (MRI) atlas for each subject. To evaluate the lesions, extensive, quantitative histological analysis was performed for each brain. The adult subjects for these studies were male rhesus monkeys who were assessed preoperatively to determine social status in their natal groups. The first study has been completed, and analysis of subject animals in the second study is still under way. The first included a cohort of adult rhesus monkeys who sustained bilateral amygdala lesions and a control group of unlesioned animals. The second study involves one group of experimental animals who have sustained amygdala lesions, a comparison group who have sustained lesions of the hippocampus, and another group of surgical control animals. To maintain some commonality of social experience, in both studies an additional group of "stimulus animals" served as partners for members of all experimental groups for some of the social interaction studies. We investigated the changes these lesions produced to the responses animals made to inanimate objects as well as to their behaviors in various social contexts. A comprehensive list of social and nonsocial behaviors (the ethogram) was used to assess the behavioral repertoire of all animal groups (Capitanio et al. 1998). The behavioral observers were blind to the lesion status of the animals, and the ethogram allowed the detection of increases or decreases in either affiliative or agonistic behaviors.

EFFECTS OF AMYGDALA LESIONS ON EMOTIONAL AND SOCIAL BEHAVIOR IN THE ADULT RHESUS MONKEY

We first evaluated the subjects' emotional responsivity to a variety of stimuli, including novel objects (W.A. Mason, J. Ruys, C. Machado, J.P. Capitanio, and D.G. Amaral, "The Response of Macaque Monkeys With Amygdala Lesions to Complex Objects and Humans," manuscript in preparation, 2003). Some of the objects, such as rubber replicas of snakes, provoke intense fear responses in normal monkeys. In one such study, the latency to retrieve a food reward (usually a grape or piece of another desirable fruit) from a position in front of the stimulus items was measured. For normal animals, the latency to retrieve the food reward depended on whether there was a stimulus object present and on the fear-provoking qualities of the stimulus. With the amygdala-lesioned animals, in contrast, a fear-eliciting stimulus such as a snake did not appreciably increase the latency to retrieve the food. The lesioned animals would even tactually explore such objects, which the normal animals were never observed to touch. These observations were consistent with findings in the literature involving destructive lesions that bilateral damage to the amygdala produces a subject that is less fearful and less emotionally responsive (Zola-Morgan et al. 1991).

The same animals were then tested in a variety of social situations with a group of either two animals (dyad) or four animals (tetrad) present in a large chain-link enclosure. In a condition that we have called "unconstrained dyads," either the amygdala-lesioned animals or age-, sex-, and dominance-matched control animals interacted with stimulus monkeys (two males and two females). Each experimental animal interacted with each stimulus animal for six 20-minute periods. In another test of dyadic social interaction (the round-robin format), each of the experimental animals interacted with each of the other 11 experimental animals (in the first study) for one 20-minute episode. The results from both tests of dyadic interaction were striking and consistent. Rather than exhibiting social apathy or social awkwardness, the amygdala-lesioned monkeys generated qualitatively similar types of social interactions and responded to social gestures from the stimulus animals in an entirely species-typical manner. In fact, the amygdala-lesioned animals generated significantly greater amounts of affiliative social behavior toward the stimulus monkeys or toward the other experimental monkeys. On closer analysis, it appeared that the most striking alteration in behavior occurred at the early stages of social interaction. Whereas the control animals were initially reluctant to interact with the stimulus monkeys, the amygdala-lesioned animals initiated affiliative social behavior almost immediately. The lesioned monkeys appeared to be socially uninhibited in that they did not go through the normal period of evaluation of the social partner before engaging in social interactions. These results, of course, were entirely inconsistent with our initial hypothesis that the amygdala is essential for normal social communication.

An equally surprising result was how the control animals interacted with the lesioned monkeys. One can imagine that the inappropriate social interaction of the lesioned monkeys with the stimulus monkeys might have been interpreted as "pathological" by the stimulus animals and could have resulted in their avoiding the lesioned animals. However, the stimulus monkeys actually generated more affiliative social behaviors toward the amygdala-lesioned animals than toward the control animals. Even in the round-robin format, in which the animals had only one 20-minute period of social interaction, the control animals immediately identified the amygdala-lesioned animals as different and generated more social behavior toward them. We have not yet determined what it is in the amygdala-lesioned animals' demeanor or behavior that signals their approachability to the other animals. Because aggression was rarely observed in our experimental animals, it was not a lack of aggression that made them more appealing. A detailed description of the dyadic social interaction studies has been published (Emery et al. 2001).

Thus, contrary to our original premise, it appears that monkeys with extensive bilateral lesions of the amygdala can interpret and generate social gestures and initiate and receive more affiliative social interactions than normal control animals. They are clearly not critically impaired in carry-ing out social behavior. In fact, it appears that the lesions have produced a socially uninhibited monkey, with the normal reluctance to engage a novel animal apparently eliminated.

Based on the apparent lack of fear that these monkeys demonstrate to-ward inanimate objects and the uninhibited social interaction in the dyad studies, we have hypothesized that a primary role of the amygdala is to evaluate the environment for potential threats. Without a functioning amygdala, macaque monkeys do not evaluate novel conspecifics as poten-tial dangers, and whatever systems are involved in mediating social inter-actions are freed of the inhibitory influence of the amygdala. This, of course, could lead to devastating consequences in a more challenging en-vironment. We expect that the amygdala-lesioned animals, for example, would approach a predator as readily as they approach a novel conspecific in the dyadic social interaction studies.

EFFECTS OF NEONATAL LESIONS OF THE AMYGDALA ON THE EMERGENCE OF SOCIAL BEHAVIOR

As these results were obtained, we began to consider whether even though the amygdala is not necessary for generating social behavior in the adult, it may be essential for learning appropriate social behaviors. This line of thinking came from the literature on the hippocampal formation and mem-ory. The hippocampal formation is clearly essential for the establishment of long-term episodic or declarative memories. However, analysis of well-known amnesic patients, such as H.M. or R.B., who have marked bilateral damage to the hippocampal formation indicate that it is not essential for the retrieval of memories stored prior to the hippocampal damage. One inter-pretation of these findings is that declarative memories must be stored in brain regions other than the hippocampal formation (Squire 1993).

We have carried out a series of studies in which the amygdala is le-sioned bilaterally in primates at 2 weeks of age (Bauman et al. 2004, in press; Prather et al. 2001). This is a time when infant macaque monkeys are mainly found in ventral contact with their mothers and there is virtu-ally no play or other types of social interactions with other animals. One issue that was a concern in designing these studies was how the infants were raised following the neurosurgical procedure. The issue is of enormous signif-icance in interpreting any behavioral pathology in animals who have received brain manipulations. When animals are reared other than by their mother or by an adoptive mother, a variety of aberrant behaviors are observed. Sackett et al. (2002) have described some of these behaviors and demonstrated that extraordinary measures are necessary to mitigate the deleterious effects of nursery rearing on psychosocial behavior. This laboratory has provided substantial evidence that pair rearing leads to socioemotional pathologies such as excessive clinging (Novak and Sackett 1997). Early-nonmaternal-rearing situations also negatively impact an animal's ability to respond to environmental challenges (Suomi 1991). More recently, Parr et al. (2002) demonstrated that peer-reared rhesus monkeys have higher baseline levels of fear-potentiated startle than mother-reared age-matched controls. Moreover, as Wallen (1996) has pointed out, the ability to express species-typical sexual behavior "results from hormonally induced predispositions to engage in specific patterns of juvenile behavior whose expression is shaped by the specific social environment experienced by the developing monkey" (p. 364). Rearing conditions have also been shown to have a profound influence on the development of monoaminergic systems (Clarke et al. 1996), leading the authors to conclude that primate mothers influence the psychobiological development of central nervous system neurotransmitter systems in their infants. Finally, Coe and colleagues (Lubach et al. 1995) have produced overwhelming evidence that rearing in the absence of the mother severely affects several aspects of cellular immunity. For example, nursery-reared monkeys have significantly lower proportions of CD8 cells and lower natural killer cell activity than mother-reared monkeys.

Given these behavioral and physiological alterations due to rearing condition, it is difficult to interpret previous lesion studies with infant monkeys. Are the behavioral alterations due to rearing, to the lesion, or to some complex interaction of the two? To circumvent these interpretive problems, strategies were developed to allow the postsurgical return of the infant to its biological mother for rearing. Moreover, all mother-infant pairs engaged in daily 3-hour "play groups" with other mother-infant pairs and an adult male to allow the possibility of experiencing and learning normal conspecific social interactions.

In our population of infant animals who received bilateral lesions of the amygdala, we found that the interactions of the lesioned animals with their mothers was similar to those of control animals. Moreover, we found that, like adult animals with bilateral amygdala lesions, they showed little fear of normally fear-provoking objects such as rubber snakes. However, they showed increased fear, as indicated by more fear grimaces, more screams, and less social interactions, in novel dyadic social interactions. An intriguing, unsolved puzzle with this finding is the elucidation of which brain region is subserving the social fear since the amygdala was entirely eliminated. More germane to this discussion, however, is the finding that the lesioned animals generated substantial social behavior that could not be distinguished from that of age-matched control subjects. The quality and quantity of social interactions of the neonatally lesioned animals in a number of social formats is currently being investigated. Although the amygdala-lesioned animals may demonstrate subtle differences in their social interactions, the inescapable conclusion from observation of these animals is that none are markedly impaired in generating species-typical social behaviors such as grooming, play, and facial expressions (Bauman et al. 2004).

Our conclusion from this series of studies is that the amygdala is not essential for learning of social knowledge. The ability to perceive and produce typical types of social communication appears to be intact in these animals with neonatal lesions. Their behavior, however, has been substantially altered by the lesions. As in the adults, the main consequence of the lesions appears to be a dysregulation of the fear system. However, the outcome is more complex than in the adult. The infant lesioned animals appear to be less fearful of inanimate objects even if, like snakes, they normally elicit an innate fear response. In this respect, the infants are similar to the adults. However, compared with the adults, the infants appear to be more fearful in novel social situations. We are currently conducting additional studies with these animals to determine which conditions are and are not fear eliciting in these animals and whether other facets of social behavior are affected by the lesions.

In one of these studies, we have evaluated whether the lesioned animals demonstrate a normal preference for their biological mothers over other females that they are familiar with (Bauman et al., in press). The test is designed such that the infant is released into the large cage used for dyadic social testing with the adults, and the mother and another female are randomly placed in the start boxes located at either end of the enclosure. This experiment is conducted just after the normal weaning of the infant, and we record the amount of time that the infant spends in proximity to the mother versus the other female. We also record the behaviors that the infant carries out during the 2 minutes in which it is allowed to explore the cage. We found, consistent with the literature, that the control infants demonstrated a strong preference for their mothers. We found that infant animals with lesions of the hippocampus also demonstrated a strong preference for their mothers. However, the amygdala-lesioned infants did not demonstrate a preference for proximity to their mothers. At first blush, this result might make one think that the amygdala-lesioned infants had failed to form a normal attachment with their mothers. However, all other available information, including the amount of time that the infants spent in ventral contact both in the home cage and in the social play groups, indicated that the amygdala-impaired infants spent more time with their mothers. The reason for the amygdala-lesioned animals' behavior became clear when we analyzed what the animals were doing during the 2-minute test. We found that both the control and hippocampal-lesioned animals were producing large numbers of screams and fear grimaces, indicating that they were stressed by exposure to the novel enclosure. The amygdala-lesioned animals produced significantly fewer screams and other indications of stress. We interpret our findings by suggesting that both the control and hippocampal-lesioned animals were stressed by the novel enclosure and sought the comfort of their mothers. The amygdala-lesioned animals, in contrast, were much less stressed or fearful of the novel enclosure and therefore were less inclined to seek the comfort of their mothers.

BEHAVIORAL CONSEQUENCES OF BILATERAL LESIONS OF THE AMYGDALA IN HUMAN SUBJECTS

It is rare to find a human patient with a selective and complete bilateral lesion of the amygdaloid complex. There are, however, reports of a few patients with Urbach-Wiethe syndrome, a congenital disorder that can lead to cystic lesions of the temporal lobe. Adolphs and colleagues have studied such a patient, S.M., who appears to have fairly complete damage bilaterally to the amygdala with relatively little involvement of surrounding structures (Adolphs et al. 1995b, 1998, 1999). This woman has been married, is raising a family, and has held various jobs. Despite the complete absence of her amygdala, she appears to have a remarkably normal daily life. She clearly does not demonstrate significant social pathology. She is impaired, however, in her ability to judge facial emotions. Although she can reliably interpret happy faces, she has difficulty seeing fear in a face. Moreover, she is markedly impaired in attributing "trustworthiness" to an individual on the basis of facial appearance. These findings are consistent with the notion that the amygdala is active in surveying the environment for danger signals, and in S.M. these signals are not detected.

CONCLUSIONS

Nonhuman primates with bilateral lesions of the amygdala are capable of species-typical social interactions. This is true regardless of whether the lesions are performed near birth or in the mature animal. These findings suggest that the amygdala is not an essential component of the neural system that mediates social cognition. These animals do, however, demonstrate abnormal fear responses to environmental stimuli. We interpret these findings by hypothesizing that the amygdala plays a primary role in evaluating the environment for potential dangers. Once such a danger is detected, the amygdala plays an organizing role in mounting an appropriate response. This function has obvious adaptive significance to the preservation of the organism, and dysfunction of the amygdala might contribute to psychopathologies such as anxiety disorders and social phobia.

REFERENCES

Adolphs R, Tranel D, Damasio H, et al: Fear and the human amygdala. J Neurosci 15:5879–5891, 1995

Adolphs R, Tranel D, Damasio AR: The human amygdala in social judgment. Nature 393:470–474, 1998

Adolphs R, Tranel D, Hamann S, et al: Recognition of facial emotion in nine individuals with bilateral amygdala damage. Neuropsychologia 37:1111–1117, 1999

Aggleton JP, Passingham RE: Syndrome produced by lesions of the amygdala in monkeys (Macaca mulatta). J Comp Physiol Psychol 95:961–977, 1981

Baram TZ, Yi S, Avishai-Eliner S, et al: Development neurobiology of the stress response: multilevel regulation of corticotropin-releasing hormone function. Ann N Y Acad Sci 814:252–265, 1997

Baron-Cohen S, Ring HA, Bullmore ET, et al: The amygdala theory of autism. Neurosci Biobehav Rev 24:355–364, 2000

Bauman MD, Lavenex P, Mason WA, et al: The development of mother-infant interactions after neonatal amygdala lesions in rhesus monkeys. J Neurosci 24:711–721, 2004

Bauman MD, Lavenex P, Mason WA, Capitanio JP, Amaral DG: The development of social behavior following neonatal amygdala lesions in macaque monkeys. J Cogn Neurosci (in press)

Bremner JD, Narayan M: The effects of stress on memory and the hippocampus throughout the life cycle: implications for childhood development and aging. Dev Psychopathol 10:871–885, 1998

Buckley MJ, Gaffan D: Impairment of visual object-discrimination learning after perirhinal cortex ablation. Behav Neurosci 111:467–475, 1997

Capitanio JP, Mendoza SP, Lerche NW, et al: Social stress results in altered glucocorticoid regulation and shorter survival in simian acquired immune deficiency syndrome. Proc Natl Acad Sci U S A 95:4714–4719, 1998

Clarke AS, Hedeker DR, Ebert MH, et al: Rearing experience and biogenic amine activity in infant rhesus monkeys. Biol Psychiatry 40:338–352, 1996

Davis M, Whalen PJ: The amygdala: vigilance and emotion. Mol Psychiatry 6:13–34, 2001

Dicks D, Myers RE, Kling A: Uncus and amygdala lesions: effects on social behavior in the free-ranging rhesus monkey. Science 165:69–71, 1968

Emery NJ: The eyes have it: the neuroethology, function and evolution of social gaze. Neurosci Biobehav Rev 24:581–604, 2000

Emery NJ, Capitanio JP, Mason WA, et al: The effects of bilateral lesions of the amygdala on dyadic social interactions in rhesus monkeys (Macaca mulatta). Behav Neurosci 115:515–544, 2001

Erickson CA, Desimone R: Responses of macaque perirhinal neurons during and after visual stimulus association learning. J Neurosci 19:10404–10416, 1999

Gorno-Tempini ML, Pradelli S, Serafini M, et al: Explicit and incidental facial expression processing: an fMRI study. Neuroimage 14:465–473, 2001

Haxby JV, Hoffman EA, Gobbini MI: Human neural systems for face recognition and social communication. Biol Psychiatry 51:59–67, 2002

Herman JP, Dolgas CM, Carlson SL: Ventral subiculum regulates hypothalamo-pituitary-adrenocortical and behavioural responses to cognitive stressors. Neuroscience 86:449–459, 1998

Jarrard LE: Use of excitotoxins to lesion the hippocampus: update. Hippocampus 12:405–414, 2002

Kalin NH: The neurobiology of fear. Sci Am 268:94–101, 1993

Kalin NH, Shelton SE, Davidson RJ, et al: The primate amygdala mediates acute fear but not the behavioral and physiological components of anxious temperament. J Neurosci 21:2067–2074, 2001

Killgore WD, Yurgelun-Todd DA: Sex differences in amygdala activation during the perception of facial affect. Neuroreport 12:2543–2547, 2001

Kling A: Effects of amygdalectomy on socio-affective behavior in non-human primates, in Neurobiology of the Amygdala. Edited by Eleftheriou BE. New York, Plenum,1972, pp 511–536

Kling AS, Brothers LA: The amygdala and social behavior, in The Amygdala: Neurobiological Aspects of Emotion, Memory, and Mental Dysfunction. New York, Wiley-Liss, 1992, pp 353–377

Kling A, Cornell R: Amygdalectomy and social behavior in the caged stumped-tailed macaque (*Macaca speciosa*). Folia Primatol (Basel) 14:190–208, 1971

Kling A, Lancaster J, Benitone J: Amygdalectomy in the free-ranging vervet (*Cercopithecus aethiops*). J Psychiatr Res 7:191–199, 1970

Kluver H, Bucy PC: An analysis of certain effects of bilateral temporal lobectomy in the rhesus monkey, with special reference to "psychic blindness." J Psychol 5:33–54, 1938

LeDoux JE: Emotion: clues from the brain. Annu Rev Psychol 46:209–235, 1995

Lubach GR, Coe CL, Ershler WB: Effects of early rearing environment on immune responses of infant rhesus monkeys. Brain Behav Immun 9:31–46, 1995

Miyashita Y, Kameyama M, Hasegawa I, et al: Consolidation of visual associative long-term memory in the temporal cortex of primates. Neurobiol Learn Mem 70:197–211, 1998

Morris RG, Frey U: Hippocampal synaptic plasticity: role in spatial learning or the automatic recording of attended experience? Philos Trans R Soc Lond B Biol Sci 352:1489–1503, 1997

Morris JS, Frith CD, Perrett DI, et al: A differential neural response in the human amygdala to fearful and happy facial expressions. Nature 383:812–815, 1996

Novak MF, Sackett GP: Pair-rearing infant monkeys (*Macaca nemestrina*) using a "rotating-peer" strategy. Am J Primatol 41:141–149, 1997

Parr LA, Winslow JT, Davis M: Rearing experience differentially affects somatic and cardiac startle responses in rhesus monkeys (*Macaca mulatta*). Behav Neurosci 116:378–386, 2002

Prather MD, Lavenex P, Mauldin-Jourdain ML, et al: Increased social fear and decreased fear of objects in monkeys with neonatal amygdala lesions. Neuroscience 106:653–658, 2001

Rosvold HE, Mirsky AF, Pribram KH: Influence of amygdalectomy on social behavior in monkeys. J Comp Physiol Psychol 47:173–178, 1954

Sackett GP, Ruppenthal GC, Davis AE: Survival, growth, health, and reproduction following nursery rearing compared with mother rearing in pigtailed monkeys (*Macaca nemestrina*). Am J Primatol 56:165–183, 2002

Sapolsky RM, Zola-Morgan S, Squire LR: Inhibition of glucocorticoid secretion by the hippocampal formation in the primate. J Neurosci 11:3695–3704, 1991

Squire LR, Zola SM: Memory, memory impairment, and the medial temporal lobe. Cold Spring Harb Symp Quant Biol 61:185–195, 1996

Squire LR, Zola-Morgan S: The medial temporal lobe memory system. Science 253:1380–1386, 1991

Squire LR, Knowlton B, Musen G: The structure and organization of memory. Annu Rev Psychol 44:453–495, 1993

Suomi SJ: Early stress and adult emotional reactivity in rhesus monkeys. Ciba Found Symp 156:171–188, 1991

Sweeten TL, Posey DJ, Shekhar A, et al: The amygdala and related structures in the pathophysiology of autism. Pharmacol Biochem Behav 71:449–455, 2002

van Haarst AD, Oitzl MS, de Kloet ER: Facilitation of feedback inhibition through blockade of glucocorticoid receptors in the hippocampus. Neurochem Res 22:1323–1328, 1997

Wallen K: Nature needs nurture: the interaction of hormonal and social influences on the development of behavioral sex differences in rhesus monkeys. Horm Behav 30:364–378, 1996

Young AW, Aggleton JP, Hellawell DJ, et al: Face processing impairments after amygdalotomy. Brain 118:15–24, 1995

Zola-Morgan S, Squire LR, Alvarez-Royo P, et al: Independence of memory functions and emotional behavior: separate contributions of the hippocampal formation and the amygdala. Hippocampus 1:207–220, 1991

Reproduction of Color Figures

7
Neuroanatomy of Panic Disorder
Implications of Functional Imaging in Fear Conditioning

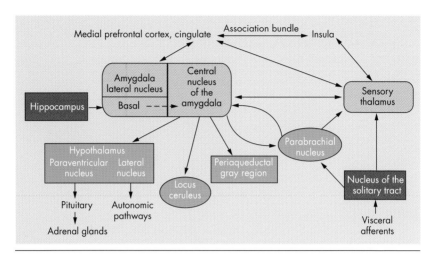

FIGURE 7–1   Neuroanatomical pathways of viscerosensory information in the brain.

Viscerosensory information is conveyed to the amygdala by two major pathways: downstream, from the nucleus of the solitary tract via the parabrachial nucleus or the sensory thalamus; and upstream, from the primary viscerosensory cortices and via corticothalamic relays allowing for higher-level neurocognitive processing and modulation of sensory information. Contextual information is stored in memory in the hippocampus and conveyed directly to the amygdala. Major efferent pathways of the amygdala relevant to anxiety include the following: the locus ceruleus (increases norepinephrine release, which contributes to physiological and behavioral arousal), the periaqueductal gray region (controls defensive behaviors and postural freezing), the hypothalamic paraventricular nucleus (activates the hypothalamic-pituitary-adrenal axis, releasing adrenocorticoids), the hypothalamic lateral nucleus (activates the sympathetic nervous system), and the parabrachial nucleus (influences respiratory rate and timing).

Source.   Adapted from Gorman JM, Kent JM, Sullivan GM, et al.: "Neuroanatomical Hypothesis of Panic Disorder, Revised." *American Journal of Psychiatry* 157:493–505, 2000. Used with permission.

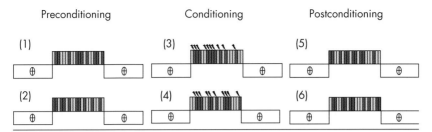

Preconditioning   Conditioning   Postconditioning

FIGURE 7–2   Sequence of imaging runs.

Forty-six images of the whole brain were acquired during each run (21 contiguous slices/image), which lasted 3 minutes and 4 seconds. A standard block design was used, in which 13 images (52 seconds) were acquired during an initial baseline epoch, followed by a task epoch of 20 images (80 seconds) and a recovery baseline epoch of 13 images (52 seconds). A total of six runs were acquired. Each baseline consisted of a crosshair. Each task epoch consisted of a randomized presentation of 10 *red* (CS+ [reinforced stimulus]) and 10 *green* (CS– [nonreinforced stimulus]) squares. Each square was presented for 3 seconds with an interstimulus interval of 0.5 seconds, during which a crosshair was presented. During the task epochs of runs 3 and 4, an aversive auditory stimulus was paired with the CS+ for 2.5 seconds.

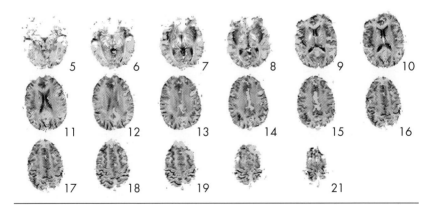

FIGURE 7–3   Classical conditioning with an auditory US and a visual CS.

Each colored region indicates a significant increase in the fMRI T2* signal from baseline ($P \leq 0.0001$, $P \leq 0.0003$, and $P \leq 0.0005$; depicted as *yellow, orange,* and *red,* respectively, on brain images).

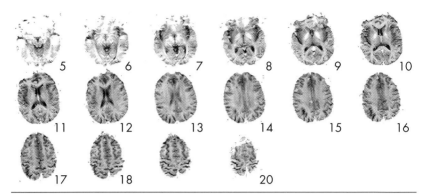

FIGURE 7–4 Classical conditioning with a visual US and an auditory CS.

Each colored region indicates a significant increase in the fMRI T2* signal from baseline ($P \leq 0.0001$, $P \leq 0.0003$, and $P \leq 0.0005$; depicted as *yellow, orange,* and *red,* respectively, on brain images).

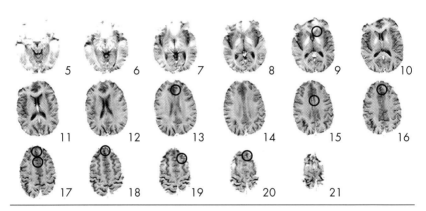

FIGURE 7–5 Long-range cortical networks activated by classical conditioning with an aversive unconditioned stimulus (a cross–sensory modality conjunction).

Active areas are highlighted with a circle. Each colored region indicates a significant increase in the fMRI T2* signal from baseline ($P \leq 0.0001$, $P \leq 0.0003$, and $P \leq 0.0005$; depicted as *yellow, orange,* and *red,* respectively, on brain images).

13

The Anatomy of Fear
Microcircuits of the Lateral Amygdala

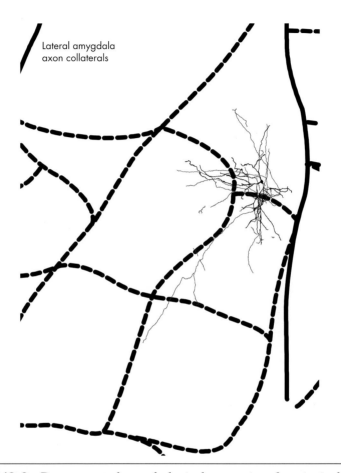

Lateral amygdala
axon collaterals

FIGURE 13–3   Reconstructed morphological properties of a principal neuron of the lateral amygdala.

The neuron is shown to scale against a brain atlas of the lateral amygdala (LA). Soma, dendrites, and dendritic spines are shown in *black*. Axon and axonal boutons are shown in *red*. (Neuron recorded and labeled in vitro from the rat LA.) Axon can be seen projecting ventrally into the basal nucleus of the amygdala. In addition, extensive axon collaterals can be seen ramifying within the LA. Individual LA neurons can possess up to 18 mm of axon. The LA contains approximately 488 m of principal neuron dendrites and 372 m of principal neuron local axons. *Source.*   Atlas outline adapted from Paxinos and Watson 1998.

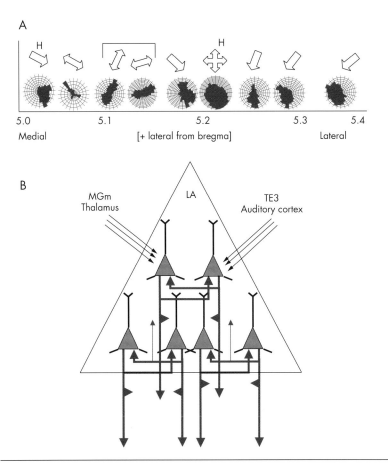

FIGURE 13–4   Polar histograms and schematic of intra–lateral amygdala local axon projection patterns.

A: Polar histograms of axon projection patterns from individual lateral amygdala (LA) projection neurons. LA principal neurons send their major projection in a ventral direction, with some collateral projections dorsally. Histograms are arranged in order along a medial to lateral axis according to the location of their soma, where an organization can be seen. In addition to ventral and dorsal axon projections, neurons located laterally send a major projection in a medial direction toward the center of the LA. Neurons located medially send a major projection in the opposite direction, laterally toward the center of the LA. (Neurons in bracket do not appear to fit this organization.) H = neurons recovered from horizontal slices; all others are coronal.

B: Schematic of axon projection patterns in the LA. Axon collaterals are arranged such that most neurons send axons ventrally and toward the center of the LA. Many also possess a component of dorsally projecting neurons. All LA principal neurons are potentially extensively interconnected. MGm = medial geniculate, medial division.

Index

*Page numbers printed in **boldface** type refer to tables or figures.*

Nonhuman primate studies *(continued)*
  neuroimaging studies of VFD
    primates, 138
  proton magnetic resonance
    spectroscopic imaging, 136,
    138–140, 142–144, **143**
  of the VFD hippocampus, 144–145
  VFD model, 136–137, **143, 144**
Noradrenergic reuptake inhibitors,
    198, 201, 205
Norepinephrine, 238
Novel Fruit test, 216, **218,** 219
Nucleus tractus solitarium (NTS), 16, 28

0
Obesity, 47
Obsessive-compulsive disorder (OCD)
  antidepressants to treat, 196
  cognitive-behavioral therapy for,
    182, 205
  SSRIs to treat, 196, 203
Occasion setters, 13
Oklahoma City bombing, 105
  implications of, 114–116
  mental health treatment following,
    114
  posttraumatic stress disorder
    following, 113
  study of, 110–115
  symptoms following, 111–112, **112**
  See also Posttraumatic stress disorder
Orbitofrontal cortex (OFC), 16, **155**
Oregon National Primate Research
    Center (ONPRC), 216–217

P
Pain, tolerance for, 3, 228
Panic, defined, 186
Panic attacks
  as conditioned fear, xiv
  cues during, 120
  fear in, 1
  laboratory-induced, 173, 181, 199
  nocturnal, 120
  and premenstrual dysphoric
    disorder, 199
Panic disorder
  amygdala in, xiv
  antidepressants as treatment for, 196

brain changes in, 50
carbon dioxide inhalation and,
    198–199
cognitive-behavioral therapy for,
    12, 25, 121, 182–185, **185**
classical conditioning as a model for,
    120
cues and, 120
defined, 119
fear in, 9
functional imaging studies to
    identify, 119–120
genetic factors in, 212
hypersensitivity to threat of
    suffocation, 95
MAT for, 188
medication for treating, 119–120, 182
and posttraumatic stress disorder
    compared, 107
psychoeducation for, 182
respiratory stimulation paradigms to
    study, 95
and separation anxiety in children,
    89
SSRIs as treatment for, 15, 196
startle reflex in, 76–77
symptoms of, 119
treatment of, experiments in,
    176–177
Panic disorder with agoraphobia
    (PDA), 173, 177
Papez's circuit, 140
Paragigantocellularis, 157
Paranoia, 228, 231, 239
Paroxetine, 12, 196, 197, 202, 203
Passive avoidance learning, 27
Passive coping, 15
Pathological anxiety, 2
Pathological fear, 9–10, 229
Pavlov, Ivan, 3, 120
Pavlovian conditioning. *See* Classical
    conditioning
Pediatric generalized anxiety disorder
    (GAD), 152–153
  behavioral inhibition as
    predisposition for, 155
  neurodevelopment of, 155–156
  and pediatric PTSD compared, 153
  symptoms of, 153